Fetus and Neonate is a series of practical, focused texts which concentrate on that critical period of human development, from late fetal to neonatal life. Each volume in the series examines a particular body system, looking at the physiological mechanisms which underlie the transition from intrauterine to extrauterine life, the pathophysiological processes which may occur, and the application of new basic scientific knowledge to the clinical situation.

This volume, prepared by an authoritative team of internationally renowned contributors, looks in depth at the growth of the fetus and neonate. It is introduced with an overview of physiology and endocrinology of normal growth, before considering new insights into the pathophysiology of growth impairment and their clinical applications.

Several chapters focus on fetal growth retardation and the challenges this poses for the clinician. The measurement and assessment of fetal growth and well-being are also fully addressed. An important theme is the role of disturbances in 'programming' of growth in the early development of the fetus in producing adult diseases. This stimulating book brings together all the disciplines relevant to this important scientific and clinical area.

GROWTH

Fetus and Neonate: Physiology and Clinical Applications

Volume 1: The Circulation
Volume 2: Breathing
Volume 3: Growth

GROWTH

Edited by

MARK A. HANSON
JOHN A. D. SPENCER
CHARLES H. RODECK
Department of Obstetrics and Gynaecology,
University College London Medical School, UK

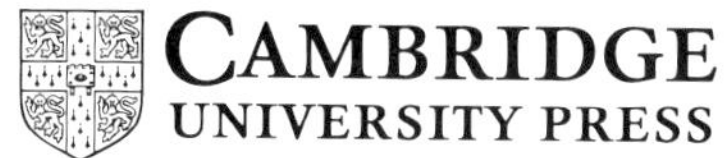
CAMBRIDGE
UNIVERSITY PRESS

Published by the Press Syndicate of the University of Cambridge
The Pitt Building, Trumpington Street, Cambridge CB2 1RP
40 West 20th Street, New York 10011-4211, USA
10 Stamford Road, Oakleigh, Melbourne 3166, Australia

First published 1995

Printed in Great Britain at the University Press, Cambridge

A catalogue record for this book is available from the British Library

Library of Congress cataloguing in publication data

Growth/edited by Mark A. Hansen, John A. D. Spencer, Charles H. Rodeck.
p. cm. – (Fetus and neonate; v. 3)
Includes index.
ISBN 0-521-45522-7 (hardback)
1. Fetus–Growth. 2. Fetal growth retardation. I. Hanson, Mark A.
II. Spencer, John A. D. III. Rodeck, Charles H. IV. Series.
[DNLM: 1. Fetal Development–physiology. 2. Fetal Growth
Retardation. WQ 210.5 G879 1995]
RG13.G76 1995
612.6′47—dc20
DNLM/DLC
for Library of Congress 95-6496 CIP

ISBN 0 521 45522 7 hardback

PN

Contents

Preface to the series

The factual burden of a science varies inversely with its degree of maturity
P. Medawar 'Two Conceptions of Science': 'Anglo-Saxon Attitudes', Henry Tizard Memorial Lecture, Encounter 143, August 1965

The idea for a series on the applications of fetal and neonatal physiology to clinical medicine came from the need of our students for something intermediate between a textbook and review articles. Textbooks provide breadth of coverage but tend to lack critical discussion. Reviews can provide such discussion but represent the view of one authority and may need a balance. For the student, such reviews are not a substitute for original papers and are better taken after consumption of a full course of such papers rather than as hors d'oeuvres to them.

We envisage the readership of the series as 'students' of the subject in the widest sense, from undergraduates learning about fetal and neonatal physiology as part of a basic science degree or preclinical medical students, to postgraduate and postdoctoral scientists and clinicians specializing in obstetrics, neonatology or paediatrics. We decided that all needs would best be met by producing a series of multiauthored volumes. This will allow rapid production of short texts that will keep the material focused whilst still allowing the subject to be reviewed from several points of view. None the less, we have decided to adopt a 'systems' approach because it has the advantages of simplicity and conformity to textbooks of physiology.

The chapters in each volume of the series are arranged in sections: Physiology, Pathophysiology and Clinical Applications. They are not intended to be all-inclusive but rather to demonstrate the applications of basic scientific research to clinical medicine via improved understanding of pathophysiological processes.

The series concentrates on late fetal and neonatal life (the perinatal period). In late gestation the fetus must have established the mechanisms which will permit it to make the transition to becoming a neonate, whilst still being highly adapted to the peculiar intrauterine environment in which it remains. The importance of making the transition successfully is underlined by the fact that this is one of the most dangerous periods of human life. In the course of it, some physiological processes continue, whilst others cease to function, undergo drastic change, or are initiated. The understanding of the underlying controlling processes constitutes one of the greatest challenges in physiology.

Our feeling that such a series is necessary has been reinforced by the increasing number of students who are keen to learn more about this fascinating area. They are aware of the possibility of obtaining biological information from the human fetus using non-invasive methods, but as they see the difficulties of interpreting such information in clinical practice, they perceive the need for a greater understanding of fundamental physiological processes. We hope that this series will stimulate some of them to take up research in this field.

Finally, the series stands for two things which seem temporarily out of fashion. First, by illustrating the clinical applications of basic research, it demonstrates how advances in modern medicine are based on animal research. We cannot, in setting out to improve the care of the human fetus or neonate, have one without the other. Secondly, we believe and teach that the knowledge gained using techniques from a range of disciplines (biochemistry, molecular biology, physics, etc.) must ultimately be integrated into concepts of how the body works as a whole. Such integration is precisely the realm of physiology; nowhere is the power of the method more clearly evident than in the fetus and neonate. This synthesis into a whole is not to generalize, but to push our understanding to greater depths.

Mark Hanson
John Spencer
Charles Rodeck

University College London

Contributors

David J.P. Barker
MRC Environmental Epidemiology Unit, Southampton General Hospital, Southampton SO16 6YD, UK.

John M. Bassett
Growth and Development Unit, University Field Laboratory, Wytham, Oxford OX2 8QJ, UK.

Tou Choong Chang
Kandang-Kerbau Hospital, 1 Hampshire Road, Singapore.

Ian M. Doughty
Department of Child Health, St Mary's Hospital, Manchester M13 0JH, UK.

Abigail L. Fowden
Physiological Laboratory, Downing Street, Cambridge CB2 3EG, UK.

Peter D. Gluckman
Research Centre for Developmental Medicine and Biology, University of Auckland, Private Bag 92019, Auckland, New Zealand.

David J. Hill
Lawson Research Institute, St Joseph's Health Centre, 268 Grosvenor Street, London, Ontario N6A 4V2.

T.Y. Khong
Department of Histopathology, Women's and Children's Hospital, 72 King William Road, North Adelaide, South Australia 5006.

Rodolfo Montemagno
Department of Obstetrics and Gynaecology, University College London Medical School, 86–96 Chenies Mews, London WC1E 6HX, UK.

Julie A. Owens
Department of Obstetrics and Gynaecology, University of Adelaide, Adelaide, South Australia 5005.

P.C. Owens
Department of Obstetrics and Gynaecology, University of Adelaide, Adelaide, South Australia 5005.

James F. Pearson
Department of Obstetrics and Gynaecology, University of Wales College of Medicine, Heath Park, Cardiff CF4 4XN, UK.

Jeffrey S. Robinson
Department of Obstetrics and Gynaecology, University of Adelaide, Adelaide, South Australia 5005.

Stephen C. Robson
Department of Fetal Medicine, Royal Victoria Infirmary, Leazes Wing, Richardson Road, Newcastle upon Tyne, UK.

Colin P. Sibley
Department of Child Health, St Mary's Hospital, Manchester M13 0JH, UK.

Peter W.S. Soothill
Fetal Medicine Research Unit, University of Bristol, St Michael's Hospital, Southwell Street, Bristol BS2 8EG, UK.

Yasmin Sultan
Darwin College, Cambridge CB3 9EU, UK.

Michael E. Symonds
Department of Biochemistry and Physiology, University of Reading, Whiteknights, PO Box 228, Reading, Berkshire, UK.

Gerard H.A. Visser
Department of Obstetrics and Gynaecology, University Hospital, PO Box 85500, 3508 GA Utrecht, The Netherlands.

Part One

Physiology

1
Placental transfer

IAN M. DOUGHTY and COLIN P. SIBLEY

Introduction

Belief that the placenta is involved with fetal nutrition was first recorded by Aristotle (Boyd & Hamilton, 1970), although he knew nothing of its microscopic structure or the circulation of fetal and maternal blood through the organ. With current knowledge, it is accepted that the human placenta provides the interface between maternal and fetal circulations across which maternofetal and fetomaternal transfer of nutrients, respiratory gases and waste products occurs. Despite this, understanding of the physiological mechanisms by which transplacental transfer of specific substances occurs is at present limited when compared with understanding of transfer mechanisms in other organs. The purpose of this chapter is, first, to review the functional anatomy of the placenta and the underlying theory of transfer mechanisms which may be applied to the structural model. Current understanding of mechanisms of transfer of selected gases and nutrients is then briefly reviewed. Space limitations prevent an exhaustive bibliography and, for a more comprehensive coverage the reader is referred to Sibley and Boyd (1992) and Morriss, Boyd and Mahendran (1994).

Structure

The mature human placenta has a multivillous architecture (Fig. 1.1*a*). The term placentome is used to describe one villous tree together with its related maternal circulation. The trunk of the tree is the stem villus from which arise the loosely arranged intermediate villi. Transfer is thought to occur mainly across the outer cell layer, or syncytiotrophoblast, of the more peripherally located mature intermediate villi with their abundant terminal villi. For completeness it may be noted that, on gross inspection,

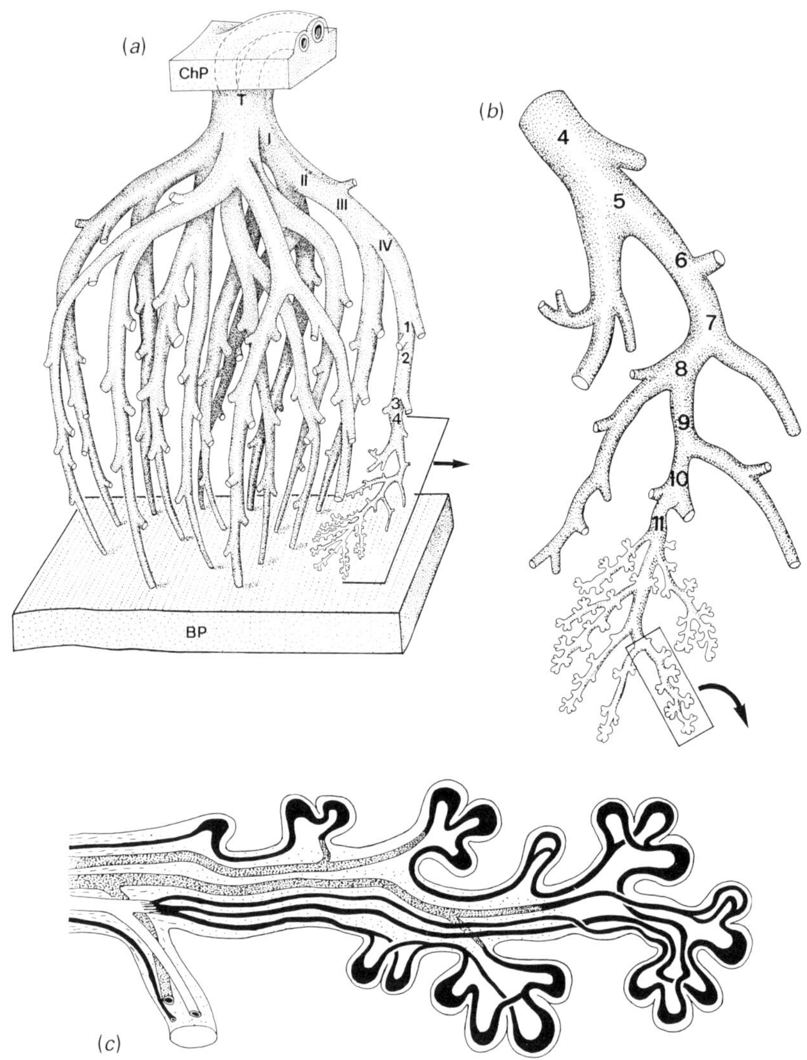

Fig. 1.1.(a),(b). Schematic drawing of the branching patterns of the villous tree. ChP = chorionic plate; BP = basal plate; T = truncus chorii; I–IV = four generations of rami; 1–11 = 11 generations of ramuli. (c). Fetal vessel architecture of an ending stem villus of the last ramulus (line hatched) and a terminal convolute composed of one mature intermediate villus (slightly point shaded) together with its terminal villi (unshaded). Arterioles are point shaded, capillaries are black and venules are unshaded. Note the long capillary loops supplying several terminal villi in series. (From Kaufmann et al. (1992), published by kind permission of Steinkopff Verlag GmbH, Darmstadt.).

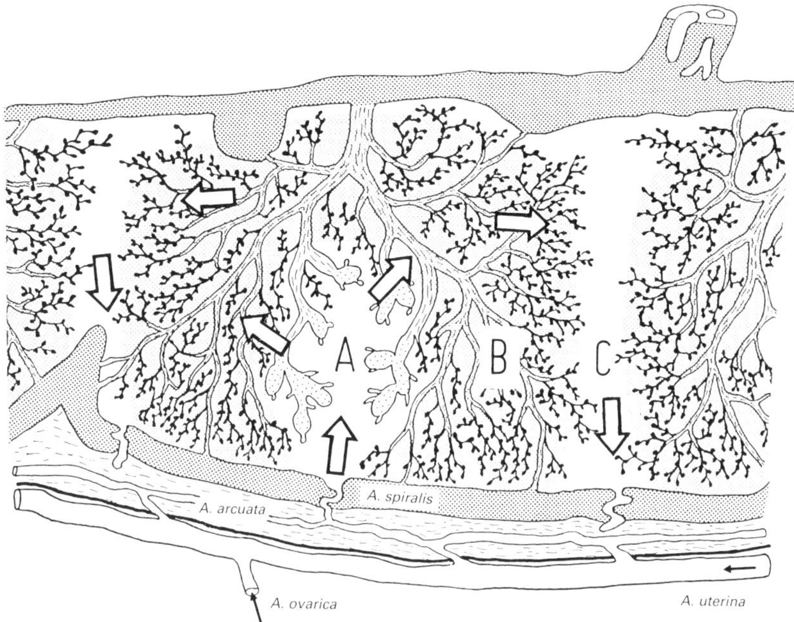

Fig. 1.2. Spatial relations between villous tree, villous types and maternal bloodstream. The maternal blood enters intervillous space near the centre (A) of the villous tree and leaves it near the clefts (C) between neighbouring villous trees. In the term placenta, the larger stem villi (line shaded), the immature intermediate villi (point shaded) and their tiny sprouting mesenchymal branches (unshaded) are concentrated in the centres of the villous trees, surrounding the central cavity (A) as maternal inflow area. The mature intermediate villi (black) together with their terminal branches (black, grape-like) make up the periphery of the villous tree (B). Due to the densely packed villi in this area, this is the high-resistance zone for the maternal circulation and the main exchange area. (From Kaufmann et al. (1992), published by kind permission of Steinkopff Verlag GmbH, Darmstadt.)

the placenta is anatomically subdivided by rudimentary septa into 10–40 lobes or cotyledons. These cotyledons contain from one to a small number of placentomes, the peripheral villous trees often overlapping.

On the maternal side, blood enters an intervillous pool from about 100 spiral arteries at a moderate filling velocity of a few centimetres per second. Spiral arteries are related anatomically to the centre of villous trees and the decidual veins lie peripherally, suggesting a directional blood flow as depicted in Fig. 1.2 (Leiser, Kosanke & Kaufmann, 1991). The blood is then thought to circulate through the intervillous space in a slow centrifugal manner before leaving via decidual veins. On the fetal side, one stem villous artery successively branches within each of about 50

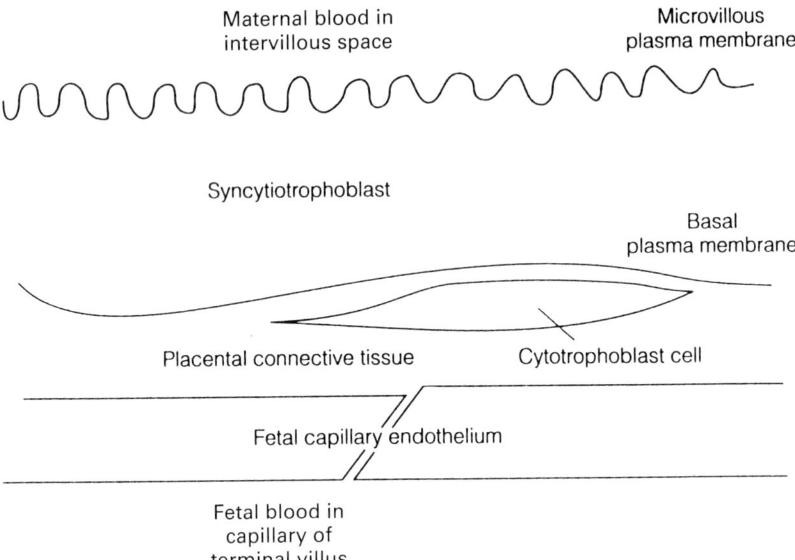

Fig. 1.3. Diagrammatic representation of the cellular layers that constitute the barrier to transplacental exchange in human placenta.

dichotomously branching villous trees, eventually forming richly branching terminal capillary beds in the intermediate villi (Fig. 1.1). The capillaries lie in close apposition to the vasculosyncytial membrane within the terminal villi and it is thought that this is the main site across which transfer occurs.

The human placenta is haemochorial, meaning that maternal blood is in direct contact with the placental trophoblast. It is also monochorial having, by term, only one continuous layer of trophoblast, i.e. the syncytiotrophoblast, separating the maternal blood from the fetal vasculature. Other tissue layers lying between the two circulations are a discontinuous layer of cytotrophoblast (although this does form another continuous cellular layer in the first trimester), a thin layer of loose placental connective tissue and the fetal capillary endothelium (Fig. 1.3). It is generally accepted that the syncytiotrophoblast is the functional barrier to both maternofetal and fetomaternal transfer of small solutes although the fetal capillary endothelium probably provides a barrier to molecules of the size of albumin and larger.

The human syncytiotrophoblast is a continuous, multinuclear cellular layer covering the whole villous structure (total surface area around $10\,m^2$) with a microvillous, maternal-facing plasma membrane and a smooth, fetal-facing basal plasma membrane. The microvillous nature of the outer-facing membrane provides a large surface area in direct contact with circulating maternal blood. It is generally accepted by physiologists, though not clearly morphologically proven, that there is an extracellular, water filled route extending across the syncytiotrophoblast, so that molecules up to the size of albumin may diffuse across the placental barrier (see below).

Mechanisms of transfer

Transfer across the syncytiotrophoblast may occur via simple diffusion, facilitated diffusion, active transport, endocytosis/exocytosis or bulk flow. All solutes can diffuse across the placenta to a greater or lesser extent and the principles underlying such diffusion are therefore outlined in some detail here. The other mechanisms of transfer are illustrated with regard to specific molecules later in this chapter.

Diffusion

Net diffusion of molecules occurs when there is an electrochemical gradient between two compartments. The net flux (J_{net}) of maternofetal diffusional transfer of a given uncharged solute across the placenta may be calculated from a derivation of Fick's law (see Sibley & Boyd, 1992):

$$J_{net} = P \cdot S\,[C_m - C_f] \tag{1}$$

where P is a proportionality constant (permeability), S is surface area available for diffusion, and C_m and C_f are the mean concentrations of the unbound solute in plasma water in maternal and fetal blood, respectively, flowing past the exchange area. The units of J_{net} are mass/time, usually moles/minute. J_{net} is the sum of the unidirectional maternofetal (J_{mf}) and fetomaternal (J_{fm}) fluxes:

$$J_{net} = J_{mf} - J_{fm} \tag{2}$$

and,

$$J_{mf} = P \cdot S\,[C_m] \tag{3}$$

$$J_{fm} = P \cdot S\,[C_f]. \tag{4}$$

Therefore, the diffusional capacity of any given solute depends upon a permeability·surface area product and concentration. For a charged solute, an extra term would need to be added to Equation 1 to account for the effects of any electrical potential difference between the intervillous space and fetal capillary. Such a potential difference, if present, would differentially affect the net flux of cations and anions.

Flow limitation

Respiratory gases and other lipophilic substances have high permeability constants because they pass freely across both lipid–bilayer cell membranes of the syncytiotrophoblast. In the situation where maternofetal J_{net} of a substance at the arterial end of the exchange barrier is high due to high $P \cdot S$ values, there is a rapid fall in C_m, rise in C_f and therefore fall in J_{net} as the venous end of the exchange barrier is approached (Fig. 1.4). Therefore, maternofetal rate of transfer of the substance is said to be flow limited and dependent upon the rate of maternal and fetal blood flows and the geometrical relationships between the two flows.

Optimal transfer of lipophilic solutes occurs across areas where maternal and fetal flow rates are matched and of high velocity. Also, if maternal and fetal blood flow is in opposite directions, i.e. are countercurrent across the exchange area, then efficiency of transfer is greater than if their flows are in the same direction, i.e. are concurrent (Fig. 1.4). In the human placenta, with its loose multivillous arrangement into placentomes, it is thought that both matching of blood flows and directional relationship of blood flows vary greatly between individual terminal villi, leading to wide differences in their transfer efficiencies. Also, the hairpin-like terminal capillary loops have opposite flow directions in each limb which would suggest a mixture of concurrent and countercurrent exchange for each individual villus.

Although the anatomical relationship of blood flows within the placenta is fixed, modulators of vascular tone within the maternal and fetal vasculatures may be involved in changing total blood flow or redirecting flow between exchange areas, thereby altering matching of the two circulations and total placental transfer efficiency. The rate of uteroplacental blood flow is known to increase throughout gestation, studies using the guinea pig suggesting that the mechanism for this may be a restructuring of collagen within the walls of blood vessels, controlled by maternal oestrogen levels (Moll et al., 1991). The uteroplacental blood velocity is thought to be affected acutely by neural, humoral and local vasoactive mechanisms, beta-adrenoceptor agonists, angiotensin II, endothelins, other vasoactive peptides and prostaglandins all possibly playing a role in determining vascular resistance, as they do in other tissues (Lunell & Nylund, 1992). Whether autoregulation of human uteroplacental circulation occurs is unknown; there appears to be no autoregulation of uteroplacental blood flow in the sheep near term, although autoregulation does occur in the rabbit near term (Rankin & Mclaughlin, 1979). With regard to modulation of fetoplacental circulation, there is no autonomic innervation of the placenta, and regulation must be effected by other means, such as autocrine or paracrine systems (for review see Macara, Kingdom & Kaufmann, 1993). There is now evidence that nitric oxide, a labile endothelium-derived relaxing factor known to reduce vascular tone in a number of tissues, is involved in maintenance of basal vascular tone and in counteracting the effects of the vasoconstrictors endothelin and thromboxane in the human, in the in vitro perfused cotyledon (Myatt, Brewer & Brockman, 1991; Myatt et al., 1992). There is also evidence that transplacental vasoregulatory mechanisms exist, modifying blood flow on one side of the placental barrier in response to changes in blood flow on the other side. In experimental animal models, when fetal circulatory flows to certain regions of the placenta were reduced or increased, there followed a corresponding reduction or increase in the maternal blood flow to that region. Similarly, fetal circulation to an area supplied by a maternal vessel was reduced when the latter was tied off (Rankin & Mclaughlin, 1979)

Membrane limitation

Most nutrients are hydrophilic and the two plasma membranes of the syncytiotrophoblast have very low permeabilities to these solutes. Because of this, transfer of these solutes across the placenta is slower than transfer of lipophilic substances and is much less dependent on blood flow; transfer is said to be membrane limited.

Despite the syncytiotrophoblast being a true syncytium with no intercellular spaces and therefore no obvious extracellular water-filled route across it, small inert hydrophilic solutes, which are known not to cross plasma membranes, do cross the placenta at rates proportional to their diffusion coefficients in water (Bain et al., 1988, 1990). This suggests that a paracellular route, through which hydrophilic solutes diffuse, does exist. Although a matter of considerable and continued debate, normally occurring discontinuities in the syncytiotrophoblast may be one such paracellular route (Edwards et al., 1993). The fetal capillary endothelium has large (approximately 15 nm radius) intercellular spaces which provide for paracellular diffusion of small solutes but might considerably restrict diffusion of solutes the size of albumin and larger (Leach & Firth, 1992).

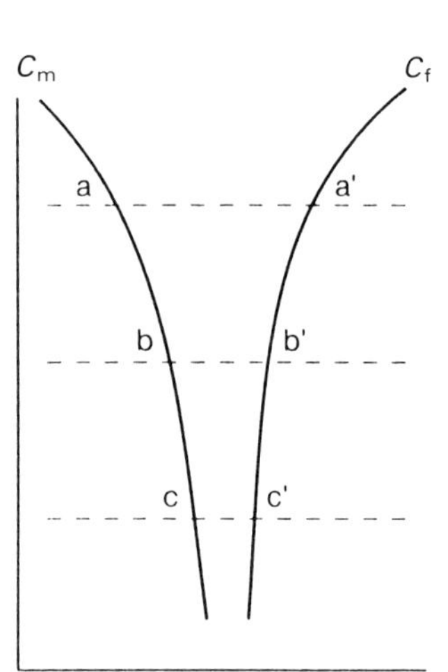
C_m
C_f
a
a'
b
b'
c
c'
increase ← Concentration → decrease

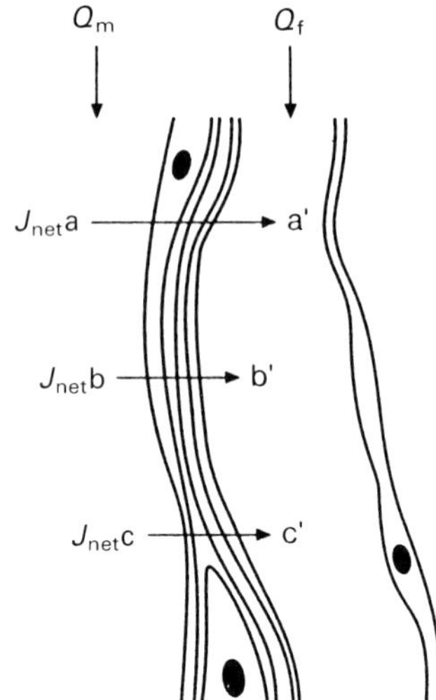
Q_m
Q_f
J_{net}a
a'
J_{net}b
b'
J_{net}c
c'

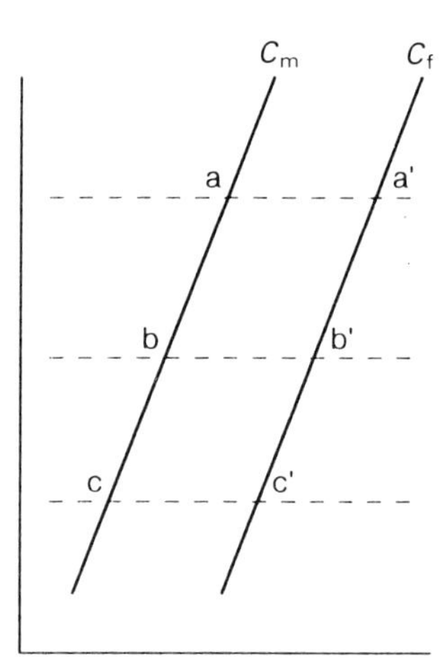
C_m
C_f
a
a'
b
b'
c
c'
increase ← Concentration → decrease

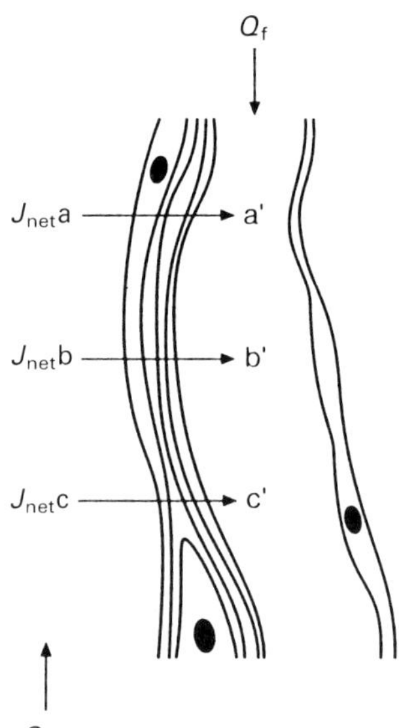
Q_f
J_{net}a
a'
J_{net}b
b'
J_{net}c
c'
Q_m

Experimental approaches and species differences

Clues to the mechanism of placental transfer of selected substances may be gained from serial analysis of their concentrations in maternal and cord blood at delivery (Faber & Thornburg, 1981) or, more recently at cordocentesis. For instance, concentrations of certain amino acids are higher in fetal blood than in maternal blood throughout second and third trimesters, and this implies that there may be active transport of these amino acids in the maternofetal direction (McIntosh, Rodeck & Heath, 1984).

Traditionally, in vivo experimentation has centred around quantitative comparison between maternofetal flux of a nutrient and calculated fetal accretion (net flux) of that nutrient, and quantitative comparison between maternofetal and fetomaternal fluxes, allowing calculation of net flux of the nutrient. If maternofetal flux and fetal accretion of a nutrient are of similar magnitude, this would suggest that fetomaternal flux is much lower than maternofetal flux, that there is transfer asymmetry across the placental barrier which might include specific and possibly active transcellular mechanisms, and that the rate of placental transfer of this substance might be critical to the normal growth and development of the fetus. Alternatively, if maternofetal and fetomaternal fluxes of a nutrient are quantitatively similar and much higher

---

Fig. 1.4. Effect of directional relationships of maternal (Q_m) and fetal (Q_f) blood flows on relative concentration differences and net fluxes of a substance crossing the placenta by diffusion under flow-limited conditions. **Top**: Concurrent maternal and fetal flows. *Left*: The maternal (C_m) and fetal (C_f) plasma concentration profiles are shown along the length of the exchange vessel that includes points a, b, and c on the maternal side of the vessel and corresponding points a′, b′, and c′ within the lumen of the fetal vessel. *Right*: The results in net fluxes, J_{net}. The net flux decreases from point a–a′, to point b–b′, to point c–c′ along the length of the exchange vessels. C_m declines along the length of the exchange vessel, and C_f increases along the length of the exchange vessel until the concentration difference that drives net diffusion decreases to almost zero. **Bottom**: Countercurrent maternal and fetal blood flows. *Left*: C_m declines along the length of the exchange vessel, and C_f increases along the length of the exchange vessel. The maternal–fetal concentration difference is constant along the exchange vessel. *Right*: The net fluxes remain uniform along the length of the capillary. Not illustrated is the membrane-limited situation in which the maternal–fetal concentration difference as well as the individual maternal and fetal concentration profiles remain approximately uniform along the length of the capillary; this will be true regardless of the directional relationship of maternal and fetal blood flows. (From Morriss, Boyd & Mahendran (1994), published by kind permission of Raven Press, New York.)

than fetal requirements, diffusional mechanisms of transfer might be more likely. However, this conceptual approach may well lead to a misunderstanding of the true situation. For instance, both unidirectional maternofetal and fetomaternal fluxes of potassium across the rat placenta are considerable when compared to the rate of accretion of this cation by the rat fetus. However, in this species it has been shown that maternofetal potassium flux occurs predominantly by transcellular, active, transport (Mohammed et al., 1993).

In vivo investigation of placental transfer in the human has been limited by the potentially harmful consequences to the mother and fetus of available techniques. In the 1940s, Flexner and colleagues measured in vivo maternofetal flux of sodium across the placenta of the human and six other species, by injection of ^{22}Na into the maternal circulation prior to delivery and counting of maternal blood and fetal specimens postpartum (Flexner et al., 1948). These experiments yielded valuable information, allowing quantitative comparison between the maternofetal flux of sodium across the placenta and the calculated fetal sodium requirements, at different gestational ages for all the species studied. However, concern about the potentially harmful effects of radioisotopes has limited subsequent human transfer in vivo work to studying the flux of non-toxic, assayable substances, such as insulin and mannitol. Therefore, most currently available information about in vivo transfer comes from animal studies. There are significant structural differences between the human placenta and those of other species (see Table 1.1), and there are interspecies variations in length of gestation and fetal constitution. Therefore, mechanisms of transplacental transfer of nutrients for different species may be different, and this should be considered when extrapolating from the animal to the human model. An exciting new technique that might allow more understanding of human transfer in vivo is the use of mass spectroscopy to analyse transplacental transfer of stable isotopes (Chien et al., 1993).

In vitro, transplacental transfer of substances in the human may be studied by dual perfusion of a placental cotyledon (Schneider, Panigel & Dancis, 1972). In this technique, matching branches of umbilical artery and vein are cannulated and perfused with oxygenated buffer, and the corresponding area of the intervillous space is perfused with the same medium via cannulae piercing the basal plate. By addition of a particular substance to either side, its clearance can be measured in either the maternofetal or the fetomaternal direction in freshly delivered placenta. Although studies have, by necessity, been limited to placenta at term,

Table 1.1 *Species differences in the tissue layers which provide a barrier in maternofetal exchange*

	Maternal endothelium	Maternal uterine epithelium	Fetal trophoblast		Fetal endothelium	Other exchange areas
			Number of layers	Type		
Human	No	No	1	Syncytial	Yes	No
Rhesus monkey	No	No	1	Syncytial	Yes	No
Sheep	Yes	Syncytial (part fetal)	1	Cellular	Yes	Haemophagus organ
Pig	Yes	Cellular	1	Cellular	Yes	No
Guinea pig	No	No	1	Syncytial	Yes	Yolk sac
Rat and mouse	No	No	3	Cellular–syncytial–syncytial	Yes	Yolk sac
Rabbit	No	No	2	Syncytial–cellular	Yes	Yolk sac

(Adapted from Morriss, Boyd & Mahendran, 1994).

they have yielded valuable information on mechanisms of transfer of selected membrane-limited substances, importantly glucose and amino acids. It might be argued that, following labour, delivery, and time delay to perfusing, structure and function of the syncytiotrophoblast are irreparably damaged altering both passive permeability and transport mechanisms. However, permeability data from this preparation compares, favourably with those obtained in vivo (Bain et al., 1988, 1990; Edwards et al., 1993).

Other in vitro techniques for studying the human placenta focus on the function of the syncytiotrophoblast and its plasma membranes and are listed in Table 1.2. From use of these techniques, it has been shown that the microvillous and basal syncytiotrophoblast membranes each contain specific transport proteins for a wide range of substances. These transporters may be concerned solely with cellular homeostasis of the syncytiotrophoblast but may also be involved in transcellular transport. For net transcellular transport to occur for a specific hydrophilic substance, there must be an entry and an exit step to the syncytiotrophoblast and an asymmetrical distribution of transport protein activity.

Transport of specific substances

Respiratory gases

Oxygen

The driving force for diffusion of oxygen in solution is its partial pressure and PO_2 correctly replaces concentration of solute in the Fick equation.

It seems probable that oxygen transfer across the human placenta is flow limited as it is in the sheep. When sheep uterine blood flow was reduced by partial occlusion of the maternal abdominal aorta, flux of oxygen to the umbilical circulation was reduced and the reduction correlated with reduction in uterine flow rates (Wilkening & Meschia, 1983). In a second series of experiments, it was shown that maternofetal oxygen flux was also reduced by partial occlusion of the fetal abdominal aorta, reducing blood flow through both umbilical arteries, but only when umbilical flow rates were 50% below those of controls (Wilkening & Meschia, 1989). When a reduction in umbilical blood flow was effected by occlusion of a single umbilical artery, as opposed to both, there was a greater reduction in maternofetal oxygen flux (Wilkening & Meschia, 1991). This demonstrates the importance of the equal matching of maternal and fetal circulations in optimizing flow-limited transfer.

Table 1.2 *In vitro methods used to assess solute transfer into and out of the syncytiotrophoblast*

Method	Variables measured	Comment
Incubation of placental slices or fragments	Uptake or efflux studies demonstrating kinetics of individual systems, their relative affinities for different solutes and effects of metabolic or specific transport protein inhibitors	Not a 'pure' preparation, contains red cells, stromal cells and endothelium
Membrane vesicles prepared from microvillous or basal syncytiotrophoblast membrane	Kinetics of individual systems, their relative affinities for different solutes and the effects of specific transport protein inhibitors on solute transfer across individul membranes	A pure membrane preparation. Activity of transport proteins studied may be changed in vivo by intracellular mechanisms
Cultured trophoblast cells	Uptake or efflux studies, similar to those using placental slices and fragments	Transport properties of fully differentiated syncytiotrophoblast may well be very different
Isolation of transport proteins. Patch-clamping of membranes of syncytiotrophoblast or cultured cells	Identification and quantification of individual transporters, and their biochemical and electrophysiological characterization	Allows direct comparison with transport systems present in other tissues
Microelectrode studies with placental fragments or cultured cells	Transmembrane or trans-syncytiotrophoblast potential difference	Has implications for ion movements

It should be noted that transport mechanisms described by these methods may not be involved in transcellular transport but in homeostasis of the syncytiotrophoblast which is subject to differing extracellular bathing fluids on its two sides.

In an ideal countercurrent exchange model, uterine venous PO_2 would relate to umbilical arterial PO_2, and umbilical venous PO_2 would be greater than either. Alternatively, with an ideal concurrent model, the umbilical venous PO_2 would be the same as uterine venous PO_2 and cannot be greater. Data from sheep and monkeys show that umbilical venous PO_2 in both species is lower than uterine venous PO_2. However, significant placental oxygen consumption and shunting of maternal blood complicate the interpretation of this data and the directional relationship of fetal and maternal blood flows cannot be inferred from this data. Interestingly in the human, PO_2 values from the umbilical vein appear to be equal to, or higher than, those from the intervillous pool (Nicolaides et al., 1986); this suggests that, in the human, there is at least some degree of countercurrent blood flow of the circulations.

Oxygen transfer is complicated by oxygen carriage by haemoglobin, and the different affinities of fetal and adult haemoglobin for oxygen. Due to the left shift in the oxygen dissociation curve of fetal haemoglobin, more oxygen is transported at a given PO_2 value in fetal blood than in maternal blood. As evidence for this effect, replacement of fetal haemoglobin by adult haemoglobin in the fetus of the sheep halves the umbilical venous oxygen saturation and reduces transplacental oxygen transfer. The situation is further complicated by the rise in fetal haemoglobin concentration throughout gestation which leads to an increase in maternofetal oxygen transfer at a given fetal PO_2. This explains why, in the human, fetal blood oxygen content normally remains constant despite PO_2 gradually falling during the second and third trimester (Soothill et al., 1986).

Factors governing oxygen transfer are therefore the uteroplacental and umbilical blood flows, the matching and geometrical relationships of these flows and the different oxygen binding capacities (concentration and affinity of haemoglobins) of the two blood supplies. Rurak et al. (1987) have calculated fetal oxygen consumption relative to oxygen delivery for both the human and the sheep; the ratio of O_2 consumption to delivery is termed fetal oxygen extraction. They found that, for a given PO_2, fetal oxygen extraction is higher in the human than in the sheep but suggest that in utero fetal oxygen extraction in the human is comparable to that of the sheep because human umbilical PO_2 is higher than that of the sheep. They propose that efficient oxygen transfer is brought about by different mechanisms in the two species: in the sheep by high fetal cardiac output and umbilical blood flow; in the human, which has relatively lower umbilical blood flow, by more efficient transplacental exchange leading to a higher PO_2, and also by higher fetal haemoglobin concentrations increasing oxygen carriage at a given PO_2.

Carbon dioxide

In solution in blood, carbon dioxide is in dynamic equilibrium with hydrogen ions and bicarbonate ions, the reaction catalysed by red cell carbonic anhydrase. About one-half of the carbon dioxide produced by the fetus is transported as bicarbonate ions within red cells (Hatano, Leichtweiss & Schröder, 1989). Therefore, carbon dioxide may be transferred across the placenta in the form of the gas itself or its ionic derivatives, although data from sheep and guinea pigs suggest that the majority of carbon dioxide is transferred across the placenta in its gaseous form (Hatano et al., 1989; Van Neen et al., 1984). In the guinea pig, in vitro perfusion studies suggest that carbonic anhydrase is present on the syncytiotrophoblast surface, which would catalyse conversion of bicarbonate to CO_2. Presence of acetazolamide (a carbonic anhydrase inhibitor) in the perfusate of the guinea pig preparation reduced fetomaternal transfer of bicarbonate/CO_2 more than maternofetal transfer of bicarbonate/CO_2, suggesting that the siting of carbonic anhydrase within the syncytiotrophoblast might selectively facilitate fetomaternal carbon dioxide transfer. The same series of experiments also suggested that, in the guinea pig, there are bidirectional trans-syncytiotrophoblast transport systems for bicarbonate ions but that these provide little, if any, overall contribution to carbon dioxide transfer (Hatano et al., 1989).

Transfer of carbon dioxide is further complicated by the fact that it binds reversibly to haemoglobin, this reaction competing with oxygen binding. Therefore maternofetal oxygen transfer enhances fetomaternal carbon dioxide transfer across the placenta by displacement of carbon dioxide from the haemoglobin molecule on the fetal side, with the reverse situation occurring on the maternal side – a 'double' Haldane effect.

Acid/base balance

Discussion of respiratory gas exchange would not be complete without reference to placental transfer mechanisms involved in acid/base regulation of the fetus. Fetal acid load has two components: respiratory due to carbon dioxide load, and metabolic due to production of lactic acid and other organic and inorganic acids. Cordocentesis has shown that, in the uncompromised human fetus, there is a gradual fall in pH and corresponding rise in PCO_2 throughout the second and third trimester (Soothill et al., 1986). This gestational effect may be related to increasing carbon dioxide production by both the fetus and the placenta. With regard to metabolic acid load, we do not know the amounts of acid generated by the uncompromised human fetus or placenta, nor do we know its disposal route, although lactic acidosis is known to be present in the human growth-retarded fetus (Soothill, Nicolaides & Campbell, 1987). In the sheep it has been shown that lactic acid is produced in the placenta and then transferred to both maternal and fetal circulations which implies that the sheep fetus metabolizes more lactate than it produces (Burd et al., 1975).

Both the microvillous and basal membranes of human syncytiotrophoblast contain Na^+/H^+ and probably Cl^-/HCO_3^- exchangers (Kulanthaivel et al., 1992; Vanderpuye et al., 1988). Also, data from in vitro human perfusion experiments suggest that the syncytiotrophoblast contains stereospecific pathways for lactate transport by facilitated diffusion (Carstensen, Leichtweiss & Schröder, 1983; Illsley et al., 1986). The role, if any, of these placental transporters in regulation of fetal acid/base balance is unknown, although the study of Illsley et al. strongly suggests that lactate transfer is predominantly by non-facilitated diffusion. It has been noted in the guinea pig that a hydrogen ion gradient across the placenta can lead to transfer of lactate against its concentration gradient, which implies that it is transported in the form of lactic acid as well as lactate (Moll, Girard & Gros, 1980).

Fatty acids and triglycerides

In the human, free fatty acid concentrations are higher in maternal blood than fetal blood suggesting net maternofetal transfer by diffusion. The exception to this is arachidonic acid which is found in higher concentrations in fetal than maternal plasma. In vitro perfusion experiments, assessing maternofetal clearance of radiolabelled palmitic acid and linoleic acid, support the idea that these fatty acids are transferred by simple diffusion (Booth et al., 1981). Also in this set of experiments, arachidonic acid concentration in both maternal and fetal outflows increased, suggesting placental production of this fatty acid. In the guinea pig, maternofetal transfer across in situ perfused placenta has been shown to be dependent on the flow rate of perfusate on the fetal side and the concentration of albumin within that perfusate which suggests that, in this species, transfer of fatty acid is flow limited as would be expected for a lipophilic substance and illustrates the importance of protein binding (Thomas et al., 1983).

In the guinea pig, triglycerides do not cross the placenta intact but the free fatty acid from the triglyceride does appear in the fetal circulation (Thomas & Lowy, 1983). It is suggested that lipoprotein lipase present on the maternal but not fetal aspect of the syncytiotrophoblast may be involved in de-esterifying triglycerides, following which there is diffusional maternofetal transfer of fatty acids. Interestingly, transfer of palmitic and linoleic acid across the sheep placenta occurs in only trace amounts and there is no detectable concentration difference between umbilical arterial and venous concentrations of these fatty acids (Elphick, Hull & Broughton-Pipkin, 1979). This is consistent with the finding that fetal sheep adipose tissue is practically devoid of essential fatty acids, whereas the fetuses of the human and guinea pig are both born with high body fat content.

In the human there is evidence that low density lipoproteins are incorporated into the syncytiotrophoblast by endocytosis although the subsequent fate of the vesicles is unknown (Malassine et al,. 1986).

Glucose

There is a facilitated diffusion mechanism for glucose transfer across the human placenta. Facilitated diffusion is a transcellular mechanism of transfer employing membrane transport proteins which is independent of direct energy input, the driving force being the concentration gradient of the solute across the cell. In the presence of such a mechanism, the rate of transfer of a solute across an epithelium is increased above that expected by simple diffusion. However, at high concentrations of solute, the rate of facilitated diffusion becomes saturated due to a combination of the kinetics of the transport proteins and the numbers of carriers present within the plasma membranes.

The evidence for facilitated diffusion of glucose across the placenta is as follows.

1. Fetal plasma glucose concentration is generally below that of maternal plasma, providing a diffusional gradient from mother to fetus (Faber & Thornburg, 1981).
2. In the isolated, perfused human placental cotyledon, net rate of maternofetal glucose transfer is directly proportional to maternal glucose concentration, until maternal glucose concentration rises well above normal physiological glucose concentrations, when rate of transfer becomes saturated (Rice, Rourke & Nesbitt, 1976*a*).

3. Glucose transfer in the perfused, isolated cotyledon is not reduced by presence of a metabolic inhibitor (Rice, Rourke & Nesbitt, 1979).
4. Again from in vitro perfusion studies, the rate of transfer of D-glucose is significantly higher than that of L-glucose, suggesting stereospecific carrier transport, and the presence of high concentrations of non-metabolizable glucose analogues on the maternal side reduces maternofetal glucose transport and may even stimulate net fetomaternal transfer against its concentration gradient (Rice, Nesbitt & Rourke, 1976*b*).
5. D-Glucose transport proteins have been identified in both the microvillous and basal membranes of the human syncytiotrophoblast; their affinities for glucose are in agreement with the linear relationship between glucose transfer and physiological transplacental concentration gradients (see Morriss et al., 1994 for further details).

Insulin does not appear to directly affect glucose transfer across the perfused placenta or microvillous membrane vesicles. Specific receptors for insulin are, however, present on the human syncytiotrophoblast, their function presently being unknown, although an insulin effect on metabolism of a glucose analogue by rat placenta has been described. As well as providing for facilitated diffusional transfer of glucose, the placenta also uses glucose for its own metabolic needs; the relationship between these demands has not been systematically studied in the human.

Amino acids

Human umbilical venous plasma concentrations of most amino acids are significantly higher than maternal concentrations at mid-gestation and at term (McIntosh et al., 1984). Placental tissue concentrations of free amino acids appear to be higher than in either maternal or fetal plasma, presumably owing to a high syncytiotrophoblast concentration (Pearse & Sornson, 1969). For these concentration gradients to be maintained, energy is required which implies active transport of amino acids across the syncytiotrophoblast in the maternofetal direction. The high placental concentration of amino acids suggests that the amino acids are actively transported from maternal blood into the syncytiotrophoblast across the microvillous membrane. Amino acids might then 'leak' down their concentration gradient from the syncytiotrophoblast to the fetal circulation across the basal plasma membrane by a process which does not require energy. Passive leak from the syncytiotrophoblast back to the maternal circulation must be much lower than the syncytiotrophoblast–fetal circulation leak for effective functioning of this model.

Uptake of amino acids into human placental slices in vitro is inhibited by the presence of metabolic inhibitors, consistent with active transport (Dancis et al., 1968). The presence of an asymmetrical leak predominantly in the fetal direction has been demonstrated in the dually perfused guinea pig. In these studies amino acid uptake by the placenta was similar from both the maternal and fetal circulations, suggesting that there is also active uptake of amino acids from fetal blood and that it is the asymmetry in passive leak that is primarily responsible for net maternofetal transport (Eaton & Yudilevich, 1981). Similar asymmetrical transfer of selected amino acids has been shown to occur in the human in vitro dually perfused cotyledon; stereospecific transport of neutral amino acids L-leucine and L-alanine occurs in the maternofetal but not in the fetomaternal direction (Schneider, Möhlen & Dancis, 1979), and faster maternofetal than fetomaternal transfer of L-leucine, L-lysine and aminoisobutyric acid (AIB, a non-metabolizable amino acid analogue) has also been demonstrated (Schneider et al., 1987). In the latter series of experiments, fetomaternal flux of the amino acids was half the magnitude of maternofetal flux and was also comparable to fetomaternal transfer of L-glucose, an extracellular marker, suggesting transfer in this direction was mainly via paracellular diffusion. Assuming paracellular permeability of the human in vitro perfusion model is unchanged compared to that in vivo, these results suggest that transcellular active transport of these amino acids would also be required to compensate for net fetomaternal paracellular diffusion down the prevailing concentration gradient.

Uptake studies of amino acids by human placental microvillous membrane vesicles have identified a number of amino acid transport systems analogous to those described for other epithelia. These transporters may each translocate a number of different amino acids which compete for transfer, or they may be specific to transfer of a single amino acid. A number of the transporters are sodium dependent, which implies that the energy needed for transport against the concentration gradient is derived from the sodium gradient across the microvillous membrane. This sodium gradient is maintained by the activity of Na^+/K^+ ATPase mainly present in the basal plasma membrane. Other amino acid transporters appear to be sodium independent and must harness energy by other means. Further details of these transporters are to be found in the review by Morriss et al. (1994).

Cations and inorganic anions

Human umbilical venous plasma concentrations of sodium, potassium, chloride, calcium (ionized and total), magnesium and phosphate are significantly higher than their respective concentrations in maternal venous blood at term (Faber & Thornburg, 1981). These concentration gradients may result from an electrical potential difference (p.d.) across the placental barrier or active transcellular transport mechanisms across the syncytiotrophoblast.

As regards p.d. there is a small (3 mV) fetal side negative maternofetal p.d. at mid-gestation in the human (Štulc et al., 1978), and this is similar to the recent in vitro measurement of trans-syncytiotrophoblast p.d. in term human placental villi (Greenwood, Boyd & Sibley, 1993). However, Mellor et al. (1969) reported that there was no maternofetal p.d. at term delivery. If a fetal side negative trans-syncytiotrophoblast p.d. does exist at term, then this could explain the fetomaternal concentration gradient for cations, but not for anions.

As regards active transport, there is evidence, particularly from studies on the rat and guinea pig, that there is primary, active, transplacental transport of sodium, potassium, calcium, magnesium phosphate and probably chloride (Štulc, Štulcová & Švihovec, 1982; Štulc & Švihovec, 1984; Štulc & Štulcová, 1986; Štulc et al., 1992; Štulc, Štulcová & Sibley, 1993; Mohammed et al., 1993; Shaw et al., 1990). The human syncytiotrophoblast certainly seems to have most of the transport proteins in its microvillous and basal plasma membranes which would enable active transport of these ions, but direct evidence that such transplacental active transport occurs is currently lacking. As mentioned previously, transport proteins may be involved in cellular homeostasis as well as transcellular transfer.

The work of Flexner and colleagues (Flexner et al., 1948), previously referred to, shows that the unidirectional maternofetal flux of sodium across human placenta is considerably greater than its net maternofetal flux calculated from fetal accretion of the ion. Again using data from Flexner's experiments, the maternofetal flux of sodium at term appears to be of comparable magnitude to the estimated unidirectional diffusional flux of the ion, calculated from the data on in vivo maternofetal clearance of membrane-impermeable, inert substances (e.g. insulin, mannitol and sucrose; Bain et al., 1988, 1990), strongly suggesting that a considerable proportion of transplacental sodium transfer occurs by diffusion.

In summary, we do not yet know how the slightly higher fetal than maternal plasma inorganic ion concentrations are generated in the human. A reasonable working model of ion transfer is that, in the near term woman, it is primarily by paracellular diffusion with a much smaller transcellular component.

Proteins

The human placenta has a low but finite permeability to proteins and large macromolecules. Small amounts of alphafetoprotein do cross from fetus to mother and, in normal pregnancy, this fetomaternal transfer may well be transplacental. Raised amniotic fluid concentrations of serum alphafetoprotein in the presence of fetal congenital abnormality, such as spina bifida, lead to raised maternal serum levels of alphafetoprotein, suggesting protein transfer may also occur from fetus to mother across the chorion laeve and amnion.

Immunoglobulin G (IgG) is transferred from mother to fetus in significant amounts in women, and has been reported to be present in higher concentrations in fetal as compared to maternal plasma at term (Kohler & Farr, 1966). This is a larger molecule than either albumin or alphafetoprotein, and its rate of paracellular diffusion across the placenta must be extremely low. Therefore a specific transport mechanism is implicated. IgG transfer across the yolk sac (but not the chorioallantoic) placenta of rodents has been demonstrated to occur by a specific endocytosis/exocytosis mechanism. Specific Fc receptors for IgG are present in coated pits along the maternal-facing plasma membrane of the endoderm. These pits then invaginate to form coated vesicles, and cross the endoderm, avoiding fusion with lysosomes, exocytosing their contents by fusion with the fetal-facing membrane of the endoderm (Jollie, 1986). In the human chorioallantoic placenta, there is evidence for the presence of Fc receptors on the microvillous membrane of the syncytiotrophoblast, and for the presence of coated pits and coated vesicles containing IgG within the syncytiotrophoblast (Johnson & Brown, 1981). Histochemical techniques suggest that these vesicles may fuse with each other, or with phagolysosomes within the cell, but have not clearly shown exocytosis on to the basal membrane (Lin, 1980; King, 1982; Leach et al., 1989). However, some of their contents is present in the villous core suggesting that trans-syncytiotrophoblast transfer is achieved. The fetal capillary endothelium must present a significant barrier to maternofetal transfer of such a large molecule and it is most likely that endocytosis/exocytosis is also involved here (King, 1982; Leach et al., 1989).

Water

The net flux of water to the fetus is greater than that of any other substance, including oxygen. In vivo studies at term, using deuterium oxide as a marker, show that unidirectional flux of water across the human placenta is some 10 000 times that of net flux (Hutchinson et al., 1959), unidirectional fluxes between mother and fetus across amniotic fluid accounting for only 5% of the total flux in either direction (Wilbur, Power & Longo, 1978). Therefore, there appears to be a considerable bidirectional flux of water across the placental barrier. The driving forces for net flux are likely to be hydrostatic and osmotic pressure gradients between the fetal and maternal circulations and there is experimental evidence from animal studies to support this (Anderson & Faber, 1982; Bruns et al., 1964).

To calculate the effective osmotic pressure gradient, we would need to know the reflection coefficients across the placenta of all the individual solutes. For instance, inorganic ions pass more freely across the human placenta than the larger macromolecules and therefore have lower reflection coefficients, contributing less to osmotic pressure than proteins and large macromolecules. So, although the concentration of many solutes, and apparent overall osmolarity of fetal umbilical venous blood is higher than that of maternal venous blood, it is currently not possible to assess the relevant osmotic gradient across the placental barrier governing water movement. Hydrostatic pressure gradients between the umbilical circulation and the intervillous space are thought overall to favour fetomaternal water flux, the hydrostatic pressure in the umbilical vein being higher than that estimated in the intervillous space (Reynolds et al., 1968). However, we do not know the hydrostatic pressure within the capillary beds of individual mature terminal villi.

Štulc and Štulcová (1993) have recently proposed a model for combined bidirectional water and solute transfer across the haemotrichorial rat placenta, elements of which may apply to the human situation. In vivo studies of the rat placenta showed an asymmetrical transfer of inert hydrophilic solutes, fetomaternal transfer being greater than maternofetal transfer. In the proposed model, this asymmetry in transfer is accounted for by fetomaternal bulk flow of water containing the solutes down a hydrostatic pressure gradient through wide extracellular channels. Water moves in a maternofetal direction through smaller extracellular channels, impermeable to larger inert molecules, down an osmotic gradient created by transcellular transport of ions and other solutes. Our current knowledge of the term human placenta suggests that solute transfer has a large diffusional component, but if a maternofetal osmotic gradient is generated by active transcellular transfer, then a similar model might apply.

References

Anderson, D. & Faber, J. (1982). Water flux due to colloid osmotic pressures across the haemochorial placenta of the guinea pig. *Journal of Physiology*, **332**, 521.

Bain, M.D., Copas, D.K., Landon, M.J. & Stacey, T.E. (1988). In vivo permeability of the human placenta to inulin and mannitol. *Journal of Physiology*, **399**, 313–19.

Bain, M.D., Copas, D.K., Taylor, A., Landon, M.J. & Stacey, T.E. (1990). Permeability of the human placenta in vivo to four non-metabolised hydrophilic molecules. *Journal of Physiology*, **431**, 505–13.

Booth, C., Elphick, M.C., Hendrickse, W. & Hull, D. (1981). Investigation of linoleic acid conversion into arachidonic acid and placental transfer of linoleic and palmitic acids across the perfused human placenta. *Journal of Developmental Physiology*, **3**, 177–89.

Boyd, J.D. & Hamilton, W.J. (1970). *The Human Placenta*. Heffer, Cambridge.

Bruns, P.D., Hellegers, A.E., Elmore Seeds, A., Behrman, R.E. & Battaglia, F.C. (1964). Effects of osmotic gradients across the primate placenta upon fetal and placental water contents. *Pediatrics*, **34**, 407–11.

Burd, L.I., Jones, M.D., Simmons, M.A., Makowski, E.L., Meschia, G. & Battaglia, F.C. (1975). Placental production and fetal utilisation of lactate and pyruvate. *Nature*, **254**, 710–11.

Carstensen, M.H., Leichtweiss, H-P. & Schröder, H. (1983). Lactate carriers in the artificially perfused human placenta. *Placenta*, **4**, 165–75.

Chien, P.F.W., Smith, K., Watt, P.W., Scrimgeour, C.M., Taylor, D.J. & Rennie, M.J. (1993). Protein turnover in the human fetus studied at term using stable tracer amino acids. *American Journal of Physiology*, **265**, E31–5.

Dancis, J., Money, W.L., Springer, D. & Levitz, M. (1968). Transport of amino acids by placenta. *American Journal of Obstetrics and Gynecology*, **101**, 820.

Eaton, B.M. & Yudilevich, D.L. (1981). Uptake and asymmetric efflux of amino acids at maternal and fetal sides of the placenta. *American Journal of Physiology*, **241**, C106.

Edwards, D., Jones, C.J.P., Sibley, C.P.S. & Nelson, D.M. (1993). Paracellular permeability pathways in the human placenta: a quantitative and morphological study of maternal–fetal transfer of horseradish peroxidase. *Placenta*, **14**, 63–73.

Elphick, M.C., Hull, D. & Broughton-Pipkin, F. (1979). The transfer of fatty acids across the sheep placenta. *Journal of Developmental Physiology*, **1**, 31–45.

Faber, J.J. & Thornburg, K.L. (1981). The forces that drive inert solutes from water across the epitheliochorial placentae of the sheep and the goat and the hemochorial placentae of the rabbit and the guinea pig. In *Placental Transfer: Methods and Interpretations, Placenta Suppl. 2* ed. Young et al. pp. 203–14. W.B. Saunders, London.

Flexner, L.B., Cowie, D.B., Hellman, L.M., Wilde, W.S. & Vosburgh, G.J. (1948). The permeability of the human placenta to sodium in normal and abnormal pregnancies and the supply of sodium to the human fetus as determined with radioactive sodium. *American Journal of Physiology,* **55**, 469–80.

Greenwood, S.L., Boyd, R.D.H. & Sibley, C.P. (1993). Transtrophoblast and microvillous membrane potential difference in mature intermediate human placental villi. *American Journal of Physiology*, **265**, C460–6.

Hatano, H., Leichtweiss, H-P. & Schröder, H. (1989). Uptake of bicarbonate/ CO_2 in the isolated guinea pig placenta. *Placenta*, **10,** 213–23.

Hutchinson, D.L., Gray, M.J., Plentl, A.A., Alvarez, H., Caldeyro-Barcia, R., Kaplan, B. & Lind, J. (1959). The role of the fetus in the water exchange of the amniotic fluid of normal and hydramniotic patients. *Journal of Clinical Investigation*, **38**, 971–80.

Illsley, N.P., Wootton, R., Penfold, P., Hall, S. & Duffy, S. (1986). Lactate transfer across the perfused human placenta. *Placenta*, **7,** 209–21.

Johnson, P.M. & Brown, P.J. (1981). Review article: Fc receptors in the human placenta. *Placenta*, **2**, 355–70.

Jollie, W.P. (1986). Review article: ultrastructural studies of protein transfer across rodent yolk sac. *Placenta*, **7**, 263–81.

Kaufmann, P., Kosanke, G., Leiser, R., Schweikhart, G. & Scheffen, I. (1992). Morphologische und morphometrische Grundlagen der Gefässversorgung der menschlichen Plazenta; In *Perinatale Dopplerdiagnostik, Grenzen der Methodik und Neue Aspekte*, ed. H. Fendel et al. Steinkopf Verlag, Darmstadt.

King, B.F. (1982). Absorption of peroxidase-conjugated immunoglobulin G by human placenta: an in vitro study. *Placenta*, **3**, 395–406.

Kohler, P.F. & Farr, R.S. (1966). Elevation of cord over maternal IgG immunoglobulin: evidence for an active placental IgG transport. *Nature*, **210**, 1070.

Kulanthaivel, P., Furesz, T.C., Moe, A.J., Smith, C.H., Mahesh, V.B., Leibach, F.H. & Ganapathy, V. (1992). Human placental syncytiotrophoblast expresses two pharmacologically distinguishable types of Na^+/H^+ exchangers, NHE-1 in the maternal-facing (brush border) membrane and NHE-2 in the fetal-facing (basal) membrane. *Biochemical Journal*, **284**, 33–8.

Leach, L., Eaton, B.M., Firth, J.A. & Contractor, S.F. (1989). Immunogold localisation of endogenous immunoglobulin-G in ultrathin frozen sections of the human placenta. *Cell Tissue Research*, **257**, 603–7.

Leach, L. & Firth, J.A. (1992). Fine structure of the paracellular junctions of terminal villous capillaries in the perfused human placenta. *Cell Tissue Research*, **268**, 447–52.

Leiser, R., Kosanke, G. & Kaufmann, P. (1991). Human placental vascularisation. Structural and quantitative aspects. In *Placenta: Basic Research for Clinical Application,* ed. H. Soma. pp. 32–45. Karger, Basel.

Lin, C-T. (1980). Immunoelectron microscopic localisation of immunoglobulin G in human placenta. *Journal of Histochemistry and Cytochemistry*, **28**, 339–46.

Lunell, N-O. & Nylund, L. (1992). Uteroplacental blood flow. *Clinical Obstetrics and Gynecology*, **35(1)**, 108–18.

Macara, L.M., Kingdom, J.C.P. & Kaufmann, P. (1993). Control of placental circulation. In *Fetal and Maternal Medicine Review*, **5**, 167–79.

McIntosh, N., Rodeck, C.H. & Heath, R. (1984). Plasma amino acids of the mid-trimester human fetus. *Biology of the Neonate*, **45**, 218–24.

Malassine, A., Roche, A., Elsat, E., Rebourcet, R., Mondon, F., Goldstein, S. & Cedard, L. (1986). Ultrastructural visualisation of gold low density lipoprotein endocytosis by human term placental cells (abstract). *Placenta,* **7**, 485.

Mellor, D.J., Cockburn, F., Lees, M.M. & Blagden, A. (1969). Distribution of ions and electrical potential differences between mother and fetus in the human at term. *Journal of Obstetrics and Gynaecology of the British Commonwealth*, **76**, 993.

Mohammed, T., Štulc, J., Glazier, J.D., Boyd, R.D.H. & Sibley, C.P. (1993). Mechanisms of potassium transfer across the dually perfused rat placenta. *American Journal of Physiology*, **265**, R341–7.

Moll, W., Baustädter, R., Eder, R., Ruider, A., Götz, R. & Pohl, H. (1991). Adaptation of the maternal arterial system supplying the placenta. In *Placenta: Basic Research for Clinical Application,* ed. H.Soma. pp. 1–10. Karger, Basel.

Moll, W., Girard, H. & Gros, G. (1980). Facilitated diffusion of lactic acid in the guinea pig placenta. *Pflügers Archiv*, **385**, 229–38.

Morriss, F.H., Boyd, R.D.H. & Mahendran, D. (1994). Placental transport. In *The Physiology of Reproduction, Volume 2,* ed. E. Knobil, J. Neill et al. pp. 813–862. Raven, New York.

Myatt, L., Brewer, A.S. & Brockman, D.E. (1991). The action of nitric oxide in the perfused human placental cotyledon. *American Journal of Obstetrics and Gynecology*, **164**, 687–92.

Myatt, L., Brewer, A.S., Langdon, G. & Brockman, D.E. (1992). Attenuation of the vasoconstrictor effects of thromboxane and endothelin by nitric oxide in the human fetal–placental circulation. *American Journal of Obstetrics and Gynecology,* **166**, 224–30.

Nicolaides, K.H., Soothill, P.W., Rodeck, C.H. & Campbell, S. (1986). Ultrasound guided cord and placental blood sampling to assess fetal well-being. *Lancet* **i,** 1065–7.

Pearse, W.H. & Sornson, H. (1969). Free amino acids of normal and abnormal human placenta. *American Journal of Obstetrics and Gynecology,* **105**, 696.

Rankin, J.R. & Mclaughlin, M.K. (1979). The regulation of placental blood flows. *Journal of Developmental Physiology,* **1**, 3–30.

Reynolds, S.R.M., Freese, U.E., Bieniarz, J., Caldeyro-Barcia, R., Mendez-Bauer, C. & Escarcena, L. (1968). Multiple simultaneous intervillous space pressures recorded in several regions of the hemochorial placenta in relation to functional anatomy of the fetal cotyledon. *American Journal of Obstetrics and Gynecology*, **102**, 1128.

Rice, P.A., Nesbitt, R.E.L. & Rourke, J.E. (1976*b*). In vitro perfusion studies of the human placenta V. Counter transport of glucose induced by an analog. *Gynecological Investigation* **7**, 344–57.

Rice, P.A., Rourke, J.E. & Nesbitt, R.E.L. (1976*a*). In vitro perfusion studies of the human placenta IV. Some characteristics of the glucose transport system in the human placenta. *Gynecological Investigation*, **7**, 213–21.

Rice, P.A., Rourke, J.E. & Nesbitt, R.E.L. (1979). In vitro perfusion studies of the human placenta VI. Evidence against active glucose transport. *American Journal of Obstetrics and Gynecology*, **133**, 649–55.

Rurak, D., Selke, P., Fisher, M., Taylor, S. & Wittman, B. (1987). Fetal oxygen extraction: comparison of the human and sheep. *American Journal of Obstetrics and Gynecology*, **156**, 360–6.

Schneider, H., Möhlen, K-H. & Dancis, J. (1979). Transfer of amino acids across the in vitro perfused human placenta. *Pediatric Research,* **13**, 236.

Schneider, H., Panigel, M. & Dancis, J. (1972). Transfer across the perfused human placenta of antipyrine sodium and leucine. *American Journal of Obstetrics and Gynecology*, **114**, 822–8.

Schneider, H., Proegler, M., Sodha, R. & Dancis, J. (1987). Asymmetrical transfer of alpha-aminoisobutyric acid (AIB), leucine and lysine across the in vitro perfused human placenta. *Placenta*, **8**, 141.

Shaw, A.J., Mughal, M.Z., Mohammed, T., Maresh, M.J.A. & Sibley, C.P. (1990). Evidence for active maternofetal transfer of magnesium across the in situ perfused rat placenta. *Pediatric Research,* **27**, 622–5.

Sibley, C.P. & Boyd, R.D.H. (1992). Mechanisms of transfer across the human placenta. In *Fetal and Neonatal Physiology,* ed. R.A. Polin & W.W. Fox. pp. 62–74. Saunders, Philadelphia.

Soothill, P.W., Nicolaides, K.H. & Campbell, S. (1987). Prenatal asphyxia, hyperlactinemia, hypoglycemia and erythroblastosis in growth retarded fetuses. *British Medical Journal*, **294**, 1051–3.

Soothill, P.W., Nicolaides, K.H., Rodeck, C.H. & Campbell, S. (1986). The effect of gestational age on blood gas and acid-base values in human pregnancy. *Fetal Therapy,* **1**, 168–75.

Štulc, J., Husain, S.M., Boyd, R.D.H. & Sibley, C.P. (1992). Mechanisms of chloride transfer across the in situ perfused placenta of the anaesthetised rat. *Journal of Physiology*, **452**, 94P.

Štulc, J. & Štulcová, B. (1986). Transport of calcium by the placenta of the rat. *Journal of Physiology*, **371**, 1–16.

Štulc, J. & Štulcová, B. (1993). Asymmetrical transfer of inert hydrophilic solutes across rat placenta. *American Journal of Physiology*, **265**, R670–5.

Štulc, J., Štulcová, B. & Sibley, C.P.(1993). Evidence for active maternal–fetal transport of Na^+ across the placenta of the anaesthetised rat. *Journal of Physiology*, **470**, 637–49.

Štulc, J., Štulcová, B. & Švihovec, J. (1982). Uptake of inorganic phosphate by the maternal border of the guinea pig placenta. *Pflügers Archiv* **395**, 326–30.

Štulc, J. & Švihovec, J. (1984). Transport of inorganic phosphate by the fetal border of the guinea pig placenta perfused in situ. *Placenta*, **5**, 9–20.

Štulc, J., Švihovec, J., Drábková, J., Stříbrný, J., Kobilková, J., Vido, I. & Doležal, A. (1978). Electrical potential difference across the mid-term human placenta. *Acta Obstetrica Gynecologica Scandinavica*, **57**, 125–6.

Thomas, C.R. & Lowy, C. (1983). Placental transfer of free fatty acids: factors affecting transfer across the guinea pig placenta. *Journal of Developomental Physiology*, **5**, 323–32.

Thomas, C.R., Lowy, C., St Hillaire, R.J. & Brunzell, J.D. (1983). Studies on the placental hydrolysis and transfer of lipids to the fetal guinea pig. In *Fetal nutrition, Metabolism and Immunology: Role of the Placenta,* ed. R.K. Miller & H.A. Thiede. pp. 135–48. Plenum Press, New York.

Vanderpuye, O.A., Kelley, L.K., Morrison, M.M. & Smith, C.H. (1988). The apical and basal plasma membranes of the human placental syncytiotrophoblast contain different erythrocyte membrane protein isoforms. Evidence for placental forms of band 3 and spectrin. *Biochimica et Biophysica Acta*, **943**, 277–87.

Van Neen, L.C.P., Hay, W.W., Battaglia, F.C. & Meschia, G. (1984). Fetal CO_2 kinetics. *Journal of Developmental Physiology*, **6**, 359–65.

Wilbur, W.J., Power, G.G. & Longo, L.D. (1978). Water exchange in the placenta: a mathematical model. *American Journal of Physiology*, **235**, R181.

Wilkening, R.B. & Meschia, G. (1983). Fetal oxygen uptake, oxygenation, and acid–base balance as a function of uterine blood flow. *American Journal of Physiology*, **244**, H749–55.

Wilkening, R.B. & Meschia, G. (1989). Effect of umbilical blood flow on transplacental diffusion of ethanol and oxygen. *American Journal of Physiology*, **256**, H813–20.

Wilkening, R.B. & Meschia, G. (1991). Effect of occluding one umbilical artery on placental oxygen transport. *American Journal of Physiology*, **260**, H1319–25.

2

Nutrient requirements for normal fetal growth and metabolism

ABIGAIL L. FOWDEN

Introduction

Normal fetal growth and development are dependent on the adequate provision and appropriate utilization of a number of different nutrients. These nutrients are used not only for the accretion of new structural tissue and fuel reserves such as glycogen and fat but also for the provision of energy for the growing tissues. The total nutrient requirement of the fetus is therefore determined by its growth rate, body composition and rate of oxidative metabolism.

In late gestation, fetal growth rate varies between species and ranges from 0.9–30% per day (Table 2.1). There are similar species variations in body composition, particularly in body fat content (Table 2.1), which lead to large differences among species in the specific nutrients required

Table 2.1. *The growth rate, body weight and fat content of fetuses of different species during late gestation (≥85% gestation)*

		Growth rate (g/kg fetal wet wt/day)			
Species	Birthweight kg	Total	Non-fat dry wt	Fat	% body fat at term
Rat	0.06	300.0	32.4	3.0	1.1
Guinea pig	0.09	68.0	21.2	10.7	11.7
Monkey	0.50	44.0	10.0	1.4	3.0
Pig	1.20	32.8	6.6	0.5	1.0
Sheep	3.00	36.0	6.5	0.8	2.0
Human	3.50	15.0	2.3	3.5	16.0
Horse	52.00	9.2	2.8	0.4	2.6

Data from Moustagaard, 1962; Meyer & Ahlswede, 1978; Sparks, 1984.

for growth during late gestation (Battaglia & Meschia, 1988). By contrast, fetal O_2 consumption is remarkably uniform in different species during late gestation when values are expressed on a weight-specific basis (Table 2.2). The actual rate of fetal O_2 consumption depends on gestational age as does the growth rate and body composition of the fetus. In the human infant, growth rate declines from 15 g/kg/day at 36 weeks to about 6 g/kg/day at term while fat content increases from 80 g/kg to over 160 g/kg during the same period of gestation (Sparks, 1984). Hence, at any given stage of gestation, normal intrauterine growth will only occur if sufficient nutrients are supplied to meet the combined requirements of oxidation and tissue growth.

Nutrient supply

Nutrients can be supplied to the fetal tissues by three different routes. First, they may be transported across the placenta from the maternal circulation. Secondly, they can be synthesized in the placenta and released into the umbilical circulation. Finally, they may be produced endogenously by the fetal tissues themselves either by mobilization of stored reserves or by de novo synthesis. The relative importance of these different nutrient sources to the total supply varies with the specific substrate and the nutritional state of the animal. However, in the fed, unstressed state, the primary origin of most of the fetal substrates is the maternal nutrient pool.

Oxygen

Oxygen crosses the placenta by passive diffusion down the concentration gradient from maternal to fetal blood. The magnitude of this transplacental O_2 gradient varies between species and depends on a variety of factors including placental vascular architecture, blood flow, placental O_2 consumption and the O_2 affinity of the fetal blood (Silver, 1984). In the human, the drop in arterial PO_2 across the placenta is about 60–70 torr which results in a fetal arterial PO_2 of 20–25 torr in the normal infant (Longo, 1991). However, these relatively low PO_2 values do not imply fetal hypoxia or a major anaerobic component to fetal metabolism.

The rate of oxygen uptake by the uterus is 50% higher than the rate at which it is delivered to the fetus. A significant amount of O_2 is therefore consumed by the uteroplacental tissues before it reaches the fetus (Fig. 2.1). When values are expressed on a weight-specific basis, utero-

Table 2.2. *Mean (±SEM) rates (µmol/min/kg respective tissue wt) of uptake or output (†) of glucose, lactate and oxygen by the uterus plus tissue contents (uterine uptake), fetus (umbilical uptake) and uteroplacental tissues (human, placenta; other species, uterus + placenta + membranes) in sheep, horses, cows and humans during late gestation (⩾0.85% gestation)*

	Glucose			Lactate			Oxygen		
	Uterus and tissue contents	Fetus uptake	Utero-placental tissues	Uterus and tissue contents	Fetus uptake	Utero-placental tissues	Uterus and tissue contents	Fetus uptake	Utero-placental tissues
Sheep	50	30	120	15†	25	100†	440	315	630
Cow	60	30	120	20†	50	300†	380	300	560
Horse	100	45	200	–	35	–	390	315	450
Human*	160	45	430	80†	10	470†	–	350	300

*Perfused placenta or at caesarian section.
Data from Morriss et al., 1975; Comline & Silver, 1976; Hauguel et al., 1983; Hay et al., 1984; Silver, 1984.

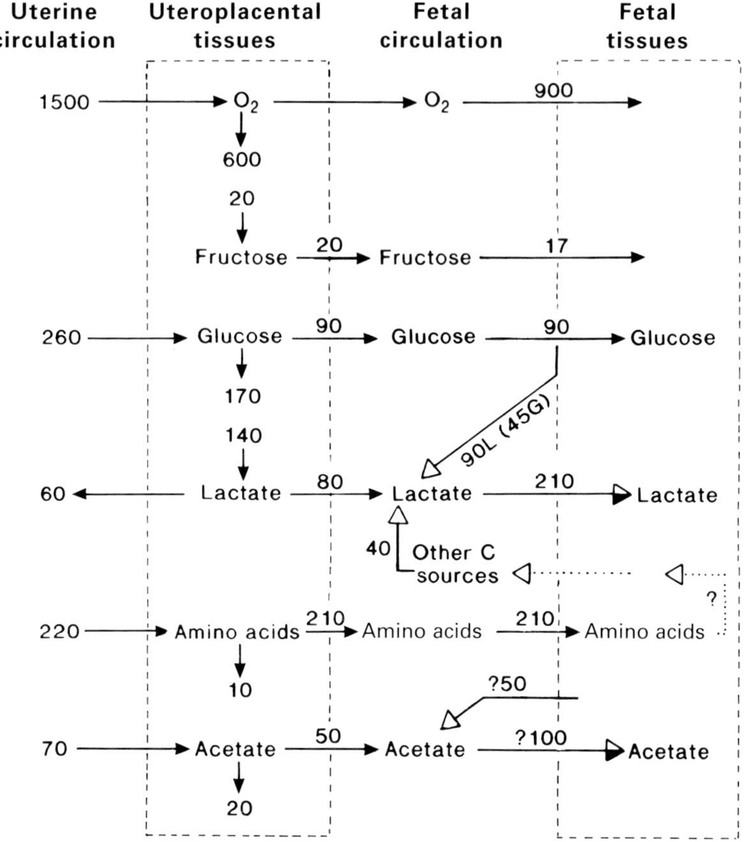

Fig. 2.1. The partitioning of substrates between the fetus (3.0 kg) and uteroplacental tissues in well-fed ewes during late gestation (≥85% gestation). Rates of flux of substrates are given in μmol/min. Origin of substrates: maternal and/or uteroplacental (——▶), fetal (——▷), mixed origin (——▷). (Data from Char & Creasy, 1976; Sparks et al., 1981; Lemons & Schreiner, 1983; Hay et al., 1984; Meznarich et al., 1987.)

placental O_2 consumption is 4–6-fold greater than the fetal rate of O_2 uptake and about 10-fold higher than adult rates of oxidative metabolism (Table 2.2).

Glucose

Glucose appears to be taken up and transported across the placenta by facilitated diffusion. This process requires carrier molecules and a glucose concentration gradient from the maternal to fetal circulations. In the ovine placenta, the carriers mediating glucose transfer have been shown to be specific for hexoses with a preference for glucose among the hexoses (Stacey, Weedon & Haworth, 1978). Glucose transporters have also been identified in the human placenta on both maternal- and fetal-facing surfaces of the trophoblast (Johnson & Smith, 1980). However, relatively little is known about the characteristics or regulation of the placental glucose transporters, although they appear to be insensitive to acute changes in insulin concentration (Hay, 1991).

The gradient for glucose transfer across the placenta is determined by the maternal and fetal glucose concentrations. In ruminants, fetal glucose levels are 25–30% of those in the mother (2.5–3.5 mmol/l) while in other, non-ruminant, species such as primates and humans fetal glucose levels are normally 60–70% of the maternal values (>4.0 mmol/l). The transplacental glucose concentration therefore also varies with species and is less in humans (0.5–1.5 mmol/l) than in the ruminant (2.0–3.5 mmol/l). However, in all species studied so far, placental to fetal glucose transfer rises with increases in the transplacental glucose concentration gradient (Comline & Silver, 1976; Simmons, Battaglia & Meschia, 1979; Silver, 1984).

In normal circumstances, the main determinant of the transplacental gradient is the maternal glucose concentration, although fetal glucose levels can rise independently of the maternal concentrations during adverse conditions (Hay, 1991). Both the uterine and umbilical glucose uptakes rise with increases in the maternal glucose level but plateau when the transport system becomes saturated at supraphysiological maternal glucose concentrations (Fig. 2.2). When fetal glucose levels are manipulated independently of the maternal glucose levels, umbilical glucose uptake varies inversely with the fetal glucose level (Hay et al., 1990). Placental to fetal glucose transfer is therefore sensitive to the fetal glucose level, and can be altered by changing the transplacental glucose gradient from either the maternal or fetal side of the placenta. This may have an important role in regulating the transplacental (or exogenous) glucose supply to the fetus during adverse conditions which activate fetal glucogenesis.

The rate of facilitated glucose transport across the placenta increases during the last half of gestation in both sheep and man (Hay, 1991). In part, this is due to an increase in the transplacental glucose concentration gradient as fetal glucose levels fall towards term in both species (Battaglia, 1991). However, when the gradient is held constant experimentally, placental glucose transfer still doubles between 100 days and term in the

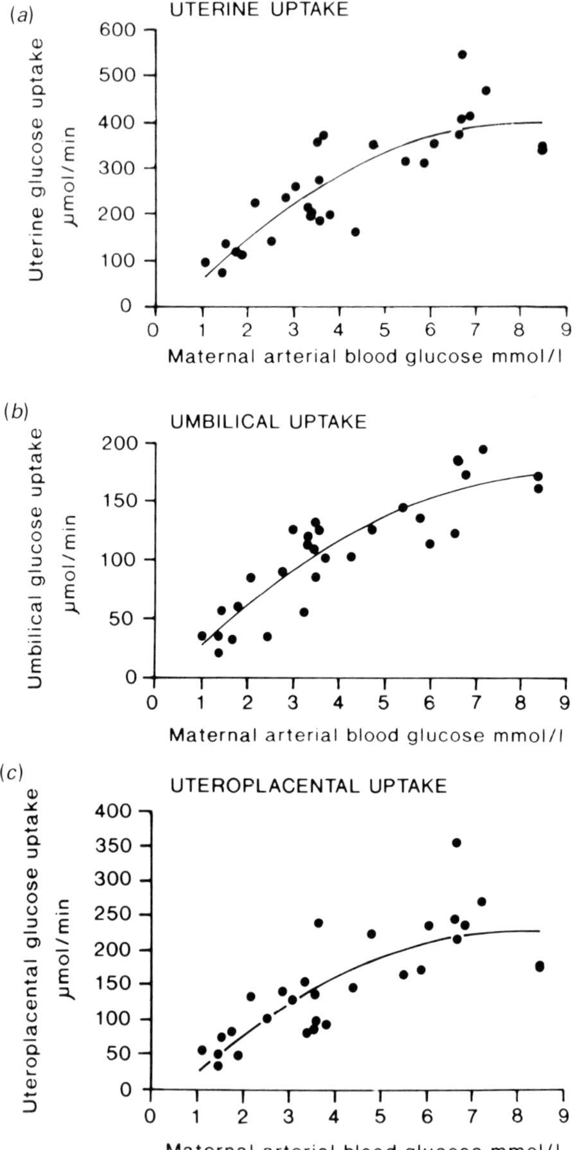

Fig. 2.2. Relationship between maternal arterial blood glucose concentrations and (*a*) uterine glucose uptake, (*b*) umbilical (or placental to fetal) glucose uptake and (*c*) uteroplacental glucose uptake (or consumption) in pregnant ewes during late gestation. (Data redrawn from Hay & Meznarich, 1989 with permission.)

sheep (Molina et al., 1991). The glucose transport capacity of the ovine placenta therefore increases towards term and accounts for about 60% of the increase in placental glucose transfer that occurs between mid- and late gestation in this species.

The explanation for the increased transport capacity of the placenta towards term remains unclear but there are changes in placental morphology during the last half of gestation that may promote glucose transfer. In the human, villus surface area increases three-fold between 25 and 36 weeks of gestation while the cross-sectional diameter of the villi decreases four-fold during the same period (Teasdale, 1980). There is therefore an increase in the placental surface area and a reduction in the diffusion distance in the human (and other species) towards term. Changes in the number of placental glucose transporters, uterine and umbilical blood flow and in placental glucose consumption may also contribute to the enhanced glucose transport capacity of the placenta that occurs towards term.

In all species, the uteroplacental tissues consume a significant proportion of the glucose leaving the uterine circulation (Table 2.2). This increases the transplacental glucose concentration gradient but significantly reduces the amount of glucose reaching the fetus. In normal fed conditions, the rate of uteroplacental glucose consumption is high and accounts for 60–75% of the total uterine glucose uptake in late gestation (Table 2.2). In mid-gestation, glucose consumption by the ovine uteroplacental tissue is lower (40 μmol/min/kg) but, because these tissues are a larger proportion of the total uterine mass earlier in gestation, the fraction of total uterine glucose uptake used by the uteroplacental tissues is higher in mid- than late gestation (Bell et al., 1986).

In sheep, uteroplacental glucose consumption rises with increases in the maternal glucose levels but reaches a plateau of 150–200 μmol/min/kg at glucose levels greater than 6.0 mmol/l (Fig. 2.2). In part, this apparent dependence of uteroplacental glucose consumption on maternal glycaemia is due to the concommitant changes in glucose concentration in the fetal circulation. When maternal and fetal glucose levels are identical, 80% of glucose used by the uteroplacental tissues is derived from the fetal glucose pool (Simmons et al., 1979). More recent studies using glucose clamp techniques have shown that uteroplacental glucose consumption is regulated by the fetal glucose level and is virtually independent of the maternal glucose concentration (Hay et al., 1990). Uteroplacental glucose consumption is therefore primarily accounted for by tissues, such as the placenta, which have direct access to the fetal circulation.

Table 2.3. *The rates of substrate uptake (+) or output (−) and of protein synthesis in individual tissues of the sheep fetus from well-nourished ewes near term*

	Oxygen	Glucose	Lactate	Protein synthesis	
	μmol/min/100 g	μmol/min/100 g	μmol/min/100 g	g/day	% day
Brain	+180	+25.0	+1.3	1.01	37
Heart	+400	+22.0	+73.0	0.40	14
Liver	+180	+0.6	+37.0	9.06	78
Kidney	+123	−5.2	+18.0	1.02	45
Gut	+50	+3.5	+7.5	12.90	93
Carcass*	+22	+3.0	−1.2	12.93	26
Lung	+57	+6.0	−8.0	5.92	65

*Calculated with data from the fetal hindlimb.
Data from Jones et al., 1975; Charlton et al., 1979; Fisher et al., 1980; Schaefer & Krishnamuti, 1984; Singh et al., 1984; Gleason et al., 1985; Iwamoto, Oh & Rudolph, 1985; Simmons & Charlton, 1988.

The glucose taken up by the uteroplacental tissue is either oxidized or used for non-oxidative processes such as lipogenesis, glycogenesis and conversion to lactate, fructose and amino acids. Since some of these products (e.g. lactate) are released into the umbilical circulation, not all the glucose carbon taken up by the uteroplacental tissues is lost to the fetus. However, the factors regulating uteroplacental metabolism and the distribution of glucose between the oxidative and non-oxidative metabolic pathways in the placenta remain unclear.

Glucose can also be supplied to fetal tissues by glucogenesis (Hay et al., 1984). In the fetus, the main sites of endogenous glucose production are the liver and kidneys (Table 2.3). In late gestation, these tissues show no net consumption of glucose and contain all the enzymes necessary for glucogenesis (Fowden, Mijovic & Silver, 1993; Table 2.3). In the fetus as a whole, the rate of endogenous glucose production is negligible in normal basal conditions (Hay et al., 1984). However, significant glucogenesis is observed in fetuses close to term during adverse intrauterine conditions such as placental insufficiency and undernutrition, which compromise the transplacental nutrient supply (Hay, 1991). During prolonged hypoglycaemia, the fetal liver can produce glucose at a rate of 8–15 μmol/min/kg fetal bodyweight which accounts for 50% or more of the actual rate of fetal glucose utilization in these circumstances (Hay et al., 1984; Fowden, 1989; Hay, 1991). Glucogenesis can therefore ameliorate the effects of a reduced umbilical glucose uptake and help to maintain a supply of glucose to essential fetal tissues such as the brain, heart and placenta. It also reduces the drain on the maternal glucose pool when the maternal nutritional supply is limited.

Glucose can be produced by glycogenolysis from hepatic glycogen or by gluconeogenesis from precursors such as lactate and amino acids. Both processes can occur in utero but their relative contribution to hepatic glucose output remains unclear. Hepatic glycogen and gluconeogenic enzyme levels rise towards term and, hence, the fetal capacity for glucogenesis is enhanced during late gestation (Fowden et al., 1993). In the sheep fetus, these changes are dependent on the prepartum rise in fetal plasma cortisol but relatively little is known about the mechanisms that actually activate the gluconeogenic pathways in the fetus. Insulin appears to be involved in regulating hepatic glucose production but hypoinsulinaemia per se is insufficient to trigger glucogenesis in the sheep fetus (Fowden, 1989). A change in the insulin to glucagon molar ratio or an increase in fetal catecholamine concentrations may be required to actually initiate glucogenesis in the fetus. Glucagon and adrenaline have both been shown to increase glucose output by the fetal liver and their concentrations rise in the sheep fetus during adverse conditons which are known to stimulate fetal glucogenesis (Apatu & Barnes, 1991; see Bassett this volume, Chapter 9).

Lactate

Lactate is produced by the uteroplacental tissues in all species in relatively large amounts (Table 2.2). The amount of lactate produced in utero and its distribution between the fetal and maternal circulations varies with species and gestational age (Table 2.2). Between mid- and late gestation, lactate production by the ovine uteroplacental tissues increases 4–5-fold on a weight-specific basis (Sparks et al., 1981; Bell et al., 1986). In mid-gestation, the lactate is released almost entirely into the uterine circulation whereas, in late gestation, it is partitioned preferentially into the umbilical circulation of the fetal lamb (Bell et al., 1986). By contrast, in vitro studies with perfused human placenta suggest that, in this species, lactate is released solely into the maternal circulation, even at term (Hauguel et al., 1983). In sheep, uteroplacental lactate production does not appear to be influenced by the rates of uteroplacental glucose or oxygen consumption, at least over the physiological range of values observed in utero (Hay & Meznarich, 1989). However, umbilical lactate uptake is inversely related to the arterial O_2 content in fetal sheep which suggests that the distribution of uteroplacental lactate production may be affected by the fetal metabolic state.

In sheep, the uteroplacental tissues are not the only source of lactate for fetal metabolism. It is also produced by fetal tissues, such as muscle and lung (Table 2.3), at nearly double the rate of umbilical (or exogenous) supply (Fig. 2.1). About 60–70% of this endogenous lactate production is derived from glucose with the remaining lactate carbon coming from other sources such as fructose and amino acids (Fig. 2.1). Certainly, fetal lactate levels rise during fetal hyperglycaemia whether induced by fetal hypoinsulinaemia or by exogenous glucose infusion in the sheep fetus (Fowden, 1993). Fetal lactate production therefore appears to be determined, at least in part, by fetal glucose availability but relatively little is known about its regulation at a cellular level.

Amino acids

Amino acids are essential for oxidation, protein synthesis and as a source of carbon and nitrogen for other metabolic processes in the fetus (Carter, Moores & Battaglia, 1991). They are supplied to the fetus either transplacentally or by synthesis within the feto-placental tissues. Non-essential amino acids may be derived by either route, but essential amino acids, which cannot be synthesized de novo, must be maternal in origin. Fetal amino acid levels are higher than those in the mother throughout the later part of gestation, in a wide variety of species including man, but the precise ratio of fetal to maternal concentrations varies between species and with physiological state. In sheep, the fetal to maternal ratio of amino acid concentrations is less in conscious (1.5–2.0) than anaesthetized animals (2.0–3.0) and rises during fasting in chronically catheterized ewes (2.0–2.5). Amino acid transport across the placenta therefore appears to be active although relatively little is known about the specific characteristics of the placental amino acid transporters (Carter et al., 1991). Placental amino acid levels are higher than those in either the fetal or maternal plasma in sheep which suggests that it is the uterine and not the umbilical uptake that is the active process.

Umbilical venous–arterial concentration differences in individual amino acids have only been measured in chronically catheterized fetal sheep and in human infants sampled by intrauterine cordocentesis or from the cord at Caesarean delivery (Lemons & Schreiner, 1983; Cetin et al., 1988; Bell et al., 1989). These studies have shown a net fetal uptake of the neutral and basic amino acids but not of acidic ones in both mid- and late gestation. In fact, there were significant effluxes of glutamate and serine from the fetus to the placenta despite their accumulation in fetal protein. These two amino acids may therefore be used to excrete nitrogen from the fetus or provide substrates for amino acid synthesis by the placenta itself. Certainly, more glutamine and glycine are released into the umbilical circulation than are removed from the uterine circulation in the pregnant ewe (Lemons & Schreiner, 1983). Significant amounts of ammonia are also released by the placenta into both the fetal and maternal circulations in the sheep (Battaglia & Meschia, 1988; Battaglia, 1991). Hence, umbilical uptake of an amino acid does not establish that it was derived from the maternal circulation. Even essential amino acids are not simply transported across the ovine placenta. Leucine, for instance, is deaminated within the placenta to give rise to α-ketoisocaproic acid which is released into both the umbilical and uterine circulations of the ewe (Loy et al., 1990). The placenta is therefore not only transporting amino acids but is also metabolizing them by deamination and transamination reactions throughout the second half of gestation.

In sheep, placental amino acid metabolism appears to alter with increasing gestational age. At mid-gestation, the weight-specific uptake of nitrogen from amino acids is also four times higher than in late gestation and the net effluxes of glutamate and serine from the fetal circulation to the placenta are 2- and 20-fold greater, respectively, than at term (Bell et al., 1989). There may also be changes in amino acid uptake and metabolism by the ovine uteroplacental tissues during placental insufficiency and in response to variations in the maternal nutritional state (Lemons & Schreiner, 1983; Carter et al., 1991). However, umbilical uptake of total as well as individual amino acids does not change during short-term fasting of the ewe (Lemons & Schreiner, 1983).

The placenta is not the only source of amino acids in the fetus. The fetal liver and muscle can also deliver amino acids to the fetal circulation in certain circumstances (Liechty & Lemons, 1984; Marconi et al., 1989). The fetal liver takes up most individual amino acids from the umbilical venous blood but has a net output of glutamate and serine into the hepatic venous drainage, even in normal basal conditions. Since these are the two amino acids that are lost from the umbilical circulation to the placenta, an interorgan system of amino acid transport appears to exist between the fetal liver and placenta in well-nourished animals (Marconi et al., 1989). Fetal muscle, on the other hand, appears to contribute to the fetal amino acid pool only during nutrient restriction. In ewes fasted for 4–5 days, the fetal hind limb releases the two gluconeogenic amino acids, glutamine and alanine, into the fetal circulation whereas, in fed conditions, there is a net uptake of these two and most other amino acids (Liechty & Lemons, 1984). The source and amount of specific amino acids available to fetal tissues therefore appears to vary with nutritional state even though there is little, if any, change in the umbilical supply of amino acids in these circumstances (Lemons & Schreiner, 1983).

Lipid

Lipid is present in a number of different forms in the fetus. Significant amounts of triglycerides (TG), phospholipids, free fatty acids (FFA) and volatile short chain fatty acids have been detected in the fetal circulation, but the absolute concentrations and relative proportions of each vary between species and with nutritional state (Kimura, 1991). The FFA detected in the fetal plasma may come from the mother by direct placental transfer, from de novo synthesis within the feto-placental tissue or from breakdown of TG and phospholipids.

Fetal FFA levels are lower than those in the mother in a number of different species including man (Hull, 1976). But, despite this transplacental gradient, placental permeability to FFA varies widely between species (Hull, 1976). Changes in maternal dietary lipid have been shown to affect FFA levels and fat deposition in rabbit, guinea pig and human fetuses but have little effect on the fatty acid profile of the sheep fetus (Kimura, 1991). In rats and rabbits, labelled FFA injected into the mother appears rapidly in the fetal circulation while, in the human infant, there is a significant venous–arterial concentration difference in FFA across the umbilical circulation at elective Caesarean section (Hendrickse, Stammers & Hull, 1985). However, in sheep, only a very small FFA concentration difference can be detected across the umbilical circulation which suggests there is little, if any, net flow of FFA to the fetus from the ovine placenta (James, Meschia & Battaglia, 1971). Maternal FFA is therefore likely to contribute to the fetal FFA pool in the human and must account for, at least, the essential FFA in other species.

Placental transfer of maternal FFA appears to be dependent on the transplacental FFA gradient. In the human infant, FFA levels and the umbilical venous–arterial concentration difference in FFA rise in parallel with maternal FFA concentrations (Hendrickse et al., 1985). There is also an increase in FFA transfer across perfused placenta when fetal FFA levels are effectively lowered by increasing the perfusion rate or albumin concentration on the fetal side of the placenta (Kimura, 1991). In addition, in vitro studies have shown that the placenta itself can saturate, elongate and liberate FFA from maternal TG in the human, sheep and guinea pig (Hull, 1976; Kimura, 1991). Thus, placental lipid metabolism may also alter the transplacental FFA gradient and affect the amount and type of FFA reaching the fetal circulation.

Estimation of the umbilical supply of maternal FFA suggests that the mother can only provide 20–50% of the FFA stored in the human infant at term. In species with lower body fat contents at term, the mother may supply a greater proportion of the total fetal FFA requirement but, even in these species, there must be other sources of FFA in late gestation when fat accumulation rises in the fetus. In in vitro experiments, synthesis of FFA has been demonstrated in the placenta, fetal liver, brain and adipose tissue from a number of different species (Kimura, 1991). There is also no significant venous–arterial concentration difference in TG across the umbilical circulation of the human infant at elective Caesarean section, which suggests that the TG present in the fetal circulation is synthesized by the fetus (Hendrickse et al., 1985). The enzymes required for FFA and TG synthesis are present in high levels in the fetal liver of the human, monkey, rat and guinea pig near term (Hull, 1976). However, in other species such as the pig, which have very little fat at birth, fetal lipogenesis is limited and occurs at a very low rate, even close to term (Moustagaard, 1962). In the fetal lung, liver and adipose tissue, the main precursor for de novo lipid synthesis appears to be carbohydrate (glycogen, lactate and glucose) but small amounts of ketone bodies have also been shown to be incorporated into lipid in the fetal rat brain (Kimura, 1991).

Nutrient utilization

Nutrient utilization by the fetal tissues is dependent on the rates of umbilical uptake and fetal production of the nutrient. Measurement of umbilical nutrient uptake will therefore underestimate the actual rate of nutrient utilization if there is significant endogenous production by the fetal tissues. The relative contributions of the exogenous (umbilical) and endogenous (fetal) nutrient supply to the total rate of nutrient utilization varies between specific substrates (Fig. 2.1) and with nutritional state (Hay, 1991; Carter et al., 1991). For instance, umbilical glucose uptake accounts for almost all the glucose consumed by the fetal tissues in fed conditions (Fig. 2.1) but only 50–70% of that utilized during maternal undernutrition (Hay et al., 1984). By contrast, umbilical uptake of lactate provides less than 30% of the lactate used by the fetus even in normal, fed conditions (Fig. 2.1; Sparks et al., 1981).

The nutrients taken up by the fetal tissues are used either for oxidation or for tissue accretion (Fig. 2.3). The rate of nutrient oxidation and the partitioning of nutrients between the oxidative and non-oxidative pathways of metabolism can be determined by measuring the production of labelled CO_2 from labelled carbon in the nutrient. In fetal sheep, these measurements show that glucose, lactate and amino acids are all substrates for fetal oxidative metabolism but that they differ in their relative contribution to the total rate of fetal O_2 consumption (Battaglia & Meschia, 1988).

Oxygen

In late gestation, the total rate of fetal O_2 consumption is about 300 μmol/min/kg fetal body weight, irrespective of species (Table 2.2). The absolute rate of O_2 consumption (μmol/min) increases with increasing gestational age as fetal body weight rises towards term. However, when body weight is taken into account, weight specific O_2 consumption decreases from mid- to late gestation in the sheep fetus (Bell et al., 1986). Tissue-specific rates of O_2 consumption vary widely between individual organs in the sheep fetus (Table 2.3). On a weight-specific basis, O_2 consumption is highest in the heart and lowest in skeletal muscle but, when the relative mass of these tissues is taken into account, fetal skeletal muscle accounts for the largest proportion (~50%) of the total fetal O_2 consumption (Table 2.3).

Glucose

In normal, fed conditions, the rate of fetal glucose consumption varies between 20 and 70 μmol/min/kg fetal body weight depending on the species. It is lower in ruminant (20–35 μmol/min/kg) than in human (45 μmol/min/kg) or rat (70 μmol/min/kg) fetuses during late gestation (Hay, 1991). In the sheep fetus, fetal glucose utilization increases from 20–40 μmol/min/kg over the normal range of maternal glucose concentrations and can fall as low as 10 μmol/min/kg during maternal undernutrition (Fowden, 1989). Conversely, during experimentally induced fetal hyperglycaemia, fetal glucose utilization can increase to values of 50–60 μmol/min/kg (Fowden, 1993). Glucose uptake by the fetal tissues is therefore normally limited by the rate of glucose supply and not by the intracellular rate of glucose consumption.

Tissue-specific rates of glucose uptake have been measured by the Fick principle in a number of individual organs and tissues of the sheep fetus (Table 2.3). These measurements indicate that the fetal carcass (skin, bone and muscle) consumes about 75% of the glucose used by the whole fetus while the brain and visceral organs account for only 15% and 10%, respectively, of the total rate of fetal glucose utilization in fed conditions. During undernutrition, the fetal carcass uses a smaller proportion of the total glucose utilization rate and tissues such as the brain which are oligatory glucose consumers account for 30% or more of the total glucose consumption (Jones et al., 1975; Lemons & Schreiner, 1983).

Of the glucose used by the sheep fetus as whole, 50–60% is oxidized while the remaining 40–50% is consumed by the non-oxidative pathways of glucose metabolism (Hay et al., 1983). Glucose carbon is therefore oxidized at a rate of 80–100 μmol/min/kg fetal body weight which accounts for 25–30% of the total fetal oxygen consumption. The remaining, unoxidized glucose carbon is incorporated into a variety of fetal tissues and provides 40–45% of the daily carbon requirement for growth in the sheep fetus (Table 2.4). Glucose is therefore a major but not the sole source of carbon for both oxidation and tissue accretion in the sheep fetus during late gestation (Table 2.4).

Much less is known about fetal glucose utilization in the human infant although glucose provides a greater proportion of the total umbilical carbon supply in this species (Table 2.4). If all the umbilical glucose supply was oxidized, it would account for 75% of the total fetal O_2 consumption in the human infant compared with a value of 55% in the sheep fetus (Table 2.4). The human infant may therefore be more dependent on glucose as an oxidative fuel, but it must still be oxidizing carbon from other substrates to account for its total rate of CO_2 production.

Lactate

Lactate is another source of carbon to the fetus. In all species studied so far, there is a significant umbilical uptake of lactate which, if completely oxidized, would account for 14–45% of the fetal oxygen consumption depending on the species (Table 2.2). In the sheep fetus, this exogenous lactate supply is supplemented by lactate produced endogenously and, hence, the total rate of lactate utilization is three-fold higher than its rate

Table 2.4. *The metabolic balance (g/kg fetal wet wt/day) for energy, carbon and nitrogen in sheep and human fetuses during late gestation (⩾85% of gestation)*

	Sheep			Human		
	Energy	Carbon	Nitrogen	Energy	Carbon	Nitrogen
Requirement						
Accumulated in carcass	32.0	3.20	0.65	44	?	0.23
Excretion						
As CO_2	0	5.18	0	0	6.0	0
As urea	2.0	0.20	0.36	1.33	0.11	0.24
As glutamate	3.2	0.39	0.09	1.10	0.13	0.03
As serine	0.8	0.10	0.02	0	0	0
Oxidation	50.0	0	0	56	0	0
Total	88.0	9.07	1.12	102.4	(6.24+?)	0.50
Supply						
As glucose	27.4	2.90	0	44.4	4.66	0
As lactate	14.0	1.40	0	5.0	0.52	0
As acetate	7.0	0.56	0	–	–	–
As amino acids	38.0	3.08	1.34	24.4	1.98	0.54
As ammonia	0	0	0.04	0	0	0.01
Total	86.4	8.15	1.38	73.8	7.16	0.55

Data from Morriss et al., 1975; Sparks, 1984; Hay et al., 1984; Battaglia & Meschia, 1988; Lemons & Schreiner, 1983; Sparks et al., 1981.

of umbilical supply (Fig. 2.1). Of the total amount of lactate consumed by the sheep fetus, 70% is oxidized while the remainder enters the fetal carbon pool (Fig. 2.3). Lactate carbon therefore actually accounts for 40–50% of the fetal oxygen consumption rate and about 15–20% of the daily carbon requirement for tissue accretion in the sheep fetus (Table 2.4).

Several individual tissues have been shown to consume lactate in the sheep fetus (Table 2.3). It is the main carbohydrate taken up by the liver and heart and its consumption in these tissues accounts for about 30% of the lactate used by the whole sheep fetus (Table 2.3). It is the major precursor of hepatic glycogen and lipid synthesis and also contributes to hepatic glucogenesis during adverse intrauterine conditions (Fowden, 1989; Hay, 1991; Kimura, 1991).

Fructose

Fructose is found in the fetal circulation and fluid sacs of several species (ruminants, pigs, horses) but not in the human infant (Silver, 1984). Studies with labelled fructose show that it is utilized at a very low rate and can account for only 6% of the CO_2 produced by the sheep fetus (Meznarich et al., 1987). Labelled fructose can be converted into lactate in fetal sheep and is incorporated into hepatic glycogen in fetal rats and rabbits, but its role in these processes is small compared with other carbohydrates (Battaglia & Meschia, 1988). Hence, fructose does not appear to be a significant source of either energy or carbon for tissue accretion, even in those species in which it is present in relatively large amounts.

Amino acids

Amino acids are quantitatively the most important source of carbon to the fetus. They provide 50% or more of the daily carbon requirement for growth as well as 80–90% of the nitrogen accumulated in the tissue of the fetal sheep each day (Table 2.4). Much of the net umbilical amino acid uptake by the fetus is used for protein synthesis. In the sheep fetus, the whole body rate of protein synthesis varies widely among studies and ranges from 15 to 63 g/day/kg fetal bodyweight (Carter et al., 1991). It also varies with gestational age, nutritional state and oxygen delivery to the fetus. In fetal sheep, the fractional rate of whole body protein synthesis is higher at mid-gestation (23% per day) than at term (10% per day) and is reduced by hypoxia and maternal fasting for 48 h during late gestation (Bell et al., 1989; Milley, 1989). A similar decline in the fractional rate of protein synthesis is observed in fetal rats towards term, although the absolute values are higher than those in the fetal sheep (Milley, 1989).

Rates of protein synthesis have been determined in a number of individual tissues in the fetal sheep and rat (Milley, 1989). In the sheep fetus, the fractional rate of protein synthesis is highest in the gastro-intestinal tract and lowest in skeletal muscle (Table 2.3). But, because of the differences in the relative masses of the two tissues, they each contribute about 20% of the total whole body rate of protein synthesis. Other visceral tissues (e.g. liver, lungs) make smaller contributions to whole body protein synthesis in the sheep fetus (Table 2.3). In fetal rats, the liver accounts for the greatest proportion (~30%) of total body protein synthesis (Milley, 1989).

Whole body protein synthesis includes protein accretion due to growth and protein turnover due to degradation and re-synthesis of existing protein (Carter et al., 1991). Studies of tracer leucine flux in the sheep fetus show that protein breakdown accounts for 40% of the rate of fetal leucine utilization and approximately 75% of the total leucine flux which includes the leucine lost from the fetus to the placenta (Loy et al., 1990). Using this data and the average leucine content of protein, the rate of protein turnover in the sheep fetus near term can be estimated at 40 g protein per day which compares to a protein accretion rate of 10–12 g protein per day (Milley, 1989). Protein turnover is therefore a quantitatively important component of fetal protein synthesis and could account for about 15–20% of the total rate of fetal O_2 consumption.

During growth, the rate of protein synthesis must exceed the rate of protein degradation if there is to be a net gain of protein mass. In fetal sheep in the fed state, the fractional rate of protein synthesis is greater than that of protein accretion throughout the later part of gestation, irrespective of whether lysine or leucine is used to calculate the rate of protein synthesis (Kennaugh et al., 1987). In undernourished fetal sheep and rats, reduced fractional rates of protein synthesis and accretion are observed, which are accompanied by small or no reductions in the fractional rate of protein degradation (Milley, 1989). Utilization of body protein stores may therefore occur in the fetus during adverse conditions and result in a negative nitrogen balance.

The umbilical uptake of amino acids exceeds that required for tissue accretion by 50% even in fed conditions (Carter et al., 1991). Hence, a large proportion of the fetal amino acid uptake is available for catabolism and oxidative metabolism. The main deamination product of amino acids is urea and its rate of production by the fetus can be calculated from the transplacental rate of urea excretion as little urea is excreted by the fetal kidneys. Fetal urea production, estimated in this way, ranges from 3–7 μmol/min/kg fetal body weight in the cow, horse and human but gives higher values (7–10 μmol/min/kg) in the fetal sheep (Silver, 1984). These rates of fetal urea production are greater than those seen in the respective newborn animal and could account for 15%–30% of fetal O_2 consumption depending on the species. During maternal fasting, fetal urea production doubles which suggests there is increased amino acid catabolism in these circumstances (Lemons & Schreiner, 1983).

Using tracer methodology, production of labelled CO_2 has been demonstrated from labelled essential (leucine and lycine) and non-essential amino (glycine, tyrosine and alanine) acids. In the sheep fetus the rate of amino acid oxidation varies with the specific amino acid and with nutritional state: mean values are higher for leucine than for glycine or lysine and increase during maternal fasting (Battaglia, 1991; Carter et al., 1991). In the fed state, fetal oxidation of leucine, glycine and lysine accounts for 25%, 12% and 9%, respectively, of the corresponding rates of utilization (Battaglia, 1991). These observations are consistent with the finding that the umbilical uptake of lysine only exceeds its accretion rate in protein by 20% while that of leucine has a safety margin of 40–50%. The fetus therefore uses both essential and non-essential acids as oxidative fuels, and can divert amino acids from the non-oxidative to the oxidative metabolic pathways when fetal glucose availability is limited.

Tissue-specific amino acid uptakes have been determined in relatively few fetal tissues. An uptake of amino nitrogen has been demonstrated across the gut of the sheep fetus which is consistent with the high fractional rate of protein synthesis observed in this tissue (Charlton, Reis & Lofgren, 1979). Similarly, significant amino acid uptakes have also been observed across the fetal liver and hind limb (Liechty & Lemons, 1984; Marconi et al., 1989). In fed conditions, the fetal hind limb takes up most amino acids and releases ammonia into the fetal circulation whereas, during maternal fasting, there is an efflux of alanine and glutamine and an increased uptake of leucine (Liechty & Lemons, 1984). These observations suggest that fetal muscle catabolizes amino acids, even in fed conditions, and that, during undernutrition, it not only oxidizes more leucine but also transaminates amino acids to provide gluconeogenic precursors. Similar processes of amino acid oxidation and transamination occur in the liver of the sheep fetus (Marconi et al.,

1989). Hepatic tissue can account for 70% of the total fetal glycine oxidation, and is a major site of serine and glutamate synthesis in the fetus (Battaglia, 1991). The placenta, on the other hand, oxidizes relatively little leucine or glycine but does take up amino acids such as leucine from the fetal circulation despite a net efflux of the amino acid from the placenta to the umbilical circulation (Loy et al., 1990). When tracer leucine is infused into fetal sheep, 40% of the tracer enters the placenta and remains there. Some of the labelled leucine is deaminated to α-ketoisocaproic acid but the fate of all the labelled leucine carbon taken up by the placenta remains unclear as little tracer leucine is released back into the maternal circulation (Loy et al., 1990). The placenta is therefore more metabolically active than implied by the net differences in uterine and umbilical amino acid uptakes.

Lipids

There is little evidence of lipid oxidation in the fetus. Fatty acids (FA) are not taken up in excess of the fetal requirement for growth, and the enzymes needed for FA oxidation are low in activity in the fetal liver (Kimura, 1991). In vitro experiments have shown that in some species palmitate can be oxidized to CO_2 by fetal tissues but only to a limited extent. In ruminants, there is a net uptake of acetate across the umbilical circulation which is supplemented with acetate produced by the fetal tissues (Char & Creasy, 1976; Comline & Silver, 1976; Battaglia & Meschia, 1988). Acetate utilization is therefore likely to be higher than its rate of umbilical supply in these species (Fig. 2.1). It is consumed by the fetal hind limbs, and has been shown to be incorporated into fetal fatty acids (FFA), steroids and membrane lipids in the fetus (Singh et al., 1984). The only other lipid components that could contribute to fetal metabolism are glycerol and ketones. Glycerol may act as a gluconeogenic precursor and, thereby, be incorporated into hepatic glycogen. Ketones such as hydroxybutyrate are oxidized by fetal tissues in the rat, and have been shown to be taken up by the brain in the fetal rat and sheep, particularly during adverse intrauterine conditions (Battaglia & Meschia, 1988).

Fetal metabolic balance

The total fetal requirements for carbon, nitrogen and energy can be calculated for any given species from its oxygen consumption, growth rate and body composition and its rate of transplacental excretion of carbon and nitrogen. By comparing these requirements with the umbilical supply of nutrients, the metabolic balance of the fetus can be estimated. While the nutrient requirements for growth and oxidation are known for a number of different species (Sparks, 1984), much less is known about the umbilical supply of nutrients in these species. Only in the sheep fetus is there sufficient data to assess the metabolic balance with any degree of accuracy (Table 2.4).

In the sheep fetus, amino acids have the most important role in fetal metabolic balance. They provide 35–45% of the carbon, 40–45% of the energy and virtually all the nitrogen required by the sheep fetus each day (Table 2.4). Amino acid carbon also accounts for about 50% of the CO_2 produced each day. After the amino acids, the next most important nutrient in the sheep fetus is glucose. It provides about 35% of the carbon and 30% of the total energy requirement in the fed state (Table 2.4). Lactate and acetate also make small contributions to the fetal energy and carbon balances (Table 2.4). In total, carbohydrate carbon is responsible for about 50% of the fetal CO_2 production when the conversion of glucose to lactate is taken into account.

During undernutrition, the fetal nutrient requirement for oxidative metabolism does not change as fetal O_2 consumption remains at normal fed values despite a fall in the umbilical supply of oxidative substrates (Hay et al., 1984; Fowden, 1989; Hay, 1991). The balance between the supply and demand for nutrients is therefore maintained in these circumstances by reducing the fetal growth rate and by changing the contribution of glucose and amino acids to the total energy and carbon balances. In fasted ewes, glucose accounts for a smaller proportion of the fetal CO_2 production and contributes only 10–15% of the carbon required for tissue accretion by the sheep fetus each day (Fowden, 1993). Conversely, amino acids contribute a greater amount of carbon to fetal oxidative metabolism during undernutrition (Lemons & Schreiner, 1983). When the umbilical nutrient supply is severely restricted, sufficient oxidative substrates can only be provided by catabolizing body protein which may result in a negative growth rate (Milley, 1989). Amino acids therefore have an even more important role in maintaining fetal metabolic balance during adverse nutritional conditions than they do in the fed state (Carter et al., 1991).

When all the known umbilical nutrient uptakes are summed, the total supply of energy and carbon is slightly less than the amounts required each day by the sheep fetus in both the fed and fasted states. This suggests that there must be other sources of carbon and energy in the fetus that have not been identified yet. Given the high molecular weight and carbon content of fat, it seems most likely that lipid utilization accounts for the deficits in the fetal carbon and energy balances as even a very small net umbilical venous–arterial concentration difference in FFA represents a significant supply of substrate to the fetus. However, any contribution of lipid to the fetal metabolic balance will be relatively small compared to those of the carbohydrates and amino acids in the sheep fetus.

In the human infant, estimates of the fetal energy and nitrogen balance can be made using data obtained from autopsies and at Caesarean delivery (Table 2.4). These calculations indicate that glucose has a more prominent role in the fetal energy balance in this species and may account for 40% or more of the energy required by the human fetus each day. Amino acids, on the other hand, contribute only about 20% of the total energy requirement (Table 2.4). In the human infant there is a greater shortfall between the known supplies of energy and its total requirement than is observed in the sheep fetus (Table 2.4). Since the placenta is more lipid permeable in the human than the sheep, FFA may make a greater contribution to fetal metabolism in the human infant, and could account for as much as 25% of the total fetal energy requirement in this species (Table 2.4).

While calculation of the fetal metabolic balance is useful in identifying the key fetal nutrients, it provides little information about the turnover of the fetal carbon and nitrogen pools or the flux of substrates between the various nutrient pools in the fetus. Carbon in the fetal carbon pool is derived from glucose, lactate, fructose, acetate and amino acids and is used for the synthesis of protein, glycogen and fat in the sheep fetus (Fig. 2.3). Certain of these fluxes, such as those to glucose and to and from glycogen, are dependent on the nutritional state of the animal and only occur in late gestation. Glucose carbon, originally derived from the maternal glucose pool, can therefore be transferred into the lactate, fructose, FFA or amino acid pools in the sheep fetus. Similarly, nitrogen enters the fetal nitrogen pool from a variety of sources (e.g. amino acids, ammonia and adenosine) and leaves in the form of proteins, urea and other nitrogen-containing compounds such as the nucleotides (Fig. 2.3). Turnover of the fetal nitrogen pool probably decreases with increasing gestational age as the rates of protein synthesis, urea production and umbilical nitrogen uptake decline towards term (Bell et al., 1989; Kennaugh et al., 1987). In contrast, fetal nitrogen turnover increases

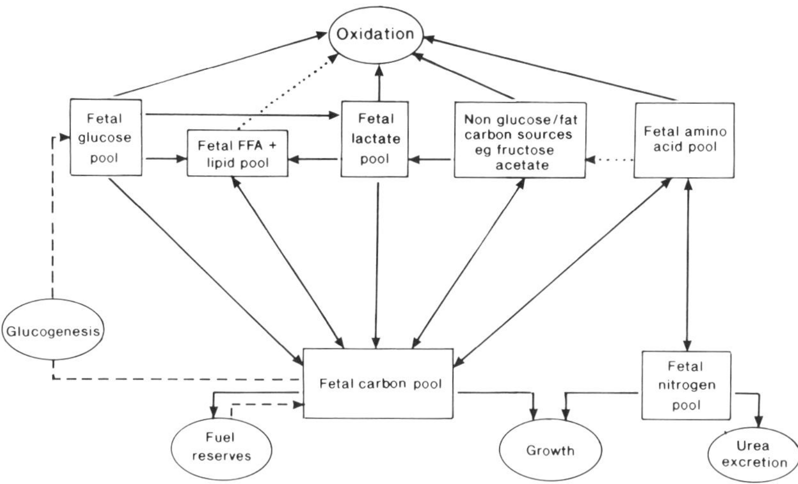

Fig. 2.3. The sources, fates and interconversion of carbon and nitrogen in the sheep fetus during late gestation (⩾85% gestation). Pathways known to occur in sheep fetuses in the fed and fasted states (——►) and in the fasted state alone (– – ►). Pathways presumed (but not actually demonstrated) to exist in the sheep fetus (····►).

during undernutrition when urea production and protein catabolism are high in the fetus (Lemons & Schreiner, 1983; Milley, 1989). These changes in nitrogen metabolism will also affect the availability of amino acid carbon for incorporation into the fetal glucose and lactate pools (Fig. 2.3). The magnitude and precise nature of the interconversions between the various fetal nutrient pools therefore depend on the gestational age and nutritional state of the animal.

Conclusions

If the fetus is to grow normally, its supply of nutrients must meet the carbon, nitrogen and energy requirements for tissue accretion. These requirements are determined by the rate and type of tissue accumulated in the fetus and vary between species and with gestational age. The supply of nutrients to the fetal tissues depends on the availability of nutrients in the fetal circulation and on the cellular uptake of these nutrients. Since most of the substrates used by the fetus are derived either directly or indirectly from the maternal nutrient pool, the transfer of nutrients from the maternal to fetal circulations has a key role in regulating fetal growth. Any changes in the transplacental nutrient supply induced, for example, by variations in maternal nutrition or placental function will lead to abnormal fetal growth. Similarly, alterations in cellular nutrient uptake caused by endocrine or other abnormalities will adversely affect growth and development in utero. Thus, it is ultimately the supply of nutrients to the fetal metabolic pathways that is critical in determining the rate and pattern of intrauterine growth.

References

Apatu, R.S.K. & Barnes, R.J. (1991). Release of glucose from the liver of fetal and postnatal sheep by portal vein infusion of catecholamines or glucagon. *Journal of Physiology*, **436**, 449–68.

Battaglia, F.C. (1991). Metabolic aspects of fetal and neonatal growth. *Early Human Development*, **29**, 99–106.

Battaglia, F.C. & Meschia, G. (1988). Fetal nutrition. *Annual Reviews of Nutrition*, **8**, 43–61.

Bell, A.W., Kennaugh, J.M., Battaglia, F.C., Makowski, E.L. & Meschia, G. (1986). Metabolic and circulatory studies of fetal lamb at mid-gestation. *American Journal of Physiology*, **250**, E538–44.

Bell, A. W., Kennaugh, J. M., Battaglia, F. C. & Meschia, G. (1989). Uptake of amino acids and ammonia at mid-gestation by the fetal lamb. *Quarterly Journal of Experimental Physiology*, **74**, 635–43.

Carter, B.S., Moores, R.R. & Battaglia, F.C. (1991). Placental transport and fetal and placental metabolism of amino acids. *Journal of Nutritional Biochemistry*, **2**, 4–13.

Cetin, I., Marconi, A.M., Bozzetti, P., Sereni, C.P., Carbetta, C., Pardi, G. & Battaglia, F.C. (1988). Umbilical amino acid concentration in appropriate and small for gestational age infants: a biochemical difference present in utero. *American Journal of Obstetrics and Gynecology*, **158**, 120–6.

Char, V.E.C. & Creasy, R.K. (1976). Acetate as a metabolic substrate in the fetal lamb. *American Journal of Physiology*, **230**, 357–61.

Charlton, V.E., Reis, B.L. & Lofgren, D.J. (1979). Consumption of carbohydrates, amino acids and oxygen across the intestinal circulation in the fetal sheep. *Journal of Developmental Physiology*, **1**, 329–36.

Comline, R.S. & Silver, M. (1976). Some aspects of foetal and utero-placental metabolism in cows with indwelling umbilical and uterine vascular catheters. *Journal of Physiology*, **260**, 571–86.

Fisher, D.J., Heyman, M.A. & Rudolph, A.M. (1980). Myocardial oxygen and carbohydrate consumption in fetal lambs in utero and in adult sheep. *American Journal of Physiology*, **238**, H399–405.

Fowden, A.L. (1989). The endocrine regulation of fetal metabolism and growth. In *Research in Perinatal Medicine VIII*, ed. P.D. Gluckman, B.M. Johnston & P.W. Nathanielsz. pp. 229–43. Perinatology Press, New York.

Fowden, A.L. (1993). Insulin deficiency: effects on fetal growth and development. *Journal of Paediatrics and Child Health*, **29**, 6–11.

Fowden, A.L., Mijovic, J. & Silver, M. (1993). The effects of cortisol on hepatic and renal gluconeogenic enzyme activities in the sheep fetus during late gestation. *Journal of Endocrinology*, **137**, 213–22.

Gleason, C.A., Rudolph, C.D., Bristow, J., Itskovitz, J. & Rudolph, A.M. (1985). Lactate uptake by the fetal sheep liver. *Journal of Developmental Physiology*, **7**, 172–83.

Hauguel, S., Challier, J.C., Cedard, L. & Olive, G. (1983). Metabolism of the human placenta perfused in vitro: glucose transfer and utilization, O_2 consumption, lactate and ammonia production. *Pediatric Research*, **17**, 729–32.

Hay, W.W. (1991). The role of placental–fetal interactions in fetal nutrition. *Seminars in Perinatology*, **15**, 424–33.

Hay, W.W. & Meznarich, H.K. (1989). Effect of maternal glucose concentration on uteroplacental glucose consumption and transfer in pregnant sheep. *Proceedings of the Society of Experimental Biology and Medicine*, **190**, 63–9.

Hay, W.W., Molina, R.A., DiGiacomo, J.E. & Meschia, G. (1990). Model of placental glucose consumption and glucose transfer. *American Journal of Physiology*, **258**, R569–77.

Hay, W.W., Myers, S.A., Sparks, J.W., Wilkening, R.B., Meschia, G. & Battaglia, F.C. (1983). Glucose and lactate oxidation rates in the fetal lamb. *Proceedings of the Society of Experimental Biology and Medicine*, **173**, 553–63.

Hay, W.W., Sparks, J.W., Wilkening, R.B., Battaglia, F.C. & Meschia, G. (1984). Fetal glucose uptake and utilization as functions of maternal glucose concentrations. *American Journal of Physiology*, **246**, E237–42.

Hendrickse, W., Stammers, J.P. & Hull, D. (1985). The transfer of free fatty acids across the human placenta. *British Journal of Obstetrics and Gynaecology*, **92**, 945–52.

Hull, D. (1976). Fetal fat metabolism. In *Fetal Physiology and Medicine*, ed. R.W. Beard & P.W. Nathanielsz. pp. 105–20. W.B. Saunders, London.

Iwamoto, H., Oh, W. & Rudolph, A.M. (1985). Renal metabolism in fetal and newborn sheep. *Pediatric Research*, **19**, 641–4.

James, E., Meschia, G. & Battaglia, F.C. (1971). A-V differences of free fatty acids and glycerol in the ovine umbilical circulation. *Proceedings of the Society for Experimental Biology*, **138**, 823–6.

Johnson, L.W. & Smith, C.H. (1980). Monosaccharide transport across microvillous membrane of human placenta. *American Journal of Physiology*, **238**, C160–8.

Jones, M.D., Burd, L.I., Makowski, E.D., Meschia, G. & Battaglia, F.C. (1975). Cerebral metabolism in sheep: a comparative study of the adult, the lamb and the fetus. *American Journal of Physiology*, **229**, 235–9.

Kennaugh, J.A., Bell, A.W., Teng, C., Meschia, G. & Battaglia, F.C. (1987). Ontogenetic changes in the rates of protein synthesis and leucine oxidation during fetal life. *Pediatric Research*, **22**, 688–92.

Kimura, R.E. (1991). Lipid metabolism in the fetal–placental unit. In *Principles of Perinatal–Neonatal Metabolism*, ed. R.M. Cowett. pp. 291–303. Springer Verlag, New York.

Lemons, J.A. & Schreiner, R.L. (1983). Amino acid metabolism in the ovine fetus. *American Journal of Physiology*, **244**, E459–66.

Liechty, E. A. & Lemons, J. A. (1984). Changes in ovine fetal hind limb amino acid metabolism during maternal fasting. *American Journal of Physiology*, **246**, E430–5.

Longo, L.D. (1991). Respiration in the fetal-placental unit. In *Principles of Perinatal–Neonatal Metabolism*, ed. R.W. Cowett. pp. 304–15. Springer Verlag, New York.

Loy, G.L., Quick, A.N., Hay, W.W., Meschia, G., Battaglia, F.C. & Fennessy, P.V. (1990). Fetoplacental deamination and decarboxylation of leucine. *American Journal of Physiology*, **259**, E492–7.

Marconi, A.M., Battaglia, F.C., Meschia, G. & Sparks, J.W. (1989). A comparison of amino acid arteriovenous differences across the liver and placenta of the fetal lamb. *American Journal of Physiology*, **257**, E909–15.

Meyer, H. & Ahlswede, L. (1978). The intrauterine growth and body composition of foals and the nutrient requirements of pregnant mares. *Animal Research and Development*, **8**, 86–112.

Meznarich, H.K., Hay, W.W., Sparks, J.W., Meschia, G. & Battaglia, F.C. (1987). Fructose disposal and oxidation rates in the ovine fetus. *Quarterly Journal of Experimental Physiology*, **72**, 617–25.

Milley, J.R. (1989). Fetal protein metabolism. *Seminars in Perinatology*, **13**, 192–201.

Molina, R.D., Meschia, G., Battaglia, F.C. & Hay, W.W. (1991). Gestational maturation of placental glucose transfer capacity in sheep. *American Journal of Physiology*, R697–704.

Morriss, F.H., Makowski, E.L., Meschia, G. & Battaglia, F.C. (1975). The glucose/oxygen quotient of the term human fetus. *Biology of the Neonate*, **25**, 44–52.

Moustagaard, J. (1962). Foetal nutrition in the pig. In *Nutrition of Pigs and Poultry*, ed. J.T. Morgan & D. Lewis. pp. 57–89. Proceedings of the Easter School in Agricultural Science, University of Nottingham.

Schaefer, A.L. & Krishnamuti, C.R. (1984). Whole body and tissue fractional protein synthesis in the ovine fetus in utero. *British Journal of Nutrition*, **52**, 359–69.

Silver, M. (1984). Some aspects of equine placental exchange and foetal physiology. *Equine Veterinary Journal*, **16**, 227–32.

Simmons, M.A., Battaglia, F.C. & Meschia, G. (1979). Placental transfer of glucose. *Journal of Developmental Physiology*, **1**, 227–43.

Simmons, R.A. & Charlton, V.E. (1988). Substrate utilization by the fetal sheep lung during the last trimester. *Pediatric Research*, **23**, 606–11.

Singh, S., Sparks, J. W., Meschia, G., Battaglia, F. C. & Makowski, E. L. (1984). Comparison of fetal and maternal hind limb metabolic quotients in sheep. *American Journal of Obstetrics and Gynecology*, **149**, 441–9.

Sparks, J. W. (1984). Human intrauterine growth and nutrient accretion. *Seminars in Perinatology*, **8**, 74–93.

Sparks, J.W., Hay, W.W., Bonds, D., Meschia, G. & Battaglia, F.C. (1981). Simultaneous measurements of lactate turnover rate and umbilical lactate uptake in the fetal lamb. *Journal of Clinical Investigation*, **70**, 179–92.

Stacey, T.E., Weedon, A.P. & Haworth, C. (1978). Feto-maternal transfer of glucose analogues by sheep placenta. *American Journal of Physiology*, **234**, E32–7.

Teasdale, F. (1980). Gestational changes in the functional structure of the human placenta in relation to fetal growth: a morphometric study. *American Journal of Obstetrics and Gynecology*, **137**, 560–8.

3

Hormonal control of fetal growth

DAVID J. HILL

Introduction

Growth in childhood is heavily dependent on classical endocrine hormones such as growth hormone, thyroid hormones, glucocorticoids and insulin. Some of the trophic actions of these hormones are mediated by peptide growth factors, especially the mediation of growth hormone action on longitudinal skeletal growth by insulin-like growth factor-I (IGF-I). However, classical endocrine hormones of fetal origin, with the exception of insulin, are not major determinants of size at birth. In some instances, as in the maturational effects of thyroid hormones on the central nervous system, transplacental passage of maternal hormones is sufficient to satisfy the basic needs of the conceptus. Other hormones, such as glucocorticoids, have defined roles in late gestation as the liver and lungs mature in preparation for postnatal existence. Insulin, however, has a fundamental role as a mitogen in the early embryo, and its absence leads to severe intrauterine growth retardation. The relevance of insulin and other hormones to prenatal development has been reviewed extensively (Gluckman & Liggins, 1984; Hill & Milner, 1989; Hill, 1992).

The fundamental drive to embryonic and fetal growth appears to be orchestrated by the widespread expression, regulation of availability, and interaction of a number of peptide growth factors. Recent studies of gene manipulation have shown peptide growth factors to be obligatory for specific events of embryonic morphogenesis, and for growth of the conceptus in toto. Since the expression of most growth factors is not restricted to individual tissues, but is widespread, prenatal development can be considered mainly as an integrated network of paracrine and autocrine events. This chapter will review recent findings on the contributions of peptide growth factors to embryogenesis and to somatic and visceral growth prior to birth. Their contributions to the growth and maturation of the central nervous system have been reviewed in detail recently (Snider, 1994).

Growth factor structure and mechanism of action

Peptide growth factors are widely expressed at both mRNA and peptide levels in developing tissues, but probably have limited access to target tissues much of the time due to high affinity binding to extracellular matrix, specific binding proteins, or cell surface molecules other than high affinity receptors. They often rely on proteolytic processing from the target tissue to become bioavailable; they mostly interact with high affinity cell membrane receptors which signal to the nucleus via tyrosine or serine/threonine-specific kinase phosphorylation events, and the *ras* proto-oncogene signalling pathway (Hill & Hogg, 1989).

The IGFs consist structurally of an A and a B chain connected by a C peptide, and share about a 40% homology with insulin. Two types, IGF-I and -II, have been purified from serum and have molecular sizes of approximately 7.6 kDa. Liver is a major site of expression both in fetal and postnatal life, although almost all tissues have been shown to express these peptides in the human and animal fetus (Brown et al., 1986; Han et al., 1988), suggesting a predominantly autocrine or paracrine role. In the fetus, the most abundant isomer is IGF-II, but in some species such as rat, but not in man, IGF-II is absent from adult serum to be replaced by IGF-I. In humans, IGF-II persists throughout life, although the relative abundance of IGF-I increases postnatally. A high affinity type-1 IGF receptor is ubiquitous in developing tissues and recognizes IGF-I with an order of magnitude greater binding affinity than it does IGF-II. Consequently, IGF-I is a more potent mitogen, with an ED_{50} of approximately 1–3 nM on most cell types. This is relatively inefficient compared to the mitogenic properties of other growth factors such as the fibroblast growth factors (FGFs) and epidermal growth factor (EGF). However, the role of IGFs may not be predominantly mitogenic. They have been shown to support the differentiated function of many cell types, including the synthesis of extracellular matrix molecules such as fibronectin, collagens and glycosaminoglycans. In postnatal life, synergy between endogenous IGF-I and trophic endocrine hormones facilitates endocrine glandular function. For instance, thyroid-stimulating hormone synergizes with IGF-I to support thyroxine synthesis, while a synergy of IGFs with follicle-stimulating hormone allows sex steroid production in the ovary

(Hill & Hogg, 1989). The type-1 IGF receptor has an intracellular tyrosine kinase domain, which is capable of phosphorylating the insulin receptor substrate protein. IGFs are able to activate the proto-oncogene *ras* in many cell types, which subsequently signals gene transcriptional changes in cell nuclei by a MAP kinase pathway, culminating in the activation of the transcriptional factors, *fos*, *jun* and *myc*. An additional high affinity receptor which specifically binds IGF-II, the type 2 or cation-independent mannose-6-phosphate receptor, is ubiquitous but has no consistent intracellular signalling pathway or biological endpoint.

The IGFs are seldom found in free form but are complexed to one of six distinct classes of specific binding protein, termed IGFBPs-1 to -6. These are found both in serum and in extracellular fluids, and serve not only as carrier proteins to extend the biological half-life of the ligands but they also modulate their biological actions by either interacting or competing with the type-1 IGF receptors. While all six IGFBPs have a conserved core structure, differences in their amino- and carboxy-termini confer individual relative binding affinities for IGF-I and -II, and an ability to interact with both extracellular matrix and the cell surface (McCusker & Clemmons, 1992). Two of these IGFBPs, IGFBP-1 and -2, contain an integrin-binding motif which allows binding to the cell surface $\alpha_5\beta_1$ integrin, which is the fibronectin receptor. The ability of these IGFBPs to potentiate IGF action is related to their integrin-binding activity which may facilitate an advantageous presentation of the ligand to its high affinity receptor. All IGFs except IGFBP-1 also contain heparin-binding domains, allowing binding to sulfated glycosaminoglycans in the extracellular matrix and on the cell membrane. The majority of IGF-I and -II in blood is carried on IGFBP-3. From the second half of fetal development IGFBP-3 is associated, together with an IGF molecule, with an acid labile subunit in the circulation to generate a tertiary complex of 150 kD. In this form, IGFs cannot leave the circulation, the fraction being accessible to extracellular fluids being carried by IGFBP-1 or -2.

A large proportion of the IGF:IGFBP complexes in extracellular fluids and stored within the extracellular matrix are probably inaccessible to the cell surface receptors. Their availability depends on modification of the IGFBPs by specific proteases resulting in a reduced binding affinity for IGFs. Such proteases have been identified for IGFBPs-2 to -5. An IGFBP-3-degrading protease appears in maternal serum from the second trimester of human pregnancy until term, which reduces the amount of IGFs carried by IGFBP-3, and increases its transcapillary passage in association with other IGFBPs (Giudice et al., 1990). A naturally occurring tissue protease can also remove the three amino-terminal amino acids from IGF-I, resulting in a much reduced binding affinity for IGFs. Thus, while IGF-I and -II are present in the circulation, this serves predominantly as an extracellular store. Controlled proteolysis of IGFBPs and extracellular matrix molecules is likely to be the key regulatory step in the bioavailability and subsequent actions of IGF-I and -II.

The fibroblast growth factors (FGFs) are a family of at least nine structurally related heparin-binding growth factors which are mitogenic for many different cell types. They are potent mitogens for vascular endothelial cells and are angiogenic in vivo (Baird & Bohlen, 1990). The two most studied of these growth factors are FGF1, or acidic FGF, and FGF2, or basic FGF. Both are unusual in that their translated products have no signal sequence peptide necessary for conventional secretion via the endoplasmic reticulum. Despite this, both FGF1 and 2 are released to the cell membrane where they bind strongly to glycosaminoglycans such as heparin sulphate, or to extracellular matrix-associated glycosaminoglycans. FGF2 is a single chain polypeptide of 16.5 kD, although larger variants of 21.5 and 23 kD are also generated through alternate translational initiation sites. The actions of FGFs are mediated by a family of at least four high-affinity receptors which are single chain peptides of 110–150 kD. These are designated FGFR1–4 and all have intracellular tyrosine kinase domains which signal via *ras* activation and *fos* and *myc* induction. Alternate exon splicing of the FGFR genes yields a variety of subtypes with differing ligand-binding affinities and the potential for some to act as secreted binding proteins. Binding of FGFs to heparin sulphate on the cell surface greatly enhances the ability of the ligands to interact with high affinity receptors, and this can be reproduced by addition of heparin during tissue culture. Since most FGFs are probably bound to extracellular glycosaminoglycans in an insoluble form, proteolysis is necessary to form small, soluble glycosaminoglycan:FGF complexes which can activate the receptor. Binding to glycosaminoglycans itself protects the FGFs from proteolytic degradation.

The epidermal growth factor (EGF) family members are all structurally related and include EGF, transforming growth factor α (TGF-α), heparin-binding EGF and amphiregulin. Mature EGF has 53 amino acids and a molecular weight of 6 kD, but is derived from a much larger precursor molecule of 130 kD. The carboxy-terminal of the precursor represents mature EGF and is followed by eight EGF-like repeat sequences before containing a hydrophobic region which may represent a cellular transmembrane domain. This suggests that the EGF precursor is a membrane-bound molecule from which EGF may be liberated by extracellular proteolysis. Alternatively, the precursor may exert EGF-like activity in its own right as a 'juxtacrine' molecule directly interacting with EGF receptors on adjacent cells. The EGF precursor may also have distinct, non-mitogenic actions including the regulation of sodium and chloride ion transport at the proximal convoluted tubular epithelium of the kidney, where it is abundant. Although mature TGF-α is of similar size to EGF, its precursor is much smaller without EGF-repeat sequences. However, a transmembranal hydrophobic region is present, suggesting a possible juxtacrine mode of action. While TGF-α is expressed by many embryonic and fetal tissues, and persists in some postnatally, EGF expression is seen in predominantly epithelial tissues in postnatal life. The high affinity EGF receptors are a glycoprotein family of at least four variants, designated ER-1 to ER-4. The ER-2 receptor is the proto-oncogene, *neu*. The monomeric EGF receptor molecules must dimerize following ligand binding to facilitate intracellular signalling, and this can occur between either identical receptor isomers, or between heterologous isomers. This is likely to provide both tissue and developmental specificity to various members of the EGF family. Alternate exon splicing can give rise to mRNA transcripts encoding truncated forms of the receptors which lack an intracellular domain, and these may be secreted as EGF-binding proteins.

Platelet-derived growth factor (PDGF) consists of two separate peptide chains, an A and a B chain, which are encoded by genes on separate chromosomes. This allows the construction of three isomers, AA, AB and BB giving molecular weights between 28 and 35 kD. Platelets are a rich source of PDGF, of which 70% is in an AB configuration. Most other tissues express the BB isomer in normal development, while AA is a product of many neoplasias. The high affinity PDGF receptor is a dimer representing separate pools of 'a' subunits which can bind either PDGF A or B chains, or 'b' subunits which can only bind PDGF B chains. In the absence of PDGF, the subunits exist as separate monomers, but upon ligand binding they dimerize to undertake mitogenic signalling via the autophosphorylation of tyrosine residues on the intracellular domain, and the activation of *ras* protein.

The transforming growth factor β (TGF-β) family is extensive and includes at least five isomers of TGF-β, designated TGF-β1–5, the inhibins, activins and bone morphogenetic proteins (BMPs). In mammals, the predominant forms of TGF-β are TGF-β1 and TGF-β2, which are of about 25 kD molecular size, and are widely distributed amongst tissues. TGF-β3 mRNA transcripts have been identified in placenta, ovary and cartilage. All TGF-βs share a well-conserved amino acid sequence, are translated as much larger precursor molecules which require proteolytic activation extracellularly to liberate the bioactive molecule, and have integrin-binding domains. Three classes of high affinity receptor have been identified. The class 1 receptor is of 65 kD and is not itself an intracellular signalling receptor. However, binding of TGF-β to this receptor allows its further recognition by a 85–95 kD class 2 receptor which has an intracellular serine/threonine kinase domain and signals changes in cell growth and differentiation. A class 3 receptor is the cell surface proteoglycan, betaglycan, which binds TGF-βs with high affinity and appears to present the ligand to the signalling receptor in an advantageous configuration. All three binding components need to complex for optimal signalling by TGF-β. TGF-β acts predominantly as a growth inhibitor for epithelial cell types and some mesenchymal cells, but has widespread effects on cell differentiation and morphogenesis.

Peptide growth factors are intimately associated with extracellular matrix molecules to provide an integrated cell signalling system. Matrix molecules not only provide for an enormous extracellular store of growth factors, due to specific binding domains within the growth factor molecules or their specific binding proteins, but the formation and subsequent remodelling of the extracellular matrix is ultimately controlled by growth factor actions. In this way, extracellular matrix is a key player in the regulation of early development. First, matrix molecule synthesis is differentially controlled by growth factors. Type IV collagen, a major component of basement membranes, and type I collagen are synthesized in response to TGF-β. Type I collagen forms a complex with decorin, a dermatan sulfate within the extracellular matrix which has a high binding affinity for TGF-β (Yamaguchi, Mann & Ruoslahti, 1990). Thus, TGF-β can theoretically increase its own extracellular storage capacity. Other growth factors will also potentiate extracellular matrix formation, the IGFs being potent inducers of type I and II collagen synthesis and of sulfated glycosaminoglycans. Since most IGFBPs will bind to highly sulfated glycosaminoglycans, ligand action on the cell will again favour the regeneration of the extracellular store. The FGFs have a tissue-specific effect on hyaluronic acid synthesis, which has been documented for muscle cell precursors migrating from trunk somites into the limb buds, and prevents muscle cell adhesion and terminal differentiation.

Tissue remodelling is dependent on the production of matrix-specific proteases and glyconases. One such ubiquitous protease is the neutral protease, plasminogen, which is enabled by plasminogen activator. FGF2 is a potent initiator of plasminogen activator expression in mesenchymal tissues, while this is suppressed by TGF-β. Since such proteases can activate and/or release growth factors during extracellular matrix reconstruction, growth factor availability can be controlled interactively by other growth factors via modulation of the extracellular matrix composition.

Growth factor expression and distribution in development

Growth factors such as IGF-II, FGF2 and TGF-β are expressed in almost every tissue of the rat and mouse embryo (Han et al., 1988; Gonzalez et al., 1990; Roberts & Sporn, 1990). Peptide growth factors appear very early in development. In the oocyte and fertilized egg mRNAs for TGF-α, FGF2 and PDGF-A chain are present as products of the maternal genome (Rappolee et al., 1988). However, shortly after fertilization these maternally encoded transcripts are rapidly degraded so that products of the embryonic genome may predominate. In the mouse embryo the fetal genomic products are first apparent at the two- to four-cell stage, and mRNAs encoding TGF-α, TGF-β, activin and IGF-II are immediately detectable following amplification by reverse transcriptase polymerase chain reaction. Two members of the FGF family, FGFs 3 and 4, are also present at the four-cell stage, and are maximally expressed prior to organogenesis. Platelet-derived growth factor-A is detected as an embryonic mRNA transcript in the eight-cell embryo. IGF-I mRNA appears later, around the time of implantation at 8–9 days gestation (Rotwein et al., 1987). Some of the first products of the activated fetal genome are therefore peptide growth factors, suggesting fundamental roles in morphogenesis.

The expression of IGF-II mRNA in human embryos was studied by Brice et al. (1989) using in situ hybridization. Blastocysts produced by in vitro fertilization did not express IGF-II, but mRNA was detectable in primitive trophoblasts obtained as early as 35 days postconception. This suggests that IGF-II may be activated concurrent with cell differentiation pathways, and this is supported by studies with embryonal carcinoma cell lines. Little IGF-II is expressed by rat embryonal carcinoma cells until differentiation is induced by exposure to retinoic acid (Nagarajan et al., 1985; Van Zoelen et al., 1989). An increase in IGF-II synthesis is accompanied by a downregulation of expression of members of the FGF family.

Preimplantation mouse embryos express IGFBPs-2, -3, -4 and -6, but not IGFBPs-1 or -5 (Hahnel & Schultz, 1994). IGFBP-2 mRNA was detected throughout the epiblast of the egg cylinder as early as day 7, at a time when IGF-II expression is limited to the trophectoderm (Wood, Streck & Pintar, 1992). On days 10 and 11, IGFBP-2 mRNA was localized to the rostral brain of the primary neural tube, and in neuroepithelium of the tail during secondary neurulation. During mid-gestation IGFBP-2 was abundant in surface ectoderm, particularly that of the branchial arches. This complemented the expression of IGF-II in the adjacent mesenchyme of the branchial arches. IGFBP-2 was seen in a restricted number of mesodermal tissues which did not express IGF-II, such as the mesonephric tubules and the notochord, and was typically seen at sites of mesodermal/ectodermal interaction which directed tissue growth and differentiation. Whether this implies intrinsic morphogenic actions for IGFBP-2, or a key role in regulating IGF availability, is not known. The distribution of IGFBP-5 mRNA in the postimplantation mouse embryo is distinct from that of IGFBP-2 (Green et al., 1994), being abundant in muscle precursor cells, all cells of the anterior pituitary, and axial regions of the neuroepithelium. During late gestation in the mouse, IGFBP-3 mRNA is seen in liver and in vertebrae, while IGFBP-4 mRNA is strongest in kidney, lung, liver and intestine (Babajko et al., 1993). IGFBP-6 mRNA can only be detected in late gestation in liver, lung, vertebrae and ribs, while IGFBP-1 mRNA is limited to liver. In summary, while the expression of IGF-II in early gestation, and both IGF-I and -II in later gestation, are ubiquitous, the expression of the IGFBP species is precisely anatomically and developmentally regulated. This strongly suggests that the major level of control of the IGF axis in development is the regulation of its bioavailability and actions by IGFBPs.

In the human fetus, in late first and early second trimester, IGF-II and much lower levels of IGF-I mRNAs are widely expressed, but are mostly localized to mesenchymal cells (Han, D'Ercole & Lund, 1987*a*). However, immunohistochemical localization of the IGF peptides showed that they are predominantly associated with epithelia of the lung, gut, kidney, liver parenchymal cells and adrenal cortex, and with differentiated muscle (Han et al., 1987*b*), suggesting disparate sites of synthesis and action. The sites of IGF peptide presence agree with the localization of mRNA or protein for IGFBPs (Hill et al., 1989; Hill & Clemmons, 1992; Delhanty et al., 1993), and suggest that the growth factors are present in vivo complexed with their specific binding proteins. The IGFBP mRNAs are most prevalent in regions of active cell replication and differentiation, such as the epidermis of skin, the crypt epithelia of developing gut and the ureteric bud of the kidney (Delhanty et al., 1993). At a cellular level, the IGF:IGFBP complexes are associated with the plasma membranes and/or extracellular matrix (Hill & Clemmons, 1992), suggesting that the specific binding of IGFBPs to matrix components demonstrated in vitro is also widespread in vivo.

Messenger RNA for TGF-β1 is found throughout the mouse embryo and is particularly abundant in bone and megakaryocytes of liver, which are also sites of TGF-β1 peptide synthesis (Pelton et al., 1990). Elsewhere in the embryo, TGF-β1 mRNA is associated predominantly with epithelia, while the peptide is localized to adjacent mesenchymal cells. This growth factor is particularly abundant at sites of mesenchymal/epithelial interaction during morphogenesis, such as in secondary palate formation and hair follicles. In the human fetus, also, TGF-β1, -β2 and -β3 have distinct spatial and temporal patterns of expression (Gatherer et al., 1990) which predominate during morphogenic events. The translocation of TGF-β1 peptide from epithelia to mesenchymal tissues suggests binding to extracellular matrix molecules such as the cell surface proteoglycan, betaglycan, and the extracellular matrix molecule decorin, which is a dermatan sulfate.

Messenger RNA for FGF2 increases steadily in the embryo during development until day 16, expression being greatest in the tail, face and developing limbs (Herbert et al., 1990). Conversely, FGF3 is expressed in parietal endoderm, primitive mesoderm, the pharyngeal pouches and neuroepithelium of the hind brain between 7.5 and 9.5 days of gestation. Different members of the FGF family appear to have distinct anatomical and ontological patterns of expression which together cover almost every embryonic and fetal tissue. However, outside of the central nervous system FGF peptides are predominantly associated with extracellular matrix, especially the basement membranes underlying epithelia, and in this form may be inaccessible to target tissues without liberation as a result of proteolysis.

Growth factors and embryogenesis

Mitogenic signalling by both IGF-I and -II appears to be exclusively via the type1 receptor on most cell types. Consequently, IGF-I is a more potent mitogen than IGF-II, with an ED_{50} of approximately 1–3 nM, on most cell types. This is relatively inefficient compared to the mitogenic properties of other growth factors such as the FGFs and EGF. However, this does not imply a secondary role for the IGFs in cell proliferation, since each growth factor may play a precise role within the cell replication cycle, as first elucidated for fibroblastic cells (Van Wyk et al., 1981). The G_1 phase of the cycle is a period when the cell acquires the necessary nutrients, proteins and enzymes to begin the preparation for DNA synthesis in the subsequent 'S' phase. Some growth factors, such as the FGFs and PDGF, have a major role at the beginning of G_1, and are called competence factors, rendering the cell capable of entering the cell cycle. Once within G_1, growth factor requirements change, such that EGF is necessary for the initial period and the IGFs for the latter half of G_1 progression. Since these peptides allow the cells to progress to S phase, they are known as progression factors. When present together, competence and progression factors are synergistic, and a change in the number of cells involved in active proliferation within any tissue can be modulated by altering the relative abundance of growth factors in the microenvironment. This allows for precise growth control without the need for de novo expression or suppression of individual growth factors. Following DNA synthesis during S phase, cells will progress to mitosis without further external stimulation, and driven by the sequential expression of cyclin genes.

A fundamental role for IGFs in the regulation of birth size, and particularly in muscle development, has been conclusively demonstrated using 'gene knockout' technology. Gene deletion by the process of homologous recombination is a powerful way of examining the morphological and anatomical implications of growth factor deficiency. Homologous recombination has been used to disrupt either the IGF-I, the IGF-II, or the type-I IGF receptor gene loci in mice. By interbreeding, combination gene 'knockouts' have then been obtained. Deletion of the IGF-I gene yielded homozygotes which had a birthweight about 60% that of normal, of which some died within 6 h of birth (Liu et al., 1993). However, some of the mutant mice survived to adulthood, but females were infertile owing to a failure of ovarian follicular development. Using a similar strategy to delete IGF-II, it was found that the IGF-II gene is parentally imprinted and is only transmitted from the male allele in the majority of tissues, exceptions being the choroid plexus and meninges where the gene is active on both alleles (De Chiara, Efstratiadis &

Robertson, 1990). IGF-II-deficient homozygotes had a similar growth deficiency at birth to animals lacking IGF-I, demonstrating that both isomers have a role in prenatal growth. However, IGF-II-deficient mice were fertile.

Deletion of the type-I IGF receptor, which is primarily responsible for the signalling of both mitogenesis and differentiation by both IGF-I and IGF-II, yielded homozygous animals which were only 45% of normal weight at delivery, and died within minutes of birth (Baker et al., 1993). This was due to a failure to breathe and probably resulted from a widespread muscle hypoplasia, including that of the respiratory muscles. There was an increase in neuronal cell density in the spinal cord and brainstem of the mutant animals, while the skin was thinner due to a reduction in the stratum spinosum, and bone ossification was delayed by about two fetal days. Double gene knockout involving both the IGF-I and type-I receptor genes resulted in a similar phenotype to that found after deletion of the receptor alone; however, codeletion of IGF-II and the type-1 receptor yielded a subgroup of animals with only 30% of normal birthweight at term and grossly retarded skeletal development. This suggests that an additional receptor to the type-1 form may also contribute to IGF-II signalling. The type-2/mannose-6-phosphate receptor is deleted in a naturally occurring gene deletion identified by the lack of the imprinted locus 'Tme', and results in lethality at the embryonic stage (Barlow et al., 1991). Whether this receptor can contribute to IGF-II signalling in vivo is not clear.

The above series of studies demonstrates that neither IGF-I or IGF-II are crucial for key morphological events in early development, but that they act as 'true' growth factors, contributing to the expansion of stem cell populations and the progression of cell differentiation. While both IGF-I and -II contribute to fetal growth, the size of the placenta was normal following deletion of the IGF-I and type-1 receptor genes while reduced after deletion of IGF-II (Baker et al., 1993). This suggests that a high expression of IGF-II in placenta may contribute to its development as an autocrine or paracrine agent.

One of the best-studied morphogenic events is the induction of mesoderm in the *Xenopus* embryo, and both FGF2 and members of the TGF-β family have been implicated. Mesoderm induction occurs from the embryonic animal pole ectoderm in response to diffusible morphogenic signals from the vegetal pole ectoderm. Basic FGF was able to induce the development of elements of the ventral mesoderm in explanted animal pole ectoderm from *Xenopus* embryos (Kimelman & Kirschner, 1987). Messenger RNA encoding FGF2 was identified in the embryo at the time of mesoderm induction (Kimelman et al., 1988), while endogenous mesoderm-inducing activity could be neutralized with antiserum against FGF2 (Slack & Isaacs, 1989). Proof that the endogenous members of the FGF family were responsible for the induction of ventral mesoderm was provided by Amaya, Musci and Kirschner (1991) who expressed a dominant negative mutant of a high affinity FGF receptor in the *Xenopus* embryo, which would bind FGFs, interfered with intracellular signalling, and which downregulated the endogenous receptors. Serious defects in gastrulation and in ventral mesoderm formation resulted, including a developmental failure of ventral somites leading to an absence of a tail.

FGF2 action is coordinated with other factors which regulate dorsal mesoderm formation, members of the TGF-β family being pre-eminent. Exogenous TGF-β2 was able to induce dorsal mesoderm formation in isolated animal pole ectoderm from the *Xenopus* embryo, while the actions of the endogenous morphogen(s) could be blocked by exposure to TGF-β2 antiserum (Rosa et al., 1988). Despite these results, the failure of the *Xenopus* embryo to express endogenous TGF-β at the appropriate time suggested that other members of the TGF-β-related family were biologically relevant. Both activin B_A and B_B chain mRNAs are expressed, the BB form first appearing in late blastulation, increasing in abundance during gastrulation, and being present in greatest amounts in the tadpole (Thomsen et al., 1990). The BA form of activin mRNA did not appear until late gastrulation. Despite this, analysis of the endogenous dorsal mesoderm-inducing activity in conditioned medium from embryonal ectodermal cells revealed this to be related to mammalian activin B_A. Clearly, one of the activins is responsible for dorsal mesoderm formation in amphibians, and parallel studies suggest that this is also so in the chick and mouse (Mitrani et al., 1990; Smith et al., 1990).

Transforming growth factor-β is an inhibitor of mitogenesis for most epithelial cell types in vitro, and for some mesenchymal cells (Roberts & Sporn, 1990). This, coupled with evidence that TGF-β has a fundamental role in embryonic morphogenesis, made it likely that disruption of TGF-β genes would have profound effects on phenotypes. Initial reports showed this not to be the case, since targeted disruption of the TGF-β1 gene resulted in homozygous mice with normal birth size and body function (Shull et al., 1992; Kulkarni et al., 1993). However, three to four weeks after birth animals underwent a widespread and lethal inflammatory response with massive infiltration of lymphocytes and macrophages into the heart, lungs and other organs. Both class I and II antigens of the major histocompatibility complex were overexpressed. A recent report shows that the lack of embryonic phenotype is likely to be due to maternal rescue, with a demonstration that radiolabelled latent TGF-β1 could cross the placenta from mother to fetus and distribute rapidly into the extracellular fluids, extracellular matrix and fetal cells (Letterio et al., 1994). TGF-β1 was also present in maternal cells within milk, and in milk fluid, and could be transferred across the neonatal gut to peripheral tissues within 15 minutes. When homozygous TGF-β1-deficient female mice were protected against autoimmune disease by glucocorticoid treatment in order to allow pregnancy and fetal development, the homozygous offspring, with no access to maternal TGF-β1, showed serious malformations of the heart. The arterioventricular junctions were poorly developed with disordered myocyte proliferation, and abnormal ventricular lumina. Earlier studies with mouse embryos showed that TGF-β1 mRNA was strongly expressed in endocardial cells, cardiac mesenchyme, and around the cardiac cushion tissue during heart formation between days 7 to 9.5 of gestation (Akhurst et al., 1990). TGF-β1 mRNA co-localized with the extracellular matrix protein, tenascin, suggesting that some of the morphogenic actions of TGF-β1 may have been indirectly mediated by selective matrix deposition.

Platelet-derived growth factor has also been implicated directly in embryonic morphogenesis. The Ph/+ mutant mouse is viable in the heterozygous condition but in the homozygous state gives rise to grossly malformed fetuses consistent with a failure of neural crest cell migration (Morrison-Graham et al., 1992). Embryos can exhibit an open neural tube, clubbed limbs, a lack of thymus, no dermal layer to the skin, a lack of connective tissue within the organs and a failure of craniofacial development. The condition has been linked to a deletion of one of the PDGF receptors, PDGF-α, suggesting an important role for PDGF in neural crest cell migration (Orrurtreger et al., 1992). Both PDGF-A and the PDGF-α receptor are known to be expressed within the neural crest area in amphibian embryos. Goustin et al. (1985) found expression of PDGF in human placenta from as early as 21 days after conception. Using in situ hybridization, the expression of the c-*sis* gene was localized to trophoblasts. Explants of first trimester placenta released radioreceptor-assayable PDGF, while cultured trophoblast cell lines were rich in high affinity PDGF receptors, and responded to exogenous PDGF with an increased expression of c-*myc*, accompanied by DNA synthesis. This may reflect an autocrine action of PDGF on trophoblast proliferation during the early invasive growth of the placenta.

In the mouse embryo, EGF receptors are present on the first differentiated cell type, the trophectoderm (Adamson & Meek, 1984). The major ligand appears to be TGF-α, although this may be available from the maternal decidua in addition to embryonic sources around and following implantation (Han et al., 1987*c*). Early in the second trimester of human fetal development peptides of the EGF family are present within cells at the base of the gastric and pyloric glands of the stomach, Brunner's glands in the duodenum, the epithelium of the distal convoluted tubules of the kidney, anterior pituitary, skin and the placental cytotrophoblasts (Kasselberg et al., 1985). Given such a widespread distribution, it was surprising that targeted disruption of the TGF-α gene resulted in largely normal embryonic and fetal development, although the neonatal mice had curly hair and whiskers, and abnormal eyelid maturation (Luetteke et al., 1993). However, it is possible that TGF-α is rendered redundant by the presence of other EGF family members, which may be upregulated as a compensatory mechanism when TGF-α is lacking. This would be supported by the failure of implantation that occurs following the disruption of the EGF receptor gene (ER-1). Use of targeted EGF antiserum in mice as a means of eliminating EGF peptide bioactivity has been shown to cause a failure of tooth eruption and poor lung morphogenesis (Slavkin et al., 1992; Yasui et al., 1993).

Limb formation

Formation of the limb buds and the subsequent skeletal structure of the limbs have been well studied in the chick embryo, and are now thought to be tightly controlled by peptide growth factors. The limb buds first develop as a thickening of the body wall mesenchyme, the surface ectoderm of which is induced by the underlying mesenchyme to form a specialized structure called the apical ectodermal ridge. The mesenchyme beneath the apical ectodermal ridge is maintained in an undifferentiated, rapidly proliferating state, and enables outgrowth of the limb to occur. Limb outgrowth is promptly arrested following removal of the apical ectodermal ridge. As mesenchyme moves distally to the progress zone, so it undergoes a condensation and morphogenic change to become cartilage. Subperiosteal bone then develops on the surface of the cartilage immediately below the perichondrium to give rise to primary ossification structures. Increase in length of the long bones then continues by epiphyseal chondrogenesis and subsequent ossification. Superimposed upon this sequence of outgrowth and differentiation is the formation of the pentadactyl pattern of the limb in the dorso-ventral plane. This is controlled by a diffusible morphogen which is released within a specialized area of mesenchyme on the ventral aspect of the progress zone called the polarizing region, whose actions include the sequential activation of homeobox genes.

In the rat embryo, Beck et al. (1987) localized IGF-II mRNA to precartilaginous mesenchymal condensations, perichondrium and immature chondrocytes, in addition to the periosteum and centres of intramembranous ossification. Both IGF-I and -II mRNAs were also localized to limb bud mesenchyme in the rat fetus by Streck et al. (1992), who additionally showed that, while IGF-II expression was strongest in the presumptive skeleton and muscle at the centre of the limbs, IGF-I mRNA was absent from these areas but strongly expressed in the peripheral mesenchyme beneath the epithelium. Neither IGF isomer was strongly expressed in the rapidly dividing mesenchymal cells of the progress zone. While IGF-II is a potent mitogen for isolated limb bud mesenchyme from the rat in vitro (Bhaumick & Bala, 1991), the above findings suggest that the role of IGFs is not primarily as mitogens but involves the initiation or progression of differentiation pathways for skeletal and muscular elements. In the first trimester human fetus, also, IGF-II mRNA was abundant in perichondrial areas (Han et al., 1987*a*). We localized IGF peptides by immunocytochemistry in the chick embryo limb buds (Ralphs, Wylie & Hill, 1990). At stages 20–24 a uniform presence of IGFs was seen in undifferentiated mesenchyme, but this disappeared in the prechondrogenic areas of condensation. As chondrocytes appeared around stage 28, so immunoreactive staining for IGFs returned. By stage 36 endochondrial calcification had begun and intense IGF staining was associated with hypertrophic chondrocytes, as well as osteoblasts in the subperiosteum of the membraneous bone.

During the early development of the limb bud, IGFBP-2 expression is seen within the anterior–posterior strip of ectoderm which will become the apical ectodermal ridge, and IGFBP-2 continues to be expressed here until outgrowth is complete (Streck et al., 1992). It is possible that the function of IGFBP-2 in the apical ectodermal ridge is to negate an IGF-II-dependent drive towards differentiation in the underlying progress zone mesenchyme, and to maintain a stem cell population.

TGF-β1, 2 and 3 isomers are all expressed within the developing skeleton of the mouse embryo. Heine et al. (1987) observed the distribution of TGF-β1 peptide by immunocytochemistry from 11 to 18 days gestation. Strong staining was seen in all mesenchyme undergoing condensation and cartilage formation, which persisted during ossification within the newly formed osteoblasts. Analysis of TGF-β1 mRNA distribution by in situ hybridization revealed a high expression in perichondrial osteocytes involved with membraneous calcification (Lehnert & Akhurst, 1988). However, differentiated cartilage contained little TGF-β1 mRNA, although this is a site of peptide synthesis. A similar pattern has been described for TGF-β2 and -β3 in developing skeletal tissues (Pelton et al., 1990). In the human embryo of 32–57 days gestation, TGF-β2 and -β3 mRNAs were localized to chondrogenic areas (Gatherer et al., 1990). TGF-β2 mRNA was located within the precartilaginous blastoma of limb bud mesenchyme, and in later development in actively proliferating chondroblasts at the epiphyseal/diaphyseal boundary. Messenger RNA for TGF-β3 was first seen in the developing intervertebral discs and in the perichondrium of cartilage associated with the vertebral column, but not with long bones. An intense site of TGF-β1 abundance was in areas of membraneous bone formation and, in fetuses of 10–12 weeks gestation, in osteogenic cells at sites of endochondrial calcification in the long bones. No TGF-β mRNA was located in the hypertrophic chondrocytes which immediately precede the area of provisional calcification. A divergent expression of TGF-β isoforms in skeletal primordia suggests distinct biological roles, and that of TGF-β2 would support a role in cartilaginous induction. Evidence for this is provided by the observations that mammalian TGF-β1 and -β2 induced the appearance of phenotypic chondrocytes, associated with increased sulfated mucopolysaccharide and type II collagen synthesis, in chick embryo mesenchyme cultures. Other members of the TGF-β family, namely bone morphogenetic proteins-2B and -3 (osteogenin), will also induce cartilage formation from embryonic mesoderm in the chick (Carrington et al., 1991; Chen et al., 1991) making the identity of the endogenous active ligand unclear. When TGF-β1 or -β2 were injected into the subperiosteal region of the femurs from newborn rats, local intramembraneous bone and cartilage formation resulted (Joyce et al., 1990). After injections were terminated, the new cartilage underwent endochondrial calcification. These results strongly suggest that TGF-β3 isomers are key players in the formation of cartilage from undifferentiated mesenchyme, and in the subsequent primary ossification process.

FGF2 was present at both mRNA and protein levels during limb bud formation in the chick and mouse (Herbert et al., 1990; Munaim, Klagsbrun & Toole, 1988), peptide levels in the chick limb being greatest on day 3 of gestation (stage 18) when the cell proliferation rate was highest. During this rapid proliferation, mesenchymal cells secrete an extracellular matrix rich in hyaluronic acid. Using isolated chick limb bud cells, FGF2 was shown to potentiate hyaluronic acid release to form pericellular coats (Munaim, Klagsbrun & Toole, 1991). A loss of hyaluronic acid synthesis in vitro coincided with the timing of condensation of mesoderm into the chondrogenic and myogenic regions of the limb bud, and a decline in FGF2 abundance, at stages 22–26. Within the mouse embryo, Gonzalez et al (1990) used immunocytochemistry to localize FGF2 at 18 days gestation. Positive staining was apparent in chondrocytes of the hyaline cartilage and in the perichondrium. Within ossification centres FGF2 was absent from hypertrophic cells but present within the extracellular matrix, osteoblasts and vascular endothelial cells. A different experimental approach was that of Liu and Nicholl (1988) who transplanted fetal rat paws, harvested on day 10 of gestation, under the kidney capsule of adult hosts which were then infused with FGF2 or anti-FGF2 antiserum via the renal artery. Infusion of FGF2 antiserum significantly retarded the growth of the explants and their ossification. Conversely, paw size was increased by administration of FGF2. Other isomers of FGF may also be involved in limb development, FGF5 mRNA appearing within the limb mesenchyme between embryonic days 12.5 and 14.5 in mouse (Haub & Goldfarb, 1991). Expression was limited to a patch of cells ventral to the presumptive femur which was undergoing cartilage formation. The above evidence suggests a mitogenic role for FGF2 in mesenchyme proliferation, and a possible morphogenic role for FGF5 during cartilage induction. However, the strongest evidence linking FGFs to limb formation does not involve the mesenchyme but the apical ectodermal ridge.

As soon as the apical ectodermal ridge is formed, at day 10 of gestation in the mouse, a high expression of FGF4 mRNA is seen in the posterior half, and expression persists until day 12 (Niswander & Martin, 1992). Several members of the FGF family can substitute for the apical ectodermal ridge and maintain limb bud outgrowth in vitro in both the mouse and chick (Niswander & Martin, 1992, 1993), suggesting that an FGF is involved in the endogenous signalling between the epithelium and the underlying mesenchyme. Recently, Niswander et al. (1993) demonstrated that recombinant FGF4 could substitute for the ridge in ovo, and not only maintain limb bud outgrowth but signal the correct spatial information to achieve normal pattern formation. This would imply that FGF4 is capable of regulating an appropriate release of morphogens from the polarizing zone within the mesenchyme. Contradictory evidence was provided by Fallon et al. (1994) who showed that only FGF2 was detectable in the chick limb bud, and that exogenous FGF2 could substitute for the apical ectodermal ridge.

It is now possible to predict which receptor types are involved in FGF signalling within both mesenchyme and ectoderm in the developing limbs. In the mouse embryo, the FGFR2 receptor was first expressed on day 9.5 in limb bud mesenchyme, with a concentration gradient increasing in a posterior and proximal direction. At this time, the expression of FGFR1 was more diffuse than that of FGFR2, within the limb bud mesenchyme, the somites and organ rudiments (Peters et al., 1992). By day 11.5, FGFR2 mRNA was localized to mesenchymal aggregates corresponding to the future bones, and in the surface ectoderm of the limb, being strongest in the interdigital web. At day 12.5 gestation FGFR2 mRNA located to chondrification centres, and at day 14.5 to the bodies of the distal bones. This temporal pattern of expression strongly suggests that FGFR2 mediates FGF actions on the chondrogenic pathways, while FGFR1 may mediate FGF actions on the surrounding undifferentiated mesenchyme. The FGFR4 receptor mRNA was found by in situ hybridization to map to areas of cartilage condensation, while FGFR3 mRNA was abundant in the resting cartilage during the subsequent process of endochondrial calcification (Stark, McMahon & McMahon, 1991; Peters et al., 1993).

Muscle development

The IGFs interact with other peptide growth factors during cellular differentiation, as seen during the differentiation of immortalized myoblast cell lines, such as rat L6 cells, into postmitotic, contractile myotubes. This will occur spontaneously as the myoblasts grow to high density, but can be precipitated prematurely by incubation with IGF-I, or high concentrations of IGF-II or insulin (Ewton & Florini, 1981). While IGF-I will initially induce cell proliferation, a commitment to terminal differentiation is invoked, which may be mediated by an IGF-dependent activation of specific genes controlling differentiation, such as myogenin and *Myo*D (Florini et al., 1991*a*). However, other studies have suggested that IGF-II regulates muscle cell differentiation at intracellular points distal to the activation of myogenin (Rosen et al., 1993). A recent report suggests that the actions of IGF-II on muscle cell differentiation may involve the type2/mannose-6-phosphate receptor, while those of IGF-I are mediated primarily by the type-1 IGF receptor (Rosenthal, Hsiao & Silverman, 1994).

In contradistinction to the actions of IGFs, incubation with FGF2 will potentiate the proliferation of myoblasts and prevent commitment to terminal differentiation (Linkhart, Clegg & Hauscha, 1981; Clegg et al., 1987). Further, FGF2 can suppress transcription of at least two of the myogenic regulatory genes, myogenin and MyoD1 (Vaidya et al., 1989; Brunetti & Goldfine, 1990), suggesting that a widespread presence in vivo serves to prevent a premature differentiation of muscle. TGF-β also prevents terminal differentiation, but has little effect on proliferative rate. The onset of differentiation can therefore be finely controlled by relative changes in the abundance of particular growth factors in the microenvironment.

These growth factor signals derive, in part, from the cells themselves. Proliferating myoblasts synthesize FGFs and high affinity FGF receptors, but synthesize little IGF-I or -II. Upon muscle differentiation the synthesis of FGF(s) and its receptor(s) decline, while the expression of IGF-II dramatically increases (Florini et al., 1991*b*; Rosen et al, 1993). This results in a downregulation of the type-1 IGF receptor. Insulin-like growth factor-II gene expression by differentiating myoblasts is down-regulated by exogenous IGF-I, IGF-II, or high concentrations of insulin (Magri et al., 1994). The actions of IGFs in muscle cell differentiation are also likely to involve endogenous IGFBPs. The mouse muscle cell line, C_2C_{12}, expresses abundant IGFBP-2 mRNA and releases IGFBP-2 peptide in the undifferentiated state, but IGFBP-2 expression declines substantially as differentiation proceeds (Ernst, McCusker & White, 1992). Conversely, IGFBP-5 expression increases during muscle cell differentiation. Overall, a change in IGF:IGFBP ratio in favour of the former during differentiation may maximize the availability of endogenously produced IGFs.

Skeletal development

Longitudinal skeletal growth arises from new bone formation as a result of epiphyseal chondrogenesis, and subsequent replacement of cartilage by bone. Adjacent to the epiphysis is a stem cell population of precursor chondrocytes, which gives rise to a zone of closely packed and highly proliferative chondrocytes. After a number of cell replications, cells are pushed towards the diaphysis within longitudinally arranged columns. Proliferative activity gradually ceases while the cells hypertrophy and increase their rate of macromolecular synthesis. As matrix synthesis increases, the cells become postmitotic and terminally differentiated. Mineralization then occurs between the columns of chondrocytes, and the chondrocytes are replaced by macrophages and osteocytes.

Cells within the proliferative zone of the rat growth plate continuously cycle with a cell cycle length of approximately 54 h (Walker & Kember, 1972). They also secrete an extracellular matrix consisting mainly of type II collagen fibrils and sulfated glycosaminoglycans, the most abundant of which are chondroitin-4 and -6 sulfates, and hyaluronic acid. Cells within the hypertrophic zone have a decreased nuclear labelling index, but an increased rate of collagen and sulfated mucopolysaccharide synthesis, with an increased ratio of protein to DNA. Increases or decreases in growth rate are predominantly due to alterations in hypertrophic activity rather than changes in chondrocyte proliferation rate (Hunziker, 1988). Terminal differentiation in the lower hypertrophic zone is characterized by a dramatic fall in mucopolysaccharide synthesis but a maintenance of collagen synthesis, the expression of a distinctive type X collagen, and the appearance of alkaline phosphatase activity. Adjacent to the diaphysis, cartilage matrix is eroded and replaced by hydroxyapatite at a similar rate to new cartilage formation as a result of proliferation and hypertrophy. The length of the diaphysis, therefore, increases while the width of the growth plate remains constant. Calcification is initiated in matrix vesicles in the lower hypertrophic zone coincident with vascular invasion by capillary sprouting, and the delivery of monocytes and chondroclasts which degrade cartilage matrix and may destroy hypertrophic chondrocytes.

Growth factors may therefore influence epiphyseal chondrogenesis by altering the rate of chondrocyte proliferation, by modulation of the synthetic rate of extracellular matrix molecules, or by changing the rate of terminal differentiation and calcification. There is substantial evidence that FGFs, IGFs and TGF-β isomers are expressed locally within the growth plates during both prenatal and postnatal epiphyseal chondrogenesis.

The presence of FGF2 within cartilage has been recognized for over 10 years (Bekoff & Klagsbrun, 1982), and its production by isolated chick growth plate chondrocytes has been described (Rosier, Landesberg & Puzas, 1991). Extensive analysis of IGF expression, control, and action within epiphyseal growth plate cartilage has provided conclusive proof for a substantial paracrine component of control in postnatal longitudinal skeletal growth. This series of studies was initiated by Isaksson and co-workers who found that pituitary growth hormone (GH) promoted the replication of isolated chondrocytes in vitro, or caused a widening of the epiphyseal growth plate of the proximal tibia when administered locally (Isaksson, Jansson & Gause, 1982; Lindahl et al., 1986). The sophistication of the model was enhanced by infusion of GH into a single femoral artery using an osmotic minipump. This, again, resulted in a local growth response in the treated limb compared to the contralateral control limb (Nilsson et al., 1987).

With the demonstration that IGF-I peptide could be visualized, using immunocytochemistry, in association with proliferative and maturing chondrocytes of the growth plates in rat long bones (Andersson et al., 1986), Isaksson performed a definitive experiment. When longitudinal sections were examined from the growth plates of hypophysectomized rats, chondrocytes no longer demonstrated immunolocalization of IGF-I, but abundant staining returned when hypophysectomized rats were treated with GH (Nilsson et al., 1986). These experiments were repeated by others and extended. The ability of locally infused GH to produce a localized epiphyseal growth response in rats could be reversed by the simultaneous infusion of blocking antibody against IGF-I (Schlechter et al., 1986). The model that emerged has shown IGF-I to be associated with the proliferative chondrocytes of the growth plate, and that its presence mediates the growth promoting actions of GH in vivo. Direct proof that GH controlled the transcription of the IGF-I gene in postnatal epiphyseal growth plate chondrocytes quickly followed (Isgaard et al., 1988). In agreement with the hypothesized growth system the distribution of GH receptors, determined by immunocytochemistry, was found to be limited to the stem cell and proliferative chondrocytic population of the rabbit growth plate, while IGF receptors were most abundant in the proliferative region but were also found on hypertrophic chondrocytes (Trippel, Van Wyk & Mankin, 1986). The latter observation is in agreement with the observed biological actions of IGFs in vitro, which include a predominantly mitogenic action in the proliferative chondrocyte region, and a stimulation of mucopolysaccharide synthesis in the postmitotic hypertrophic chondrocytes adjacent to newly formed bone (Hill, 1979).

The anabolic actions of GH on the epiphyseal growth plate may not be mediated entirely by locally produced IGF-I, since GH may synergize with IGF-I in addition to controlling its expression. Studies with the clonal growth of isolated chondrocytes in soft agar showed that the morphology of colonies induced by the addition of GH differed markedly from those resulting from exposure to IGF-I (Lindahl, Nilsson & Isaksson, 1987). Similarly, while IGF-I stimulated both DNA synthesis and proteoglycan synthesis by bovine articular chondrocytes, a much enhanced response was seen following the addition of GH. The latter peptide had no effects in the absence of IGF-I (Smith et al., 1989).

Using in situ hybridization, TGF-β1 mRNA was shown to be expressed in abundance in bone cells of the human fetus in first trimester, although relatively little was present within the growth plate (Sandberg et al., 1988). However, TGF-β immunoreactivity was seen in chondrocytes and cartilage matrix of fetal and postnatal mice (Ellingsworth et al., 1986; Heine et al., 1987), while biodetectable TGF-β was released from isolated growth plate chondrocytes from the postnatal chick, this being greater for hypertrophic cells than for cells of the proliferative zone (Rosier et al., 1989; Gelb, Rosier & Puzas, 1990). TGF-β may be stored within the matrix of bovine articular cartilage in a relatively inactive form, perhaps as the latent precursor molecule, which could then be activated by locally produced proteases.

We have studied the regulation of epiphyseal chondrogenesis in the fetus as a model of peptide growth factor interaction during cell proliferation and differentiation, our model being the proximal tibia of the ovine fetus. FGF2 and its high affinity receptor, FGFR1, were strongly expressed at both mRNA and peptide levels in the proliferative chondrocyte zone of the ovine growth plate, decreased during cell differentiation, and were absent from the hypertrophic chondrocytes. No IGF-I mRNA was observed in the fetal growth plate, but IGF-II mRNA and peptide were predominantly associated with the differentiating, but still mitotically active, chondrocytes. Unlike IGF-I in postnatal life, the expression and release of IGF-II in fetal growth plate chondrocytes were not increased in response to growth hormone. An associated expression of IGFBP-2 and IGFBP-3 was found. As chondrocytes began to hypertrophy, so mRNA for IGF-II declined and that encoding TGF-β1 appeared. The terminally differentiated chondrocytes also expressed IGFBP-5, which was not seen in other areas of the growth plate. In summary, as chondrocytes passed from proliferation to differentiation to hypertrophy, they sequentially expressed FGF2, then IGF-II, and finally TGF-β1. This anatomical distribution allowed testable hypotheses to be formulated with regard to growth factor contribution to epiphyseal chondrogenesis.

The expression of FGF2 and its receptor in stem and proliferating chondrocyte populations suggests a role as an autocrine mitogen. Using isolated chondrocyte cultures FGF2 was found to be released and to contribute to DNA synthesis, while a neutralizing antibody against FGF2 decreased endogenous DNA synthesis in cells by 50% (Hill & Logan, 1992*a*; Hill et al., 1992*a*). Exogenous FGF2 was 100–500 times more potent than IGF-I, IGF-II or insulin as a mitogen for fetal growth plate chondrocytes (Hill & Logan, 1992*b*; Hill et al., 1992*b*). Insulin had an equivalent mitogenic action to IGF-I at low nanomolar concentrations (Hill & De Sousa, 1990), and both were an order of magnitude more effective, on a concentration basis, than was IGF-II, the endogenously produced IGF isomer. Conversely, IGF-II, which was expressed by maturing chondrocytes, was a potent stimulator of glycosaminoglycan and collagen synthesis by chondrocytes, parameters of a differentiated phenotype (Hill et al., 1992*a*). It is likely that the actions of endogenous IGF-II on chondrocyte growth and maturation are modulated by endogenous IGFBPs. We found that exogenous IGFBP-2 had a biphasic effect on IGF-II stimulated chondrocyte DNA synthesis, enhancing the actions of IGF-II at concentrations which were approximately equimolar to the added growth factor, but inhibiting IGF-II action when the IGFBP was present in excess. At lower concentrations the IGFBP-2 may bind to cell surface integrins via its consensus RGD binding sequence, and may concentrate IGF-II at the cell surface where it is readily accessible to the high affinity type-I receptors. At greater concentrations of IGFBP-2, the integrin binding sites may be fully occupied, and soluble IGFBP-2 may then directly compete with the signalling receptor for ligand binding.

Finally, TGF-β1, which was located in terminally differentiated cells, inhibited chondrocyte replication in response to other mitogens yet potentiated extracellular matrix molecule production. TGF-β1 increased sulfated mucopolysaccharide synthesis and enhanced collagenous protein synthesis at the expense of non-collagenous protein (Hill et al., 1992*a*). Many of the biochemical features of epiphyseal chondrogenesis might therefore be explained by interactions between endogenously produced peptide growth factors. It seems likely that mineralization involves the further interaction with thyroxine, which was found to reverse the mitogenic actions of IGFs on chondrocytes while inducing alkaline phosphatase production, a marker of terminal differentiation (Ohlsson et al., 1992).

Organ maturation

Growth factors have key functions in the maturation of organ systems prior to birth. Of the steroidogenic tissues most information exists for the fetal adrenal gland. ACTH is a major trophic factor for the fetal adrenal cortex, in addition to regulating steroidogenesis. Much research on growth factors has focused on whether these might mediate or complement ACTH action. Han et al. (1987*a*) showed that the capsule and definitive zone of the human fetal adrenal expressed abundant IGF-II mRNA, and some IGF-I from at least 16–20 weeks gestation. The IGF type-1 receptor has been localized by autoradiography to the fetal zone and medulla of the adrenal gland of human fetuses at 26–33 weeks gestation (Shigematsu et al., 1989). An increase in the levels of IGF-II mRNA in response to ACTH by cultured human fetal zone adrenal cells in second trimester suggests that IGF-II may mediate ACTH effects on adrenal growth (Voutilainen & Miller, 1987*a,b*). However, infusion of ACTH into the adult rat caused a decrease in adrenal IGF-II mRNA content (Townsend, Dallman & Miller, 1990), while infusion of either ACTH or cortisol into the ovine fetus also reduced IGF-II mRNA and peptide content in the adrenals (Lu et al., 1994). These discrepancies may be explained by the effects of glucocorticoids on IGF-II expression. In the human tissue model, fetal zone adrenal cells were used which lack 3β dehydroxysteroid dehydrogenase and cannot, therefore, synthesize cortisol. Glucocorticoids were also blocked in vivo by infusion of metyrapone into the fetal rhesus monkey (Coulter et al., 1993). In this experiment ACTH levels would have increased, and an increase in IGF-II mRNA levels resulted. Thus, ACTH and glucocorticoids are likely to have opposing actions on IGF-II expression in the fetal adrenal. The rise in free cortisol levels which precedes parturition in the fetal sheep may precipitate a reduction in tissue IGF-II mRNA levels and circulating IGF-II, since infusion of cortisol to the fetus during the last third of pregnancy was able to reproduce this phenomenon (Li et al., 1993).

Direct evidence that IGFs exert effects on functional maturation of the adrenal have come mainly from studies in vitro. Pretreatment of ovine fetal adrenocortical cells with IGF-I for 4 days increased the accumulation of cAMP and corticosterone output in response to ACTH stimulation (Naamen et al., 1989). The effects of IGF-I were exerted not only on the ACTH-dependent adenylate cyclase pathway but at steps beyond this, since cAMP metabolites and IGF-I together also synergized to increase corticosterone release. It has been suggested that the primary action of IGF-I is to increase the uptake of the precursor of steroid synthesis, cholesterol, by adrenal cortical cells. However, work using cultured bovine adrenocortical cells has also shown that IGF-I can increase the activity of 3β-hydroxysteroid dehydrogenase (Chatelain et al., 1988). In cultured human adrenal cells, IGF-II mRNA increased in association with increases in mRNA for steroidogenic enzymes such as $P450_{scc}$ and $P450_{C17}$ in response to ACTH stimulation (Voutilainen & Miller, 1987*a*). However, the addition of IGFs to human adrenocortical cell cultures did not affect the mRNA levels of these enzymes. It is therefore unclear whether IGFs influence multiple enzymatic processes in the steroidogenic pathways, or simply maintain cholesterol uptake by the cells.

Using Northern blot hybridization, human fetal adrenal has been shown to express mRNA for FGF2 (DiBlasio et al., 1987), while studies in vitro have shown that FGF2 is mitogenic for cells of the fetal and adult zones of the human fetal gland (Crickard & Jaffe, 1981). Additionally, the expression of FGF2 mRNA was increased in response to ACTH (Mesiano et al., 1991), suggesting that FGF2 may act as an autocrine mediator of the trophic actions of the pituitary hormone. EGF is also a potent mitogen for adrenal cells, but an adrenal source of EGF has not been identified. In contrast to the above growth factors, TGF-β had an inhibitory effect on both basal and ACTH-stimulated growth and steroidogenesis by adrenal cortical cells. The effects on steroidogenesis appear to result from an inhibition of the enzyme responsible for converting cholesterol precursor to cholesterol, although more distal pathways may also be involved since Rainey et al. (1991) showed that TGF-β blocked stimulation of P450 17α-hydroxylase mRNA and protein in ovine fetal adrenocortical cells.

The pituitary is a rich source of growth factors and/or their receptors, including the IGFs, EGF, TGF-α, FGFs, and TGF-β. While many of these are mitogens for pituitary cells in vitro, some have also been demonstrated to have a role in the control of pituitary hormone release. Epidermal growth factor was found to increase ACTH secretion when infused into the fetal sheep or rhesus monkey (Polk et al., 1987; Luger et al., 1988). Immunoreactivity for EGF was seen in both the lactotroph and corticotroph cells, suggesting a paracrine action. Bondy et al. (1990)

showed that IGF-II mRNA was present in the pituitary primordia, and in Rathke's pouch in the rat embryo. Using cultures of human and ovine fetal pituitary, IGF-I or -II were shown to decrease both basal and theophylline-stimulated growth hormone release (Goodyer et al., 1986; Blanchard et al., 1988), and this is likely to result from a direct effect on growth hormone gene transcription. No effects of IGFs on ACTH release from pituitary cultures were found (Goodyer et al., 1986). IGF-I has been shown to increase cell survival and promote development of hypothalamic cells from the fetal rat (Torres-Aleman, Naftolin & Robbins, 1990), and its effects were additive to those of FGF2. Treatment of hypothalamic neuronal cells with FGF2 increased the abundance of type 1 IGF receptors, IGFBP release, and the release of IGF-I (Pons & Torres-Aleman, 1992). This would suggest that the IGF and FGF axes are interactive in the functional maturation of the hypothalamic neurons.

Members of the FGF family are potent mitogens for isolated lung pneumocytes, and both FGF2 and its receptor have been localized by immunocytochemistry to the airway epithelia of fetal rat lung (Han et al., 1992). A morphogenic role for the FGF family in lung development was shown in studies of functional ablation of the FGFR2 gene (Williams et al., 1994). In homozygous mice, no branching of the central airway occurs, and animals die at birth with an absence of lung development. FGF7, also called keratinocyte growth factor, is a potent mitogen for isolated type II pneumocytes from the rat (Ulich et al., 1994). The human fetal lung is rich in mRNA encoding TGF-α in mid-gestation (Strandjord et al., 1993), while fetal lung is rich in high affinity EGF receptors, and exogenous EGF given in the rabbit or lamb induced lung epithelial maturation and surfactant production (Catterton et al., 1979; Sundell et al., 1980). Studies with fetal rat lung explants showed that EGF increased phospholipid biosynthesis, thereby increasing surfactant production, while in the fetal monkey lung EGF caused an acceleration of maturation of type II pneumocytes (Plopper et al., 1992). The appearance of EGF receptors within fetal rabbit lung is under androgenic control (Klein & Nielson, 1993). Conversely, TGF-β inhibited pneumocyte development in explants of fetal rabbit lung, the mechanism of which was postulated to involve a reduced synthesis of fibroblast-pneumocyte factor, a lung fibroblast-derived factor which regulates the maturation of the adjacent epithelial cells (Nielson, Kellogg & Doyle, 1992).

During the embryonic development of the rat, mRNA transcripts for IGF-I and -II are detectable in the lung from at least day 16 gestation (term 22 days) (Davenport et al., 1987), with the latter being more abundant. Levels of IGF-II fall in late gestation and postnatally IGF-II is almost entirely replaced by an expression of IGF-I. The sites of expression of IGF-II were examined by in situ hybridization in mid-trimester human fetal lung (Han et al., 1987*a*). The cells containing IGF-II mRNA included the pleura, interlobular septa and fibroblast cells around the pulmonary vessels. This implies a mesenchymal source of IGF-II. However, immunocytochemistry showed a strong colocalization of IGF peptides with IGFBP mRNA and peptide distribution on or within the pulmonary epithelium of the developing airways (Hill et al., 1989; Delhanty et al., 1993). This would imply a sequestration of IGF-II by IGFBPs and the identification of the lung epithelium as a likely target site of IGF action. IGFBP-2 peptide was localized to the apical membrane of the lung epithelium in fetal rat lung (Klempt et al., 1992). A biological role for IGFs on pulmonary epithelium is supported by the identification of IGF receptors on membrane preparations from fetal porcine lungs (D'Ercole, Foushee & Underwood, 1976), and the synthesis of functional type-1 IGF receptors by canine tracheal epithelial cells in vitro.

IGFs and compromised fetal growth

Since only the IGFs, of the major growth factor classes, are found to any extent within the fetal circulation, it is only within this field that an extensive literature exists with regard to changes associated with fetal pathology. In the human infant subject to intrauterine growth retardation, IGF-I concentrations are lower than in age-matched control infants, while levels of IGF-II are unaltered (Lassarre et al., 1991). Conversely, in macrosomic infants of diabetic mothers, circulating levels of IGF-I are elevated (Delmis et al., 1992). While this suggests that fetal IGF-I expression may be closely related to growth rate in the last trimester of pregnancy, this association may not be the determining biological parameter since circulating levels of IGFBP-1 are substantially elevated in the circulation of the growth-retarded infant (Wang et al., 1991). This may limit IGF availability to its high affinity IGF receptors.

The observations in human pregnancy have been reproduced and extended in animal studies. When fetal growth in the rat is restricted, either by uterine vessel ligation or by maternal fasting, there is a reproducible reduction in IGF-I mRNA levels in fetal liver and other tissues, an increase in IGF-II mRNA, a reduction in IGF-I but an increase in IGF-II in plasma, and an increase in the hepatic expression and circulating levels of IGFBP-1 and -2 (Vileisis & D'Ercole, 1986; Unterman et al., 1990; Straus et al., 1991; Price et al., 1992). Acute hypoxia in the ovine fetus induces a rapid but selective reduction in DNA synthetic rate in a number of tissues including adrenal and lung (Hooper et al., 1991). This is associated with only small changes in the circulating levels of IGF-I or -II, but substantial and prompt increases in circulating levels of IGFBP-1 and its levels of steady state mRNA in liver and kidney (Iwamoto, Murray & Chernausek, 1992; McLellan et al., 1992). The rapid rise in circulating IGFBP-1, and its increased hepatic expression, could be reproduced in the normal ovine fetus by infusion of catecholamines, which are known to increase rapidly in the hypoxic fetus (Hooper et al., 1994). Collectively, these data suggest that tissue growth rate can be rapidly altered by a local or widespread change in IGFBP synthesis, and a limitation of the bioavailability of IGF-I and -II. A more sustained insult to the fetus may also induce a downregulation of IGF-I synthesis.

Acknowledgements

The author is grateful for financial support from the Medical Research Council of Canada for those studies cited from his own laboratory.

References

Adamson, E.D. & Meek, J. (1984). The ontogeny of epidermal growth factor receptors during mouse development. *Developmental Biology*, **103**, 62–70.

Akhurst, R.J., Lehnert, S.A., Faissner, A. & Duffie, E. (1990). TGF beta in murine morphogenetic processes: the early embryo and cardiogenesis. *Development*, **108**, 645–56.

Amaya, E., Musci, T.J. & Kirschner, M.W. (1991). Expression of a dominant negative mutant of the FGF receptor disrupts mesoderm formation in *Xenopus* embryos. *Cell*, **66**, 257–70.

Andersson, I., Billig, H., Fryklund, L., Hansson, H-H., Isaksson, O., Isgaard, J., Nilsson, A., Rozell, B., Skottner, A. & Stemme, S. (1986). Localization of IGF I in adult rats. Immunohistochemical studies. *Acta Physiologica Scandinavica*, **126**, 311–12.

Babajko, S., Hardouin, S., Segovia, B., Groyer, A. & Binoux, M. (1993). Expression of insulin-like growth factor binding protein-1 and -2 genes through the perinatal period in the rat. *Endocrinology*, **132**, 2586–92.

Baird, A. & Bohlen, P. (1990). Fibroblast growth factors. In *Peptide Growth Factors and Their Receptors*, ed. M.B. Sporn & A.B. Roberts. pp. 369–418. Springer-Verlag, Berlin.

Baker, J., Liu, J-P., Robertson, E.J. & Efstratiadis, A. (1993). Role of insulin-like growth factors in embryonic and postnatal growth. *Cell*, **75**, 73–82.

Barlow, D.P., Stoger, R., Herrmann, B.G., Saito, K. & Schweifer, N. (1991). The mouse insulin-like growth factor type-2 receptor is imprinted and closely linked to the Tme locus. *Nature*, **349**, 84–7.

Beck, F., Samani, N.J., Penschow, J.D., Thorley, B., Tregear, G.W. & Coghlan, J.P. (1987). Histochemical localization of IGF-I and -II mRNA in the developing rat embryo. *Development*, **101**, 175–84.

Bekoff, M.C. & Klagsbrun, M. (1982). Characterization of growth factors in human cartilage. *Journal of Cell Biochemistry*, **20**, 245–73.

Bhaumick, B. & Bala, R.M. (1991). Differential effects of insulin-like growth factors I and II on growth, differentiation and glucoregulation in differentiating chondrocyte cells in culture. *Acta Endocrinologica*, **125**, 201–11.

Blanchard, M.M., Goodyer, C.G., Charrier, J. & Barenton, B. (1988). In vitro regulation of growth hormone (GH) release from ovine pituitary cells during fetal and neonatal development: effects of GH-releasing factor, somatostatin, and insulin-like growth factor-I. *Endocrinology*, **122**, 2114–20.

Bondy, C.A., Werner, H., Roberts, C.T. & LeRoith, D. (1990). Cellular pattern of insulin-like growth factor-I (IGF-I) and type I IGF receptor gene expression in early organogenesis: comparison with IGF-II gene expression. *Molecular Endocrinology*, **4**, 1386–98.

Brice, A.L, Cheetham, J.E., Bolton, V.N., Hill, N.C.W. & Schofield, P.N. (1989). Temporal changes in the expression of the insulin-like growth factor II gene associated with tissue maturation in the human fetus. *Development*, **106**, 543–54.

Brown, A.L., Graham, D.E., Nissley, S.P., Hill, D.J., Strain, A.J & Rechler, M M. (1986). Developmental regulation of insulin-like growth factor II mRNA in different rat tissues. *Journal of Biological Chemistry*, **261**, 13144–50.

Brunetti, A. & Goldfine, I.D. (1990). Role of myogenin in myoblast differentiation and its regulation by fibroblast growth factor. *Journal of Biological Chemistry*, **265**, 5960–3.

Carrington, J.L., Chen, P., Yanagishita, M. & Reddi, A.H. (1991). Osteogenin (Bone morphometric protein-3) stimulates cartilage formation by chick limb bud cells in vitro. *Developmental Biology*, **146**, 406–15.

Catterton, W.Z., Escobedo, M.B., Sexson, W R, Gray, M.E., Sundell, H.W. & Stahlman, M.T. (1979). Effect of epidermal growth factor on lung maturation in fetal rabbits. *Pediatric Research*, **13**, 104–8.

Chatelain, P., Penhoat, A., Perrard-Sapori, M.H., Jaillard, C., Naville, D. & Saex, J. (1988). Maturation of steroidogenic cells: a target for IGF-I. *Acta Paediatrica Scandinavica Supplement*, **347**, 104–9.

Chen, P., Carrington, J.L., Hammonds, R.G & Reddi, A.H. (1991). Stimulation of chondrogenesis in limb bud mesoderm cells by recombinant human bone morphometric protein 2B (BMP-2B) and modulation by transforming growth factor β_1 and β_2. *Experimental Cell Research*, **195**, 509–15.

Clegg, C.H., Linkhart, T.A., Olwin, B.B. & Hauschka, S.D. (1987). Growth factor control of skeletal muscle differentiation: commitment to terminal differentiation occurs in G phase and is repressed by fibroblast growth factor. *Journal of Cell Biology*, **105**, 949–56.

Coulter, C.L., Goldsmith, P.C., Mesiano, S., Voytek, C.C., Martin, M.C. & Jaffe, R.B. (1993). In vivo regulation of growth and expression of IGF-II and steroidogenic enzymes in the rhesus monkey fetal adrenal. *40th Annual Meeting of the Society for Gynecological Investigation*, Toronto, Canada (Abstract S144).

Crickard, J., Ill, C.R. & Jaffe, R.B. (1981). Control of proliferation of human fetal adrenal cells in vitro. *Journal of Clinical Endocrinology and Metabolism*, **53**, 790–8.

Davenport, J.L., D'Ercole, A.J., Azizkhan, J.C. & Lund, P.K. (1987). SomatomedinC/insulin-like growth factor I (SM-C/IGF-I) and insulin-like growth factor II (IGF-II) mRNAs during lung development in the rat. *Experimental Lung Research*, **14**, 607–18.

De Chiara, T., Efstratiadis, A. & Robertson, E.J. (1990). A growth-deficiency phenotype in heterozygous mice carrying an insulin-like growth factor II gene disrupted by targeting. *Nature*, **345**, 78–80.

Delhanty, P.J.D., Hill, D.J., Shimasaki, S. & Han, V.K.M. (1993). Insulin-like growth factor binding protein-4, -5 and -6 mRNAs in the human fetus: Localization to sites of growth and differentiation? *Growth Regulation*, **3**, 8–11.

Delmis, J., Drazancic, A., Ivanisevic, M. & Suchanek, E. (1992). Glucose, insulin, HGH and IGF-I levels in maternal serum, amniotic fluid and umbilical venous serum: a comparison between late normal pregnancy and pregnancies complicated with diabetes and fetal growth retardation. *Journal of Perinatal Medicine*, **20**, 47–56.

D'Ercole, A.J., Foushee, D.B. & Underwood, L.E. (1976). Somatomedin C receptor ontogeny and levels in porcine fetal and human cord serum. *Journal of Clinical Endocrinology and Metabolism*, **43**, 1069–77.

DiBlasio, A.M., Voutilainen, R., Jaffe, R.B. & Miller, W.L. (1987). Hormonal regulation of messenger ribonucleic acids for P450scc (cholesterol side-chain cleavage enzyme) and P450c17 (17 alpha-hydroxylase/17, 20–1yase) in cultured human fetal adrenal cells. *Journal of Clinical Endocrinology and Metabolism*, **65**, 170–5.

Ellingsworth, L.R., Brennan, J.E., Fok, K., Rosen, D.M., Bentz, H., Piez, K.A. & Seyedin, S.M. (1986). Antibodies to the N-terminal portion of cartilage-inducing factor A and transforming growth factor β. *Journal of Biological Chemistry*, **261**, 12362–7.

Ernst, C.W., McCusker, R.H. & White, M.E. (1992). Gene expression and secretion of insulin-like growth factor binding proteins during myoblast differentiation. *Endocrinology*, **130**, 607–15.

Ewton, D.Z. & Florini, J.R. (1981). Effects of somatomedins and insulin on myoblast differentiation in vitro. *Developmental Biology*, **56**, 31–9.

Fallon, J.F., Lopez, A., Ros, M.A., Savage, M.P., Olwin, B.B. & Simandl, B.K. (1994). FGF-2: apical ectodermal ridge growth signal for chick limb development. *Science*, **264**, 104–6.

Florini, J.R., Ewton, D.Z. & Roof, S.L. (1991*a*). Insulin-like growth factor I stimulates terminal myogenic differentiation by induction of myogenin gene expression. *Molecular Endocrinology*, **5**, 718–24.

Florini, J.R., Magri, K.A., Ewton, D.Z., James, P.L., Grindstaff, K. & Rotwein, P.S. (1991*b*). Spontaneous differentiation of skeletal myoblasts is dependent upon autocrine secretion of insulin-like growth factor II. *Journal of Biological Chemistry*, **266**, 15197–293.

Gatherer, D., TenDijke, P., Baird, D.T. & Akhurst, R.J. (1990). Expression of TGF-β isoforms during first trimester human embryogenesis. *Development*, **110**, 445–60.

Gelb, D.E., Rosier, R.N. & Puzas, J.E. (1990). The production of transforming growth factor-β by chick growth plate chondrocytes in short term monolayer culture. *Endocrinology*, **127**, 1941–7.

Giudice, L.C., Farrell, E.M., Pham, H., Lamson, G. & Rosenfeld, R.G. (1990). Insulin-like growth factor binding proteins in maternal serum throughout gestation and in the puerperium: effects of a pregnancy-associated serum protease activity. *Journal of Clinical Endocrinology and Metabolism*, **71**, 806–16.

Gluckman, P.D. & Liggins, G.C. (1984). Regulation of fetal growth. In *Fetal Physiology and Medicine*, 2nd Edition, ed. R.N. Beard & P.W. Nathanielsz. pp. 511–558. Marcel Dekker, New York.

Gonzalez, A-M., Buscaglia, M., Ong, M. & Baird, A. (1990). Distribution of basic fibroblast growth factor in the 18-day rat fetus: localization in the basement membranes of diverse tissues. *Journal of Cellular Biology*, **110**, 753–65.

Goodyer, C.G., Marcovitz, S., Hardy, J., Lefebvre, Y., Guyda, H.J. & Posner, B.I. (1986). Effect of insulin-like growth factors on human foetal, adult normal and tumour pituitary function in tissue culture. *Acta Endocrinologica*, **112**, 49–57.

Goustin, A.S., Betsholtz, C., Pfeifer-Ohlsson, S., Persson, H., Rydnert, J., Bywater, M., Holmgren, G., Heldin, C-H., Westermark, B. & Ohlsson, R. (1985). Co-expression of the *sis* and *myc* protooncogenes in developing human placenta suggests autocrine control of trophoblast growth. *Cell*, **41**, 301–12.

Green, B.N., Jones, S.B., Streck, R.D., Wood, T.L., Rotwein, P. & Pintar, J.E. (1994). Distinct expression patterns of insulin-like growth factor binding proteins 2 and 5 during fetal and postnatal development. *Endocrinology*, **134**, 954–62.

Hahnel, A. & Schultz, G.A. (1994). Insulin-like growth factor binding proteins are transcribed by preimplantation mouse embryos. *Endocrinology*, **134** 1956–9.

Han, V.K.M., D'Ercole, A.J. & Lund, P.K. (1987*a*). Cellular localization of somatomedin (insulin-like growth factor) messenger RNA in the human fetus. *Science*, **236**, 193–7.

Han, V.K.M., Hill, D.J., Strain, A.J., Towle, A.C., Lauder, J.M., Underwood,L.E. & D'Ercole, A.J. (1987*b*). Identification of somatomedin/insulin-like growth factor immunoreactive cells in the human fetus. *Pediatric Research*, **22**, 245–9.

Han, V.K.M., Hunter, E.S., Pratt, R.M., Zendegui, J.G. & Lee, D.C. (1987*c*). Expression of transforming growth factor alpha mRNA during development occurs predominantly in the maternal decidua. *Molecular and Cellular Biology*, **7**, 2335–43.

Han, R.N.N., Liu, J., Tanswell, A.K. & Post, M. (1992). Expression of basic fibroblast growth factor and receptor: Immunolocalization studies in developing rat fetal lung. *Pediatric Research*, **31**, 435–40.

Han, V.K.M., Lund, P.K., Lee, D.C. & D'Ercole, A.J. (1988). Expression of somatomedin/insulin-like growth factor messenger ribonucleic acids in the human fetus: identification, characterization and tissue distribution. *Journal of Clinical Endocrinology and Metabolism*, **66**, 422–29.

Haub, O. & Goldfarb, M. (1991). Expression of fibroblast growth factor-5 gene in the mouse embryo. *Development*, **112**, 397–406.

Heine, U.I., Munoz, E.F., Flanders, K.C., Ellingsworth, L.R., Lam, H.Y.P., Thompson, N.L., Roberts, A.B. & Sporn, M.B. (1987). Role of transforming growth factor-β in the development of the mouse embryo. *Journal of Cell Biology*, **105**, 2861–76.

Herbert, J.M., Basilico, C., Goldfarb, M., Haub, O. & Martin, G.R. (1990). Isolation of cDNAs encoding four mouse FGF family members and characterization of their expression patterns during embryogenesis. *Developmental Biology*, **138**, 454–63.

Hill, D.J. (1979). Stimulation of cartilage zones of the calf costo-chondral growth plate in vitro by growth hormone dependent rat plasma somatomedin activity. *Journal of Endocrinology*, **83**, 219–27.

Hill, D.J. (1992). What is the role of growth hormone and related peptides in implantation and the development of the embryo and fetus? *Hormone Research*, **38(Suppl. 1)**, 28–34.

Hill, D.J. & Clemmons, D.R. (1992). Similar immunological distribution of insulin-like growth factor binding proteins -1, -2, and -3 in human fetal tissues. *Growth Factors*, **6**, 315–26.

Hill, D.J., Clemmons, D.R., Wilson, S., Han, V.K.M., Strain, A.J. & Milner, R.D.G. (1989). Immunological distribution of one form of insulin-like growth factor (IGF) binding protein and IGF peptides in human fetal tissues. *Journal of Molecular Endocrinology*, **2**, 31–8.

Hill, D.J. & De Sousa, D. (1990). Insulin is a mitogen for isolated epiphyseal growth plate chondrocytes from the fetal lamb. *Endocrinology*, **126**, 2661–70.

Hill, D.J. & Hogg, J. (1989). Growth factors and the regulation of pre- and postnatal growth. In *Clinical Endocrinology and Metabolism, Perinatal Endocrinology. Vol. 3 No. 3.*, ed. C.T. Jones. pp. 579–625. Baillière Tindall, London.

Hill, D.J. & Logan, A. (1992*a*). Cell cycle-dependent localization of immunoreactive basic fibroblast growth factor to cytoplasm and nucleus of isolated ovine fetal growth plate chondrocytes. *Growth Factors*, **7**, 215–31.

Hill, D.J. & Logan, A. (1992*b*). Interactions of peptide growth factors during DNA synthesis in isolated ovine fetal growth plate chondrocytes. *Growth Regulation*, **2**, 122–32.

Hill, D.J., Logan, A., McGarry, M. & DeSousa, D. (1992*a*). Control of protein and matrix molecule synthesis in isolated ovine growth plate chondrocytes by the interactions of basic fibroblast growth factor, insulin-like growth factor I, insulin and transforming growth factor β. *Journal of Endocrinology*, **133**, 363–73.

Hill, D.J., Logan, A., Ong, M., DeSousa, D. & Gonzalez, A.M. (1992*b*). Basic fibroblast growth factor is synthesized and released by isolated ovine fetal growth plate chondrocytes: potential role as an autocrine mitogen. *Growth Factors*, **6**, 277–94.

Hill, D.J. & Milner, R.D.G. (1989). Mechanisms of fetal growth. In *Clinical Paediatric Endocrinology, 2nd edn*, ed. C.G. Brook. pp. 3–31. Blackwell Scientific Publications, Oxford.

Hooper, S.B., Bocking, A.D., White, S., Challis, J.R.G. & Han, V.K.M. (1991). DNA synthesis is reduced in selected fetal tissues during prolonged hypoxemia. *American Journal of Physiology*, **261**, R508–14.

Hooper, S.B., Bocking, A.D., White, S.E., Fraher, L.J., McDonald, T.J. & Han, V.K.M. (1994). Catecholamines stimulate the synthesis and release of insulin-like growth factor binding protein-1 (IGFBP-1) by fetal sheep liver in vivo. *Endocrinology*, **134**, 1104–12.

Hunziker, E.B. (1988). Growth plate structure and function. *Pathology and Immunopathology Research*, **7**, 9–13.

Isaksson, O., Jansson, J-O. & Gause, I.A. (1982). Growth hormone stimulates longitudinal bone growth directly. *Science*, **216**, 1237–9.

Isgaard, J., Moller, C., Isaksson, O., Nilsson, A., Mathews, L.S. & Norstedt, G. (1988). Regulation of insulin-like growth factor messenger ribonucleic acid in rat growth plate by growth hormone. *Endocrinology*, **122**, 1515–20.

Iwamoto, H.S., Murray, M.A. & Chernausek, S.D. (1992). Effects of acute hypoxia on insulin-like growth factors and their binding proteins in fetal sheep. *American Journal of Physiology*, **263**, E1151–6.

Joyce, M.E., Roberts, A.B., Sporn, M.B. & Bolander, M.E. (1990). Transforming growth factor-β and the initiation of chondrogenesis and osteogenesis in the rat femur. *Journal of Cell Biology*, **110**, 2195–207.

Kasselberg, A.G., Orth, D.N., Gray, M.E. & Stahlman, M.T. (1985). Immunocytochemical localization of human epidermal growth factor/ urogastrone in several human tissues. *Journal of Histochemistry and Cytochemistry*, **33**, 315–22.

Kimelman, D., Abraham, J.A., Haarparanta, T., Palisi, T.M. & Kirschner, M.W. (1988). The presence of fibroblast growth factor in the frog egg: its role as a natural mesoderm inducer. *Science*, **242**, 1053–6.

Kimelman, D. & Kirschner, M. (1987). Synergistic induction of mesoderm by FGF and TGF-beta and the identification of an mRNA coding for FGF in the early *Xenopus* embryo. *Cell*, **51**, 869–71.

Klein, J.M. & Nielson, H.C. (1993). Androgen regulation of epidermal growth factor receptor binding activity during fetal rabbit lung development. *Journal of Clinical Investigation*, **91**, 425–9.

Klempt, M., Hutchins, A-M., Gluckman, P.D., Skinner & S.J.M. (1992). IGF binding protein-2 gene expression and the location of IGF-I and IGF-II in fetal rat lung. *Development*, **115**, 765–72.

Kulkarni, A.B., Huh, C-G., Becker, D., Geiser, A., Lyght, M., Flanders, K.C., Roberts, A.B., Sporn, M.B., Ward, J.M. & Karlsson, S. (1993). Transforming growth factor t31 null mutation in mice causes excessive inflammatory response and early death. *Proceedings of the National Academy of Sciences, USA*, **90**, 770–4.

Lassarre, C., Hardouin, S., Daffos, F., Forestier, F., Frankenne, F. & Binoux, M. (1991). Serum insulin-like growth factor binding proteins in the human fetus. Relationships with growth in normal subjects and in subjects with intrauterine growth retardation. *Pediatric Research*, **9**, 219–21.

Lehnert, S.A. & Akhurst, R.J. (1988). Embryonic expression pattern of TGF beta type1 RNA suggests both paracrine and autocrine mechanisms of action. *Development*, **104**, 263–73.

Letterio, J.J., Geiser, A.G., Kulkarni, A.B., Roche, N.S., Sporn, M.B. & Roberts, A.B. (1994). Maternal rescue of transforming growth factor β1 null mice. *Science*, **264**, 1936–8.

Li, J., Saunders, J.C., Gilmour, R.S., Silver, M. & Fowden, A.L. (1993). Insulin-like growth factor-II messenger ribonucleic acid expression in fetal tissues of the sheep during late gestation: effects of cortisol. *Endocrinology*, **132**, 2083–9.

Lindahl, A., Isgaard, J., Nilsson, A. & Isaksson, 0. (1986). Growth hormone potentiates colony formation of epiphyseal chondrocytes in suspension culture. *Endocrinology*, **118**, 1843–8.

Lindahl, A., Nilsson, A. & Isaksson, O. (1987). Effects of growth hormone and insulin-like growth factor I (IGF-I) on colony formation of rabbit epiphyseal chondrocytes of different maturation. *Journal of Endocrinology*, **115**, 263–71.

Linkhart, T.A., Clegg, C.H. & Hauscha, S.D. (1981). Myogenic differentiation in permanent clonal mouse myoblast cell lines: regulation by macromolecular growth factors in the culture medium. *Developmental Biology*, **86**, 19–30.

Liu, J-P., Baker, J., Perkins, A.S., Robertson, E.J. & Efstratiadis, A. (1993). Mice carrying null mutations of the genes encoding insulin-like growth factor I (Igf-1) and type 1 IGF receptor (Igf1-r). *Cell*, **75**, 59–72.

Liu, L. & Nicoll, C.S. (1988). Evidence for a role of basic fibroblast growth factor in rat embryonic growth and differentiation. *Endocrinology*, **123**, 2027–31.

Lu, F., Han, V.K.M., Milne, W.K., Fraser, M., Carter, A.M., Berdusco, E.T.M. & Challis, J.R.G. (1994). Regulation of insulin-like growth factor-II gene expression in the ovine fetal adrenal gland by adrenocorticotropic hormone and cortisol. *Endocrinology*, **134**, 2628–35.

Luetteke, N.C., Qiu, T.H., Pfeiffer, R.L., Oliver, P., Smithies, O. & Lee, D.C. (1993). TGF alpha deficiency results in hair follicle and eye abnormalities in targeted and waved-1 mice. *Cell*, **73**, 263–72.

Luger, A., Calogero, A.E., Kalogeras, K., Gallucci, W.T., Gold, P.N., Loriaux, D.L. & Chrousos, G.P. (1988). Interaction of epidermal growth factor with the hypothalamic–pituitary–adrenal axis: potential physiologic relevance. *Journal of Clinical Endocrinology and Metabolism*, **66**, 334–7.

McCusker, R.H. & Clemmons, D.R. (1992). The insulin-like growth factor binding proteins: structure and biological functions. In *The Insulin-like Growth Factors, Structure and Biological Functions*, ed. P.N. Schofield. pp. 110–150. Oxford University Press, Oxford.

McLellan, K.C., Hooper, S.B., Bocking, A.D., Delhanty, P.J.D., Phillips, I.D., Hill, D.J. & Han, V.K.M. (1992). Prolonged hypoxia induced by the reduction of maternal uterine blood flow alters insulin-like growth factor-binding protein-1 (IGFBP-1) and IGFBP-2 gene expression in the ovine fetus. *Endocrinology*, **131**, 1619–28.

Magri, K.A., Benedict, M.R., Ewton, D.Z. & Florini, J.R. (1994). Negative feedback regulation of insulin-like growth factor-II gene expression in differentiating myoblasts in vitro. *Endocrinology*, **135**, 53–62.

Mesiano, S., Mellon, S.H., Gospodarowicz, D., DiBlasio, A.M. & Jaffe, R.B. (1991). Basic fibroblast growth factor expression is regulated by corticotropin in the human fetal adrenal: a model for adrenal growth regulation. *Proceedings of the National Academy of Sciences, USA*, **88**, 5428–32.

Mitrani, E., Ziu, T., Thomsen, G., Shimoni, Y., Melton, D.A. & Bril, A. (1990). Activin can induce the formation of axial structures and is expressed in the hypoblast of the chick. *Cell*, **63**, 495–501.

Morrison-Graham, K., Schatteman, G.C., Bork, T., Bowenpope, D.F. & Weston, J.A. (1992). A PDGF receptor mutation in the mouse (patch) perturbs the development of a non-neuronal subset of neural crest-derived cells. *Development*, **115**, 133–42.

Munaim, S. I., Klagsbrun, M. & Toole, B.P. (1988). Developmental changes in fibroblast growth factor in the chicken embryo limb bud. *Proceedings of the National Academy of Sciences, USA*, **85**, 8091–3.

Munaim, S.I., Klagsbrun, M. & Toole, B.P. (1991). Hyaluronan-dependent pericellular coats of chick embryo limb mesoderm cells: induction by basic fibroblast growth factor. *Developmental Biology*, **143**, 297–302.

Naamen, E., Chatelain, P., Saez, J.M. & Durand, P. (1989). In vitro effect of insulin and insulin-like growth factor-I on cell multiplication and adrenocorticotropin responsiveness of fetal adrenal cells. *Biology of Reproduction*, **40**, 570–7.

Nagarajan, L., Anderson, W.B., Nissley, S.P., Rechler, M.M. & Jetten, A.M. (1985). Production of insulin-like growth factor II (MSA) by endoderm-like cells derived from embryonal carcinoma cells: possible mediator of embryonic cell growth. *Journal of Cellular Physiology*, **124**, 199–206.

Nielson, H.C., Kellogg, C.K. & Doyle, C.A. (1992). Development of fibroblast type-II cell communications in fetal rabbit lung organ culture. *Acta Biochimica et Biophysica*, **1175**, 95–9.

Nilsson, A., Isgaard, J., Lindahl, A., Dahlstrom, A., Skottner, A. & Isaksson, O. (1986). Regulation by growth hormone of number of chondrocytes containing IGF-I in the rat growth plate. *Science*, **233**, 571–4.

Nilsson, A., Isgaard, J., Lindahl, A., Peterson, L. & Isaksson, O. (1987). Effects of unilateral arterial infusion of GH and IGF-I on tibial longitudinal bone growth in hypophysectomized rats. *Calcified Tissue International*, **40**, 91–6.

Niswander, L. & Martin, G.R. (1992). *Fgf-4* expression during gastrulation, myogenesis, limb and tooth development in the mouse. *Development*, **114**, 755–68.

Niswander, L. & Martin, G.R. (1993). FGF-4 and BMP-2 have opposite effects on limb growth. *Nature*, **361**, 68–71.

Niswander, L., Tickle, C., Vogel, A., Booth, I. & Martin, G.R. (1993). FGF-4 replaces the apical ectodermal ridge and directs outgrowth and patterning of the limb. *Cell*, **75**, 579–87.

Ohlsson, C., Nilsson, A., Isaksson, O., Bentham, J. & Lindahl, A. (1992). Effects of triiodothyronine and insulin-like growth factor-l (IGF-I) on alkaline phosphatase activity, [^{3}H]thymidine incorporation and IGF-I receptor mRNA in cultured rat epiphyseal chondrocytes. *Journal of Endocrinology*, **135**, 115–21.

Orrurtreger, A., Bedford, M.T., Do, M.S., Eisenbach, L. & Lonai, P. (1992). Developmental expression of the alpha receptor for platelet-derived growth factor, which is deleted in the embryonic lethal patch mutation. *Development*, **115**, 289–97.

Pelton, R.W., Dickinson, M.E., Moses, H.L. & Hogan, B.L.M. (1990). In situ hybridization analysis of TGFβ_3 RNA expression during mouse development: comparative studies with TGFβ_1 and β_2. *Development*, **110**, 609–20.

Peters, K., Ornitz, D., Werner, S. & Williams, L. (1993). Unique expression pattern of the FGF receptor 3 gene during mouse organogenesis. *Developmental Biology*, **155**, 423–30.

Peters, K.G., Werner, S., Chen, G. & Williams, L.T. (1992). Two FGF receptor genes are differentially expressed in epithelial and mesenchymal tissues during limb formation and organogenesis in the mouse. *Development*, **114**, 233–43.

Plopper, C.G., Stgeorge, J.A., Read, L.C., Nishio, S.J., Weir, A.J., Edwards, L., Tarantal, A.F., Pinkerton, K.E., Merritt, T.A. & Whitsett, J.A. (1992). Acceleration of alveolar type II cell differentiation in fetal rhesus monkey lung by administration of EGF. *American Journal of Physiology*, **262**, L313–19.

Polk, D.H., Ervin, M.G., Padbury, J.F., Lam, R.N., Reviczky, A.L. & Fisher, D.A. (1987). Epidermal growth factor acts as a corticotropin-releasing factor in chronically catheterized fetal lambs. *Journal of Clinical Investigation*, **79**, 984–8.

Pons, S. & Torres-Aleman, I. (1992). Basic fibroblast growth factor modulates insulin-like growth factor-I, its receptor, and its binding proteins in hypothalamic cell cultures. *Endocrinology*, **131**, 2271–8.

Price, W.A., Rong, L., Stiles, A.D. & D'Ercole, A.J. (1992). Changes in IGF-I and -II, IGF binding protein, and IGF receptor transcript abundance after uterine artery ligation. *Pediatric Research*, **32**, 291–5.

Rainey, W.E., Oka, K., Magness, R.R. & Mason, J.I. (1991). Ovine fetal adrenal synthesis of cortisol: regulation by adrenocorticotropin, angiotensin II and transforming growth factor-β. *Endocrinology*, **129**, 1784–90.

Ralphs, J., Wylie, L. & Hill, D.J. (1990). Distribution of insulin-like growth factor peptides in the developing chick embryo. *Development*, **109**, 51–8.

Rappolee, D.A., Brenner, C.A., Schultz, R. & Werb, Z. (1988). Developmental expression of PDGF, TGF-α, and TGF-β genes in preimplantation mouse embryos. *Science*, **241**, 1823–5.

Roberts, A.B. & Sporn, M.B. (1990). The transforming growth factor-βs. In *Peptide Growth Factors and Their Receptors*, ed. M.B. Sporn & A.B. Roberts. pp. 419–72. Springer-Verlag, Berlin.

Rosa, F., Roberts, A.B., Danielpour, D., Dart, L.L., Sporn, M.B. & Dawid, I.B. (1988). Mesoderm induction in amphibians: the role of TGF-β_2-like factors. *Science*, **239**, 783–5.

Rosen, K.M., Wentworth, B.M., Rosenthal, N. & Villa-Komaroff, L. (1993). Specific, temporally regulated expression of the insulin-like growth factor II gene during muscle cell differentiation. *Endocrinology*, **133**, 474–81.

Rosenthal, S.M., Hsiao, D. & Silverman, L.A. (1994). An insulin-like growth factor-II (IGF-II) analog with highly selective affinity for IGF-II receptors stimulates differentiation, but not IGF-I receptor down-regulation in muscle cells. *Endocrinology*, **134**, 38–44.

Rosier, R.N., Landesberg, R.L. & Puzas, J.E. (1991). An autocrine feedback loop for regulation of TGF-β and FGF production in growth plate chondrocytes. *Journal of Bone and Mineral Research*, **6(suppl.1)**, S211.

Rosier, R.N., O'Keefe, R.J., Crabb, I.D. & Puzas, J.E. (1989). Transforming growth factor-beta: an autocrine regulator of chondrocytes. *Connective Tissue Research*, **20**, 295–301.

Rotwein, P., Pollock, K.M., Watson, M. & Milbrandt, J.D. (1987). Insulin-like growth factor gene expression during rat embryonic development. *Endocrinology*. **121**, 2141–4.

Sandberg, M., Vuorio, T., Hirvonen, H., Alitalo, K.L. and Vuorio, E. (1988). Enhanced expression of TGF-β and c-*fos* mRNAs in the growth plates of developing human long bones. *Development*, **102**, 461–70.

Schlechter, N.L., Russell, S.M., Spencer, E.M. & Nicoll, C.S. (1986). Evidence suggesting that the direct growth-promoting effect of growth hormone on cartilage in vivo is mediated by local production of somatomedin. *Proceedings of the National Academy of Sciences, USA*, **83**, 7932–4.

Shigematsu, K., Niwa, M., Kurihara, M., Yamashita, K., Kawai, K. & Tsuchiyama, H. (1989). Receptor autoradiographic localization of insulin-like growth factor-I (IGF-I) binding sites in human fetal and adult adrenal glands. *Life Sciences*, **45**, 383–9.

Shull, M.M., Ormsby, I., Kier, A.B., Pawlowski, S., Diebold, R.J., Yin, M., Allen, R., Sidman, C., Proetzel, G., Calvin, D., Annunziata, N. & Doetscham, T. (1992). Targeted disruption of the transforming growth factor-131 gene results in multifocal inflammatory disease. *Nature*, **359**, 693–9.

Slack, J.M.W. & Isaacs, H.V. (1989). Presence of basic fibroblast growth factor in the early *Xenopus* embryo. *Development*, **105**, 147–53.

Slavkin, H.C., Hu, C.C., Sakakura, Y., Diekwisch, T., Chai, Y., Mayo, M., Bringas, P., Simmer, J., Mak, G. & Sasano, Y. (1992). Gene expression, signal transduction and tissue specific mineralization during mammalian tooth development. *Critical Reviews of Eukaryotic Gene Expression*, **2**, 315–29.

Smith, J.C., Price, B.M.J., Van Nimmen, K. & Huylebroeck, D. (1990). Identification of a potent *Xenopus* mesoderm-inducing factor as a homologue of activin A. *Nature*, **345**, 729–31.

Smith, R.L., Palathumpat, M.V., Ku, C.W. & Hintz, R.L. (1989). Growth hormone stimulates insulin-like growth factor I actions on adult articular chondrocytes. *Journal of Orthopaedic Research*, **7**, 198–207.

Snider, W.D. (1994). Functions of the neurotrophins during nervous system development: what the knockouts are teaching us. *Cell*, **77**, 627–38.

Stark, K.L., McMahon, J.A. & McMahon, A.P. (1991). FGFR-4, a new member of the fibroblast growth factor receptor family, expressed in the definitive endoderm and skeletal muscle lineages of the mouse. *Development*, **113**, 641–51.

Strandjord, T.P., Clark, J.G., Hodson, W.A., Schmidt, R.A. & Madtes, D.K. (1993). Expression of transforming growth factor alpha in mid-gestation human fetal lung. *American Journal of Respiration and Cell Molecular Biology*, **8**, 266–73.

Straus, D.S., Ooi, G.T., Orlowski, C.C. & Rechler, M.M. (1991). Expression of the genes for insulin-like growth factor-I (IGF-I), IGF-II, and IGF-binding proteins-1 and -2 in fetal rat under conditions of intrauterine growth retardation caused by maternal fasting. *Endocrinology*, **128**, 518–25.

Streck, R.D., Wood, T.L., Hsu, M-S. & Pintar, J.E. (1992). Insulin-like growth factor I and II and insulin-like growth factor binding protein-2 RNAs are expressed in adjacent tissues within rat embryonic and fetal limbs. *Developmental Biology*, **151**, 586–96.

Sundell, H.W., Gray, M.E., Serenius, F.S., Escobedo, M.B. & Stahlman, M.T. (1980). Effects of epidermal growth factor on lung maturation in fetal lambs. *American Journal of Pathology*, **100**, 707–25.

Thomsen, G., Woolf, T., Whitman, M., Sokol, S., Vaughan, J., Vale, W. & Melton, D.A. (1990). Activins are expressed early in *Xenopus* embryogenesis and can induce axial mesoderm and anterior structures. *Cell*, **63**, 485–91.

Torres-Aleman, I., Naftolin, F. & Robbins, R.J. (1990). Trophic effects of insulin-like growth factor-I on fetal rat hypothalamic cells in culture. *Neuroscience*, **35**, 601–8.

Townsend, S.F., Dallman, M.F. & Miller, W.L. (1990). Rat insulin-like growth factor-I and -II mRNAs are unchanged during compensatory adrenal growth but decrease during ACTH-induced adrenal growth. *Journal of Biological Chemistry*, **265**, 22117–22.

Trippel, S.B., Van Wyk, J.J. & Mankin, H.J. (1986). Localization of somatomedin-C binding to bovine growth-plate chondrocytes in situ. *Journal of Bone and Joint Surgery*, **68–A**, 897–903.

Ulich, T.R., Yi, E.S., Longmuir, K., Yin, S., Biltz, R., Morris, C.F., Housley, R.M. & Pierce, G. F. (1994). Keratinocyte growth factor is a growth factor for type II pneumonocytes in vivo. *Journal of Clinical Investigation*, **93**, 1298–306.

Unterman, T., Lascon, R., Golway, M.B., Oehler, D., Gounis, A., Simmons, R.A. & Ogata, E.S. (1990). Circulating levels of insulin-like growth factor binding protein-1 (IGFBP-1) and hepatic mRNA are increased in the small for gestational age (SGA) fetal rat. *Endocrinology*, **127**, 2035–7.

Vaidya, T.B., Rhodes, S.J., Taparowsky, E.J. & Konieczny, S.F. (1989). Fibroblast growth factor and transforming growth factor β repress transcription of the myogenic regulatory gene MyoD1. *Molecular and Cellular Biology*, **9**, 3576–9.

Van Wyk, J.J., Underwood, L.E., D'Ercole, A.J., Clemmons, D.R., Pledger, W.M., Wharton, W.R. & Loef, E. (1981). Role of somatomedin in cellular proliferation. In *Biology of Normal Human Growth*. ed. M. Ritzen, A. Aperia & K. Hall. pp. 223–239. Raven Press, New York.

Van Zoelen, E.J., Koornneef, I., Holthuis, J.C., Ward van Osterwaard, T.M.J., Feijen, A., De Poorter, T.L., Mummery, C.L. & Van Buul-Offers, S.C. (1989). Production of insulin-like growth factors, platelet-derived growth factor, and transforming growth factors and their role in the density-dependent growth regulation of a differentiated embryonal carcinoma cell line. *Endocrinology*, **124**, 2029–41.

Vileisis, R. & D'Ercole, A.J. (1986). Tissue and serum concentrations of somatomedinC/insulin-like growth factor I in fetal rats made growth retarded by uterine artery ligation. *Pediatric Research*, **20**, 126–30.

Voutilainen, R. & Miller, W.L. (1987*a*). Coordinate tropic hormone regulation of mRNAs for insulin-like growth factor II and the cholesterol side-chain-cleavage enzyme, $P450_{scc}$, in human steroidogenic tissues. *Proceedings of the National Academy of Sciences, USA*, **84**, 1590–4.

Voutilainen, R. & Miller, W.L. (1987*b*). Developmental and hormonal regulation of mRNAs for insulin-like growth factor II and steroidogenic enzymes in human fetal adrenals and gonads. *DNA*, **7**, 9–15.

Walker, K.V.R. & Kember, N.F. (1972). Cell kinetics of growth cartilage in the rat tibia. I. Measurements in young male rats. *Cell and Tissue Kinetics*, **5**, 401–8.

Wang, H.S., Lim, J., English, J., Irvine, L. & Chard, T. (1991). The concentration of insulin-like growth factor-I and insulin-like growth factor binding protein-1 in human umbilical cord serum at delivery: relationship to birth weight. *Journal of Endocrinology*, **129**, 459–64.

Williams, L.T., Peters, K.G., Kikuchi, A., Hu, Q., MacNicol, A., Demo, S., Fields, S., Martin, S. & Muslin, A. (1994). Signalling molecules that mediate the actions of fibroblast growth factors. In *EMBO Workshop on Molecular and Cellular Aspects of Fibroblast Growth Factors and their Receptors*, Capri, Italy (Abstract).

Wood, T.L., Streck, R.D. & Pintar, J.E. (1992). Expression of the IGFBP-2 gene in postimplantation rat embryos. *Development*, **114**, 59–66.

Yamaguchi, Y., Mann, D. M. & Ruoslahti, E. (1990). Negative regulation of transforming growth factor-β3 by the proteoglycan decorin. *Nature*, **346**, 281–4.

Yasui, S., Nagai, A., Oohira, A., Iwashita, M. & Konno, K. (1993). Effects of anti-mouse EGF antiserum on prenatal lung development in fetal mice. *Pediatric Pulmonology*, **15**, 251–6.

4

Insulin-like growth factors and their binding proteins

PETER D. GLUCKMAN

Introduction

The insulin-like growth factors (IGFs) -I and -II are two single chain polypeptide hormones with marked structural and evolutional homology to each other and to proinsulin. They have molecular weights of 7649 D and 7471 D, respectively. Each is a single chain polypeptide with three intrachain disulfide bonds. Their presence was first suggested by observations that growth hormone (GH) acted to promote tibial epiphyseal growth by means of an intermediate serum factor. This factor was first termed sulfation factor and then somatomedin. Following purification and sequencing it was renamed insulin-like growth factor-I. This term originates, in part, because of its sequence homology to insulin and secondly, because of its spectrum of biological actions. IGF-II was identified following study of insulin-like activity in serum which was not suppressible by insulin antisera (non-suppressible insulin-like activity).

The study of these two peptides, their binding proteins and receptors has exploded in recent years. Their role in embryonic and fetal development has been of particular interest. One particular problem has been the methodological complexities of measurements of components of this axis: this has limited progress. For example, their measurement in plasma requires rigorous extraction and separation from the IGF-binding proteins. Many earlier conclusions have had to be revised as methodological advances have occurred. This chapter will review primarily our current understanding of the IGFs in the regulation of fetal growth.

The IGF axis

IGF-I and IGF-II

Both IGF-I and IGF-II are found in the adult human circulation: the major tissues of origin for circulating IGF-I are muscle and liver. However, essentially all tissues express mRNA for both IGF-I and IGF-II and there has been controversy over the relative role of circulating IGFs (*endocrine* hypothesis) versus that of locally produced IGFs which then act in an autocrine or paracrine manner (*paracrine* hypothesis). Both modes of action are probably important. Recent evidence also suggests that there are interactions between the endocrine and paracrine IGF systems (Butler et al., 1994).

IGF-I was discovered as the mediator of the somatogenic actions of growth hormone (GH). It has been shown, in both man and experimental animals, to promote linear growth via stimulation of prechondrocyte proliferation in the growth plate (*somatogenic* action), to promote protein synthesis (*anabolic* action) and to inhibit protein degradation (*anti-catabolic* function). In vitro it has been shown to be the universal progression factor in the cell cycle, essential for the cell to enter the S phase of DNA synthesis. The IGFs also act as potent differentiation factors. While most attention has focused on their role as somatogenic and proliferative agents there is increasing evidence that the IGFs play an important biological role in metabolic homeostasis. There is evidence that IGF-I tonically regulates protein turnover (Koea et al., 1992*b*) and that it regulates insulin sensitivity (Hussain et al., 1993). Whether it has a direct role in carbohydrate metabolism is unclear (Ballard et al., 1994). Both in vitro and at non-physiological doses in vivo, it can stimulate the cellular uptake of glucose, but this action may to a large extent reflect affinity of IGF-I for the insulin receptor.

The major factor regulating circulating IGF-I concentrations postnatally is GH. However, sex steroids and thyroid status also impact on circulating IGF-I levels. There is also experimental evidence to suggest that insulin can influence IGF-I secretion by the liver: this regulatory loop appears of prime importance in fetal life when the number of GH receptors is markedly reduced and IGF-I secretion is less GH dependent (Klempt et al., 1993). Nutritional status is the other major factor determining circulating IGF-I levels. IGF-I levels fall with either caloric or protein undernutrition. Two mechanisms are involved – there is a nutritional down-regulation of the number of high affinity GH receptors (Breier, Gluckman & Bass, 1988) but undernutrition is also associated with GH resistance at a postreceptor level via an unknown mechanism (Maes et al., 1991).

The regulation of paracrine IGF-I production varies in different tissues. For example, in the ovary, IGF-I is produced by granulosa cells in response to follicle stimulating hormone (FSH); this is important to the regulation of follicular development and granulosa cell proliferation. Local factors such as transforming growth factor beta (TGF-β) and basic fibroblast growth factor (bFGF) may be important in the induction of IGF-I in injured tissue.

The gene coding for IGF-I is particularly complex and can potentially give rise to a number of forms of mRNA, all coding for the same mature form of IGF-I peptide, although two forms of prohormone with different carboxyl terminal extensions are possible because of alternate 3' splicing. Because of multiple start sites and alternate splicing at the 5' end of the gene, several forms of prepro-IGF-I are formed with different length leader sequences. Only some of these forms of IGF-I mRNA appear GH dependent (Butler et al., 1994).

In general, IGF-II is less potent as an anabolic and somatogenic hormone than IGF-I. Less is known about the regulation of IGF-II although its transcriptional regulation appears equally as complex. It appears less GH dependent and only shifts under more extreme nutritional changes than IGF-I. It remains controversial as to whether there are any distinct biological actions mediated by IGF-II which are not also mediated by IGF-I. Administration of one IGF generally lowers the plasma levels of the other owing to competition for IGFBP-3 binding; limited evidence suggests that the two IGFs can interact in vivo, such that when IGF-II is co-administered with IGF-I it can block the actions of IGF-I (Koea et al., 1992*a*).

IGF receptors

The IGFs interact with at least four different receptor types: the type 1 IGF receptor, the type 2 IGF receptor, the so-called 'hybrid receptor' and the insulin receptor. The receptor of dominant interest is the type 1 or IGF-I receptor which has close homology to the insulin receptor and has high affinity for both IGF-I and IGF-II and low affinity for insulin. Currently, all known biological actions of IGF-I and IGF-II appear to be mediated by the type 1 receptor. There are suggestions of variant forms of the type 1 receptor which may have increased affinity for IGF-II. The type 2 receptor is structurally quite distinct. It is identical to the cation independent mannose-6-phosphate receptor which intracellularly is important in the regulation of protein trafficking. However, it is also expressed on the cell surface where it binds IGF-II, but not insulin or IGF-I, with high affinity. No biological function has, with certainty, been ascribed to the interaction of IGF-II with this receptor, and it has been argued this may simply be a clearance receptor. Both insulin receptors and IGF-I receptors have high homology and also exist as homodimers; it has recently been found that heterodimers of insulin and IGF type 1 receptors form and may represent a significant component of IGF-I receptor binding (Soos et al., 1994). It has been suggested that these 'hybrid receptors' which have high affinity for IGF-I and relatively low affinity for insulin, may mediate the insulin-like actions of the IGFs. IGF-I and IGF-II also bind to the insulin receptor but this is not likely to be relevant except when free levels of IGF-I in the circulation are very high following supraphysiological IGF-I therapy (Ballard et al., 1994).

IGF-binding proteins

The IGF system is further complicated in that little of the IGF-I or IGF-II, in either the circulation or in tissues, is in a free form. Most is bound to one of a number of specific IGF-binding proteins (IGFBPs) (Clemmons, 1993). There have been six specific IGFBPs identified – all have distant evolutionary homology with some structural commonalities. They have differing regulation and tissue sources. Some may be found in membrane-associated forms as well as in soluble forms. In addition, specific proteases have been identified that can regulate the degradation of the IGFBPs. Thus a complex system exists by which the level of IGF-I at the cell surface can be determined by soluble and membrane-associated IGFBPs, the level of IGF-I or -II, the number of receptors and the presence of specific IGFBP proteases. It is this complexity which allows these two peptides to have such important multifunctional roles in growth, development and metabolic homeostasis.

Broadly speaking, the actions of the IGFBPs can be seen to either enhance or inhibit the actions of the IGFs. Generally the membrane-bound forms enhance, and the soluble forms inhibit, IGF actions. Presumably, the membrane-bound forms serve to attract the IGFs to the region of the receptor whereas the soluble forms do the opposite. Secondly, the IGFBPs may serve to target IGFs to specific tissues or to specific cell types. There are many examples where the message of IGF may be found in one cell type but the protein is detected on the surface of a neighbouring cell due to the presence of binding protein associated with the second cell.

IGFBP-1 complexes with IGF-I or IGF-II to form a 29 kD complex. It can be present in different phosphorylation states that may determine its biological function (Jones et al., 1993). Its concentrations in the circulation are inversely regulated by insulin and glucose. It has been suggested that it plays a role in determining the metabolic actions of IGF-I (Lewitt & Baxter, 1991). IGFBP-1 can leave the circulation. This passage is under endocrine regulation and is enhanced by insulin (Bar et al., 1990) and thus it may play a role in targeting IGF-I to specific tissues.

IGFBP-2 can be found both in membrane-associated and soluble form and complexes with IGF to form a 31 kD complex. It can readily pass the endothelial barrier. Its regulation is poorly understood, but it is particularly important as a IGFBP in the fetal circulation. There is limited evidence to suggest it may be regulated by IGF-II.

IGFBP-3 has multiple glycosylation forms and can be membrane associated. It binds IGFs to form a 53 kD complex. However, in turn, this complex is non-covalently associated with a larger acid labile subunit (ALS) to form a 150 kD complex. This complex is the dominant form of IGF-I or IGF-II in the adult circulation and the molar concentration of the 150 kD complex is closely correlated with the molar concentration of IGF-I plus IGF-II. Both IGFBP-3 and ALS are GH-dependent proteins. There is controversy as to whether there is any direct regulation by IGF-I.

IGFBP-4 forms a 24 kD complex with the IGFs and is an inhibitory binding protein particularly found in bone and fibroblasts but also detectable in the circulation. There is an IGF-dependent IGFBP-4 protease which is normally latent but is activated by IGFs and acts to release IGF from IGFBP-4. This may be a local amplification system for IGF action (Conover et al., 1994).

IGFBP-5 is found mainly in connective tissues being expressed by chondrocytes, osteoblasts and fibroblasts. It forms a 31 kD complex with IGF-I or -II. It is normally tightly bound to the extracellular matrix and in this form is resistant to proteolysis. The solubilized form inhibits the action of IGFs, whereas the bound form has lower affinity for IGF-I and potentiates its effects presumably by acting to concentrate IGF-I in the region of the receptor (Clemmons et al., 1994).

IGFBP-6 is of similar size to IGFBP-4. It is expressed particularly in connective tissue but has only been investigated to a limited extent.

In addition, the type 2 IGF/mannose-6-phosphate receptor is found in the circulation. It is presumably cleaved from the cell surface receptor. It binds a significant amount of IGF-II particularly in the fetal circulation and may function as an IGF-II specific binding protein (Gelato et al., 1989).

Ontogeny of the IGF system

Expression and tissue levels

IGFs and their receptors and binding proteins can be detected from the earliest stage of embryogenesis, prior to implantation (Hahnel & Schultz, 1994). IGF-I receptors appear prior to blastocyst formation and it has been suggested that they may be responsive to maternal IGFs present in secretions in the Fallopian tubes (Smith et al., 1993). Given the central role of IGFs as proliferation factors, they may play a key role in regulating embryonic growth and differentiation.

Messenger RNA for both IGF-I and IGF-II and the binding proteins are found in essentially all fetal tissues and in the placenta. There are very distinct cell type and developmental specific patterns of expression (Lund et al., 1986; Han et al., 1988; Brice et al., 1989; Bondy et al., 1990). These patterns suggest the importance of paracrine IGF action in the regulation of tissue growth and differentiation. For example, in the rat fetus at E15, IGF-I mRNA is found mainly in undifferentiated mesenchyme and in areas of active tissue remodelling whereas IGF-II mRNAs are detectable in liver, developing muscle, vasculature and the choroid plexus (Bondy et al., 1990). In general, a higher abundance of IGF-II transcripts is seen in fetal than adult tissues.

The binding proteins appear to play specific roles in localizing IGFs. Such specific compartmentalization has been well demonstrated in tissues such as the fetal lung, the developing brain and the fetal kidney. For example, in the kidney, there are very specific changes in the expression of IGFBPs in the ureteric duct and metanephric blastema during nephrogenesis (Han et al., 1994). In the fetal rat lung, IGF-I protein is found associated with alveolar cells whereas the mRNA coding for IGF-I is detected in fibroblasts suggesting that alveolar IGFBPs have determined its location (Klempt et al., 1992).

Whereas IGF-II mRNAs are found in most fetal tissues, their expression postnatally is much more restricted. In the rodent the switch is most dramatic: from widespread fetal expression, the choroid plexus and meninges remain the only site of basal postnatal expression. In man, and in sheep, the relative change is similar but not so complete. The expression of IGF-I, particularly in the fetal liver, is at lower levels than postnatally (Lund et al., 1986). This may reflect in part the low number of GH receptors in fetal tissues (Klempt et al., 1993). Given that there is no compelling evidence for a different range of biological actions for either IGF-I or IGF-II, no teleological explanation is available for why expression of IGF-II should dominate prenatally and of IGF-I postnatally.

There is evidence that the levels of IGF-I in fetal tissues are reduced in experimental growth retardation (Unterman et al., 1993; Frampton, Jonas & Larkins, 1991; Vileisis & D'Ercole, 1986). IGFBP-1 expression is increased (Straus & Takemoto, 1990) which may reduce the bioavailability of IGF-I.

The human placenta produces both IGF-I and IGF-II (Fant, Munro & Moses, 1986). In diabetic pregnancies, the abundance of IGF-I mRNA is increased in macrosomic placentae (Wang et al., 1988). In contrast, in the placenta of women with pregnancy-induced hypertension associated with fetal growth retardation, IGF-II expression is markedly enhanced in the intermediate trophoblast cells surrounding infarcts and in the hyperplastic stem villous arterioles. This suggests that IGF-II may also play a role in the placental response to maternal disease (Han et al., 1994).

The ontogeny of IGFBP expression has primarily been studied in the rat (Pintar et al., 1994). In early development, IGFBP-1 is first expressed in the liver at E11.5 when hepatogenesis becomes rapid. IGFBP-1 expression in the adult liver similarly rises during regeneration. IGFBP-2 is expressed in most fetal tissues. IGFBP-3 is expressed by E10.5 in mesenchyme. IGFBP-4 expression parallels that of IGF-II and is found particularly in mesenchymal tissues. Han et al. (1994) have reported on the ontogeny of IGFBP expression in the sheep fetus. IGF-II and IGFBP-5 mRNAs are localized largely to mesenchymal cells. IGFBP-2,3, 4 and 6 are found both in mesenchymal and epithelial cells.

IGFs and their IGFBPs, especially IGFBP-1 and IGFBP-2 are found in amniotic fluid. It has been suggested that swallowed growth factors such as IGF-I and transforming growth factor α (TGF-α) may play a role in gut development. The levels of IGF-I and IGF-II are also high in colostrum.

Circulating IGF system

More is known of the regulation of circulating IGFs and their binding proteins in the fetus, primarily from studies in the late gestation fetal sheep. In the fetal sheep, IGF-I levels rise gradually through late gestation but at term are still somewhat lower than adult levels. In contrast, IGF-II levels are high in fetal life and fall to adult levels in the immediate peripartum period (Gluckman & Butler, 1983). There is experimental evidence that inhibition of IGF-II expression is determined by the peripartum rise in cortisol (Li et al., 1993).

Three major factors appear to determine circulating fetal IGF-I levels: hormonal, metabolic and the placenta.

It is now apparent that fetal GH deficiency is associated with a degree of linear growth failure in both man (Gluckman et al., 1992*a*) and sheep. In sheep, it has been shown that both GH and thyroid hormone affect IGF-I levels albeit that the degree of GH dependence is less than postnatally (Mesiano et al., 1989). Similarly GH dependence of IGF-I and IGF-II has been demonstrated in the fetal rat (Kim et al., 1993). Recently, we have shown that the administration of GH releasing factor to the fetal sheep leads to an elevation of IGF-I thus confirming its GH dependence even in utero (Bauer et al., 1994).

However, it is clear that the major determinant of fetal IGF-I circulatory levels is metabolic status. Starvation of the ewe leads to an abrupt and reversible fall in fetal IGF-I levels. If the fast is terminated by glucose infusion but not by amino acid infusion to the fetus, IGF-I levels are restored (Oliver et al., 1993). Similarly, if the fast is continued but insulin is infused into the fetus, IGF-I levels are restored. This demonstrates that glucose availability is a major determinant of fetal IGF-I levels but that the actions of glucose are indirect and are mediated via altered insulin release (Oliver et al., 1994). Similarly, in fetal pancreatectomy, fetal IGF-I levels are reduced (Gluckman et al., 1987). It appears likely that the increase in lean body mass found in infants of diabetic mothers is a consequence of fetal hyperinsulinism leading to enhanced IGF-I secretion either locally or systemically.

Limited evidence from several laboratories, including our own, suggests that the placenta can either secrete IGF-I or clear IGF-I from the fetal circulation (Iwamoto, Chernausek & Murray, 1991). When IGF-I levels are high in the fetal circulation, there is a positive A–V difference across the umbilical circulation (i.e. placental clearance), but the difference is reversed when fetal IGF-I levels are low. Thus the placenta appears to modulate extreme shifts in fetal IGF-I levels. This would reduce the risk of fetal overgrowth or fetal death.

Relatively little is known about the regulation of IGF-II in the fetal circulation. It appears to be reduced by maternal fasting to a lesser extent than IGF-I and to be reduced only in the most severely growth retarded fetuses. Glucose but not insulin elevates fetal IGF-II levels (Oliver et al.,

1994). It does not appear to be greatly influenced by hormonal status. We have therefore suggested that IGF-II may be a more constitutive form of IGF in the fetal circulation (Gluckman et al., 1992*b*).

There are differences in the forms of circulating IGF in the fetal circulation as a consequence of ontogenic differences in the IGFBPs. IGFBP-3 concentration in the fetal circulation is lower as a consequence of the relative GH resistance. IGFBP-2 levels are much higher than postnatally. IGFBP-1 levels are also relatively high. The pattern of IGFBP response in the fetus to undernutrition or maternal starvation is similar to that in the adult with IGFBP-1 and IGFBP-2 rising and IGFBP-3 falling (Oliver et al., 1994; Osborn et al., 1992). IGFBP-1 is particularly labile with levels rising in response to hypoxia, whereas IGFBP-2 falls. This may be mediated by catecholamines directly or be secondary to the inhibition of insulin release (Hooper et al., 1994).

It has recently been suggested that tissue from growth-retarded fetuses is resistant to IGF-I; whether this is due to a receptor defect or not is not known (Frampton et al., 1990).

The fetal IGF system and fetal growth

There is compelling evidence that IGF-I is a major determinant of fetal growth. The first suggestions came from correlations between birth size and umbilical cord IGF-I levels. Such relationships have been demonstrated in numerous clinical studies (Gluckman et al., 1983) and in some studies in experimental animals. More recently an inverse relationship has been reported between cord blood IGFBP-1 levels and birth size (Wang & Chard, 1992). This may simply be a reflection of the metabolic compromise of the growth-retarded fetus, but it might also suggest a role for IGFBP-1 in reducing the bioavailability of IGF-I. Scattered reports also raise the possibility of a relationship between birth size and umbilical cord IGF-II levels (Bennett et al., 1983).

More direct evidence of a role for IGF-I as a regulator of fetal growth has been provided in rodents. In mice selected for either high or low IGF-I levels, embryo transplanted mice from the high line growth to a larger fetal size than those from the low line. The experimental paradigm rules out any maternal confounders (Gluckman et al., 1992*c*). More recently, homologous recombination has been used to knock out the IGF-I gene. These mice have marked intrauterine and postnatal growth retardation. Interestingly, their growth retardation does not commence until E13.5 suggesting that IGF-I becomes important to fetal growth only after that age. This is consistent with studies reviewed below that show that in earlier gestation IGF-II has the dominant role. These IGF-I null mutant mice generally die at birth probably because of the very severe diaphragmatic muscle hypoplasia. Other phenotypic characteristics include organ hypoplasia and delayed ossification (Baker et al., 1993).

Lok et al. have infused IGF-I into the chronically instrumented normal fetal sheep and seen only relatively subtle effects on fetal growth and differentiation (Lok et al., 1994*a,b*). However, this might reflect other counteracting mechanisms such as inhibition of paracrine IGF-I production, as described postnatally, and increased placental clearance and alterations of IGFBPs which might restrict the risks of fetal overgrowth. Harding et al. (1994) have shown that acute administration of IGF-I to the late gestation sheep fetus leads to metabolic changes in the fetus and placenta consistent with a role in increasing fetal growth. Placental lactate production is inhibited, placental clearance of amino acids from the mother appears to be increased and that from the fetus reduced, there is greater fetal glucose uptake and a reduction in fetal urea production (i.e. increased anabolism and reduced catabolism). Taken together, these lines of evidence point to a central role of IGF-I in regulating fetal growth and placental metabolism. Metabolic and nutritional influences are major determinants of this role for IGF-I.

The role of IGF-II in fetal growth has been largely determined from various forms of knockout mice in important experiments by Efstratiadis and colleagues (Baker et al., 1993; Bassett et al., 1994; De Chiara, Efstratiadis & Robertson, 1990). Such experiments clearly show a role for IGF-II in an 'all or nothing' manner but unfortunately no experiments have yet addressed the potential role of IGF-II as a physiological regulator of fetal growth. IGF-II knockouts have significant fetal growth retardation from about E11 (see Table 4.1) but after E18 their growth rate is parallel to the control line. This suggests that IGF-II is critical to the regulation of the early stage of fetal growth but that IGF-I has a dominant role in late gestation. In contrast to IGF-I null mutants, placental growth is also impaired, but this may reflect the fact that in rodents only IGF-II mRNA is detected in the placenta: this observation may therefore not be extrapolatable to humans.

A variety of other mutants have been constructed including type 1 receptor knockouts; by cross breeding double mutants have been constructed including IGF-I/IGF-II knockouts and IGF-II/type 1 receptor

Table 4.1. *Phenotype of mice carrying null mutations of genes in the IGF axis*

Knockout	Birth size*	Placental size	Lethality at birth	Comment
IGF-II	60%	Impaired	No	Only exhibited in fetal IGF-II allele paternally derived. Onset of growth failure E11
IGF-I	60%	Normal	Usually	Onset of growth failure E13.5
IGF type I receptor	45%	Normal	Always	Respiratory failure at birth; organ and muscle hypoplasia
IGF-I/IGF type I receptor	45%	?	Always	
IGF-II/IGF type I receptor	30%	?	Always	
IGF-I/IGF-II receptor	30%	?	Always	
IGF type II receptor	110%	Normal	Lethal if maternal in origin	Studies of the Thp-mutant cross with Thp-mutant
IGF type 1 receptor/ type 2 receptor	93%	?	Variable survival	

*% of normal birthweight.
Derived from Baker et al., 1993; Liu et al., 1994; De Chiara et al., 1990.

knockouts. The Thp-mutant is a natural mutant in which the type 2 receptor allele is missing. A Thp-/IGF-II null mutant line has also been created. These observations are summarized in Table 4.1. In interpreting these observations it is essential to note that, in mice, IGF-II is paternally imprinted and the IGF type 2 receptor maternally imprinted. The Thp-mutation if maternally derived is lethal whereas if paternally derived leads only to minor phenotypic changes. However fetal size is normal in the Thp-mutant irrespective of parental origin.

These animals produced some compelling findings (see Table 4.1). The type 1 receptor null mutant and the IGF-I type 1 receptor double null mutant produced growth retardation of a greater degree than the IGF-I null mutant suggesting that a ligand other than IGF-I acted on the fetal type 1 receptor to promote fetal growth. This is certainly IGF-II. However, the IGF-II/type 1 receptor double knockout had greater growth retardation than the type 1 receptor knockout alone. Further, whereas placental size is impaired in IGF-II null mutants, this is not the case for type 1 receptor null mutants. These two observations led Baker et al. (1993) to conclude that there is another receptor mediating some growth promoting actions of IGF-II. The studies of the Thp-mutants make it unlikely that this second receptor is the type 2 receptor. The authors suggest that the type 2 receptor is acting as a clearance receptor and that, in the case of the maternally derived Thp-mutation, high levels of IGF-II may be postulated to be lethal, perhaps operating through both the type 1 receptor and potentially this second unknown receptor. Support for this hypothesis is given by the observation that the Thp-/type 1 receptor mutant is surprisingly rescued in comparison to the type 1 receptor null mutant. Unlike the type 1 receptor null mutant, this double mutant is viable and of normal birth size. The explanation proposed is that, in this situation, IGF-II levels are higher and thus can provide trophic support to the fetus acting through this unknown receptor. These animal models provide exciting paradigms for future study to address these various hypotheses.

The maternal IGF system

While IGF-I does not cross the placenta, recent evidence suggests that the maternal IGF-I system can indirectly influence fetal growth. Experiments in mice and rats demonstrated that elevated maternal IGF-I can overcome maternal constraint on fetal growth (Gluckman et al., 1992*c*) and that under some circumstances it leads to enhanced fetal and placental growth and to an alteration in the placental expression of the glucose transporter GLUT1 (Bassett et al., 1994). These studies suggest that maternally administered IGF-I can affect placental function. This possibility has been explored further in chronically instrumented fetal sheep (Liu et al., 1994). Short-term maternal IGF-I administration in late gestation leads to alterations in maternal glucose and thus indirectly to fetal hyperglycaemia, increased placental amino acid uptake and increased placental lactate production. When these changes are considered alongside those following fetal IGF-I administration reviewed earlier it is not unreasonable to propose a model whereby elevation in

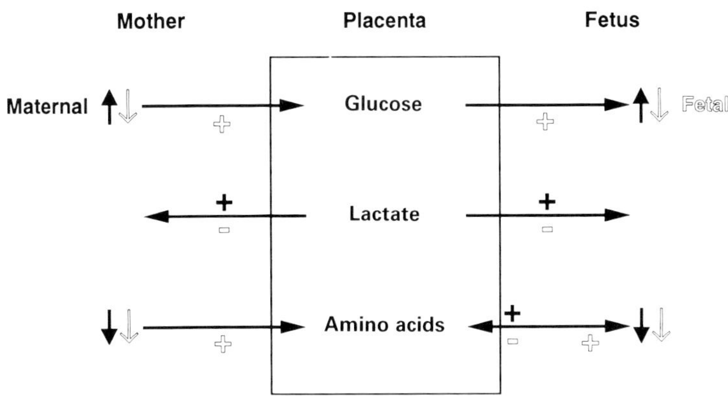

Fig. 4.1. Diagram of the hypothesized interaction between maternal and fetal IGF-I in the regulation of fetoplacental metabolism. Solid symbols indicate the effects of increased maternal IGF-I concentrations and open symbols the effects of increased fetal IGF-I concentrations. Small vertical arrows show the direction of change of the net substrate uptakes indicated by the long horizontal arrows. Increased maternal IGF-I concentrations lead to increased maternal and hence fetal blood glucose concentrations (▲) by maternal insulin suppression. Increased fetal IGF-I concentrations lead to increased fetal glucose uptake (✚), lowering fetal and maternal blood glucose concentrations (▽). Thus increased maternal and fetal IGF-I concentrations will increase net transplacental glucose transfer and fetal glucose uptake. Placental lactate production is increased by maternal (**+**) and inhibited by fetal (□) IGF-I elevation, with little effect on circulating lactate concentrations. Increased maternal IGF-I concentrations lead to decreased maternal and hence fetal blood amino acid concentrations (▼) by stimulating placental amino acid uptake (**+**). Increased fetal IGF-I concentrations lead to increased fetal amino acid uptake (✚) and inhibition of fetal protein oxidation (□), lowering fetal and maternal blood amino acid concentrations (▽). Thus increased maternal and fetal IGF-I concentrations will increase net transplacental amino acid transfer and fetal amino acid uptake. (Reprinted with permission from Liu et al., 1994.)

maternal IGF-I leads to increased glucose availability to the fetus, increased fetal IGF-I levels and thus fetal growth. Coordinate increases in fetal and maternal IGF-I levels would ensure placental metabolism and placental amino acid transfer appropriate to fetal growth (see Fig. 4.1). Preliminary evidence from studies of fetal sheep following chronic maternal growth hormone administration supports such a model (J.E. Harding, personal communication).

It is therefore of interest to note that it has been shown that maternal IGF-I levels correlate with fetal size. In pregnancies compounded by intrauterine growth retardation, maternal IGF-I levels are lowered

(Mirlesse et al., 1993). Because the levels of IGFBP-3 protease are higher in pregnancy, the levels of free IGF-I in the maternal circulation are higher than in the non-pregnant state (Binoux et al., 1994). It seems probable that placental growth hormone (hGH-v) is the dominant determinant of maternal IGF-I levels.

Significance for the future

The probable roles of IGF-I and IGF-II in fetal development are multiple and include regulation of embryogenesis, organ growth and differentiation, fetal growth and coordination of fetal and placental metabolism. As these roles become better understood, it may be possible to utilize this knowledge in clinical applications. Recombinant IGF-I is in clinical application in a variety of disease states. Already IGF-I is being considered as a potential anabolic agent in the very low birthweight infant. The recent observation, which suggests that IGF-I administered maternally can indirectly advance fetal growth, has considerable practical application if it can be applied clinically to growth retarded pregnancies.

Acknowledgements

The author's work is supported by a programme grant of the Health Research Council of New Zealand. Much of the work referred to in this review is that of my colleagues Dr Jane Harding, Dr Nicole Bassett, Dr M. Oliver, Dr M. Bauer and Dr M. Klempt.

References

Baker, J., Liu, J-P., Robertson, E.J. & Efstratiadis, A. (1993). Role of insulin-like growth factors in embryonic and postnatal growth. *Cell*, **75**, 73–82.

Ballard, F.J., Walton, P.E., Dunshea, F.R., Francis, G.L. & Tomas, F.M. (1994). Does IGF-I ever act through the insulin receptor? In *The Insulin-like Growth Factors and Their Regulatory Proteins*, ed. R.C. Baxter, P.D. Gluckman & R.G. Rosenfeld. pp. 131–8. Excerpta Medica, Amsterdam.

Bar, R.S., Boes, M., Clemmons, D.R., Busby, W.H., Sandra, A., Dake, B.L. & Booth, B.A. (1990). Insulin differentially alters transcapillary movement of intravascular IGFBP-1, IGFBP-2 and endothelial cell IGF-binding proteins in the rat heart. *Endocrinology*, **127**, 497–9.

Bassett, N.S., Currie, M.J., Woodall, S. & Gluckman, P.D. (1994). The effect of IGF-1 and bGH treatment on placental glut1 gene expression.

Proceedings of the Third International Symposium on Insulin-like Growth Factors, Sydney, Australia, 1994 Growth Regulation, **4. Suppl 1.**, I105, 72.(Abstract).

Bauer, M.K., Breier, B.H., Harding, J.E, Veldhuis, J.D & Gluckman, P.D. (1994). The fetal somatotropic axis during long-term maternal undernutrition in sheep: Evidence for nutritional regulation in utero. *Endocrinology*, in press.

Bennett, A., Wilson, D.M., Liu, F., Nagashima, R., Rosenfeld, R.G. & Hintz, R.L. (1983). Levels of insulin-like growth factors I and II in human cord blood. *Journal of Clinical Endocrinology and Metabolism*, **57**, 609–12.

Binoux, M., Lalou, C., Lassarre, C. & Segovia, B. (1994). Regulation of IGF bioavailability by IGFBP proteases. In *The Insulin-like Growth Factors and Their Regulatory Proteins*, ed. R.C. Baxter, P.D. Gluckman & R.G. Rosenfeld. pp. 217–26. Excerpta Medica, Amsterdam.

Bondy, C.A., Werner, H., Roberts, C.T., Jr. & LeRoith, D. (1990). Cellular pattern of insulin-like growth factor-I (IGF-I) and type I IGF receptor gene expression in early organogenesis: comparison with IGF-II gene expression. *Molecular Endocrinology*, **4**, 1386–8.

Breier, B.H., Gluckman, P.D. & Bass, J.J. (1988). The somatotrophic axis in young steers: Influence of nutritional status and oestradiol 17-B on hepatic high and low affinity somatotrophic binding sites. *Journal of Endocrinology*, **116**, 169–77.

Brice, A.L., Cheetham, J.E., Bolton, V.N., Hill, N.C. & Schofield, P.N. (1989). Temporal changes in the expression of the insulin-like growth factor II gene associated with tissue maturation in the human fetus. *Development*, **106**, 543–54.

Butler, A.A., Ambler, G.R., Breier, B.H., LeRoith, D., Roberts, C.T. & Gluckman, P.D. (1994). Growth hormone (GH) and insulin-like growth factor-I (IGF-I) treatment of the GH-deficient dwarf rat – differential effects on IGF-I transcription start site expression in hepatic and extrahepatic tissues and lack of effect on type I IGF receptor Mrna expression. *Molecular and Cellular Endocrinology*, **101**, 321–30.

Clemmons, D.R. (1993). IGF binding proteins and their functions. *Molecular and Reproductive Development*, **35**, 368–74.

Clemmons, D.R., Nam, T.J., Busby, W.H. & Parker, A. (1994). Modification of IGF action by insulin-like growth factor binding protein–5. In *The Insulin-like Growth Factors and Their Regulatory Proteins*, ed. R.C. Baxter, P.D. Gluckman & R.G. Rosenfeld. pp. 183–91. Excerpta Medica, Amsterdam.

Conover, C.A., Clarkson, J.T., Wissink, S., Durham, S.K. & Bale, L.K. (1994). Biological effects of IGF-regulated IGFBP in cultured human fibroblasts. In *The Insulin-like Growth Factors and Their Regulatory Proteins*, ed. R.C. Baxter, P.D. Gluckman & R.G. Rosenfeld. pp. 175–82. Excerpta Medica, Amsterdam.

De Chiara, T.M., Efstratiadis, A. & Robertson, E.J. (1990). A growth deficiency phenotype in heterozygous mice carrying an insulin-like growth factor II gene disrupted by targeting. *Nature*, **345**, 78–80.

Fant, M., Munro, H. & Moses, A.C. (1986). An autocrine/paracrine role for insulin-like growth factors in the regulation of human placental growth. *Journal of Clinical Endocrinology and Metabolism*, **63**, 499–505.

Frampton, R.J., Jonas, H.A. & Larkins, R.G. (1991). Increased secretion of insulin-like growth factor-binding proteins and decreased secretion of insulin-like growth factor-II by muscle from growth-retarded neonatal rats. *Journal of Endocrinology*, **130**, 33–42.

Frampton, R.J., Jonas, H.A., MacMahon, R.A. & Larkins, R.G. (1990). Failure of IGF-1 to affect protein turnover in muscle from growth-retarded neonatal rats. *Journal of Developmental Physiology*, **13**, 125–33.

Gelato, M.C., Rutherford, C., Stark, R.I. & Daniel, S.S. (1989). The insulin-like growth factor II/Mannose-6-phosphate receptor is present in fetal and maternal sheep serum. *Endocrinology*, **124**, 2935–43.

Gluckman, P.D., Butler, J.H., Comline, R. & Fowden, A. (1987). The effects of pancreatectomy on the plasma concentrations of insulin-like growth factors 1 and 2 in the sheep fetus. *Journal of Developmental Physiology*, **9**, 79–88.

Gluckman, P.D., Gunn, A.J., Wray, A., Cutfield, W., Chatelain, P.G., Guilbaud, O., Ambler, G.R., Wilton, P. & Albertsson-Wikland, K. (1992*a*). Congenital idiopathic growth hormone deficiency is associated with prenatal and early postnatal growth failure. *Journal of Pediatrics*, **121**, 920–3.

Gluckman, P.D., Harding, J.E., Oliver, M.H., Liu, L., Ambler, G.R., Klempt, M. & Breier, B.H. (1992*b*). Mechanisms of intrauterine growth retardation: role of fetal and maternal hormones. In *International Congress on Growth Hormone and Somatomedins During Lifespan. Milan, Italy*, ed. E.E. Muller, D. Cocchi & V. Locatelli. pp. 147–60. Springer-Verlag.

Gluckman, P.D., Johnson-Barrett, J.J., Butler, J.H., Edgar, B.W. & Gunn, T.R. (1983). Studies of insulin-like growth factor-I and -II by specific radioligand assays in umbilical cord blood. *Clinical Endocrinology*, **19**, 405–13

Gluckman, P.D., Morel, P.C.H., Ambler, G.R., Breier, B.H., Blair, H.T. & McCutcheon, S.N. (1992*c*). Elevating maternal insulin-like growth factor-I in mice and rats alters the pattern of fetal growth by removing maternal constraint. *Journal of Endocrinology*, **134**, R1–3.

Hahnel, A. & Schultz, G.A. (1994). Insulin-like growth factor binding proteins are transcribed by preimplantation mouse embryos. *Endocrinology*, **134**, 1956–9.

Han, V.K.M., Asano, H., Matsell, D.G., Delhanty, P.J.D., Hayatsu, J., Bassett, N., Phillips, I.D., Nygard, K. & Stepaniuk, O. (1994). Insulin-like growth factors (IGFs) and IGF binding proteins (IGFBPs) in fetal development: physiology and pathophysiology. In *The Insulin-like Growth Factors and Their Regulatory Proteins*, ed. R.C. Baxter, P.D. Gluckman & R.G. Rosenfeld. pp. 263–73. Excerpta Medica, Amsterdam.

Han, V.K.M., Lund, P.K., Lee, D.C. & D'Ercole, A.J. (1988). Expression of somatomedin/insulin-like growth factor messenger ribonucleic acids in the human fetus: identification, characterization, and tissue distribution. *Journal of Clinical Endocrinology and Metabolism*, **66**, 422–9.

Harding, J.E., Liu, L., Evans, P.C. & Gluckman, P.D. (1994). IGF-I alters feto-placental protein and carbohydrate metabolism in fetal sheep. *Endocrinology*, **134**, 1509–14.

Hooper, S.B., Bocking, A.D., White, S.E., Fraher, L.J., McDonald, T.J. & Han, V.K.M. (1994). Catecholamines stimulate the synthesis and release of insulin-like growth factor binding protein-1 (IGFBP-1) by fetal sheep liver in vivo. *Endocrinology*, **134**, 1104–12.

Hussain, M.A., Schmitz, O., Mengel, A., Keller, A., Christiansen, J.S., Zapf, J. & Froesch, E.R. (1993). Insulin-like growth factor-I stimulates lipid oxidation, reduces protein oxidation, and enhances insulin sensitivity in humans. *Journal of Clinical Investigation*, **92**, 2249–56.

Iwamoto, H.S., Chernausek, S.D. & Murray, M.A. (1991). Regulation of plasma insulin-like growth factor (IGF-I) by oxygen and nutrients in fetal sheep. *2nd International Symposium on Insulin-Like Growth Factors/ Somatomedins, San Francisco, California*, 48. (Abstract).

Jones, J.I., Busby, W.H., Wright, G., Smith, C.E., Kimack, N.M. & Clemmons, D.R. (1993). Identification of the sites of phosphorylation in insulin-like growth factor binding protein-1. *Journal of Biological Chemistry*, **268**, 1125–31.

Kim, J.D., Nanto-Salonen, K., Szczepankiewicz, J.R., Rosenfeld, R.G. & Glasscock, G.F. (1993). Evidence for pituitary regulation of somatic growth, insulin-like growth factors-I and -II, and their binding proteins in the fetal rat. *Pediatric Research*, **33**, 144–51.

Klempt, M., Bingham, B., Breier, B.H., Baumbach, W.R. & Gluckman, P.D. (1993). Tissue distribution and ontogeny of growth hormone receptor mRNA and ligand binding to hepatic tissue in the midgestation sheep fetus. *Endocrinology*, **132**, 1071–7.

Klempt, M., Hutchins, A.M., Gluckman, P.D. & Skinner, S.J. (1992). IGF binding protein-2 gene expression and the location of IGF-I and IGF-II in fetal rat lung. *Development*, **115**, 765–72.

Koea, J.B., Breier, B.H., Shaw, J.H.F. & Gluckman, P.D. (1992*a*). A possible role for IGF-II: evidence in sheep for in vivo regulation of IGF-I mediated protein anabolism. *Endocrinology*, **130**, 2423–5.

Koea, J.B., Gallaher, B.W., Breier, B.H., Douglas, R.G., Hodgkinson, S.C., Shaw, J.H.F. & Gluckman, P.D. (1992*b*). Passive immunization against circulating IGF-I increases protein catabolism in lambs: evidence for a physiological role for circulating IGF-I. *Journal of Endocrinology*, **135**, 279–84.

Lewitt, M.S. & Baxter, R.C. (1991). Insulin-like growth factor-binding protein-I: a role in glucose counterregulation? *Molecular and Cellular Endocrinology*, **79**, C147–52.

Li, J., Saunders, J.C., Gilmour, R.S., Silver, M. & Fowden, A.L. (1993). Insulin-like growth factor-II messenger ribonucleic acid expression in fetal tissues of the sheep during late gestation: effects of cortisol. *Endocrinology*, **132**, 2083–9.

Liu, L., Harding, J.E., Evans, P.C. & Gluckman, P.D. (1994). Maternal insulin-like growth factor-I infusion alters feto-placental carbohydrate and protein metabolism in pregnant sheep. *Endocrinology*, **135**, 895–900.

Lok, F., Owens, J.A., Mundy, L., Owens, P.C. & Robinson, J.S. (1994*a*). Insulin-like-growth factor-I promotes internal organ growth in fetal sheep. *Proceedings of the Third International Symposium on Insulin-like Growth Factors, Sydney, Australia, 1994 Growth Regulation*, **4, Suppl 1.**, I101, 71. (Abstract).

Lok, F., Owens, J.A., Mundy, L., Owens, P.C. & Robinson, J.S. (1994*b*). Effect of insulin-like growth factor-I (IGF-I) on growth of fetal sheep.

Proceedings of the Twelfth Annual Congress of the Australian Perinatal Society in conjunction with the New Zealand Perinatal Society, A25. (Abstract).

Lund, P.K., Moats-Staats, B., Hynes, M.A., Simmons, J.G., Jansen, M., D'Ercole, A.J. & Van Wyk, J.J. (1986). Somatomedin-C/insulin-like growth factor-I and insulin-like growth factor-II mRNAs in rat fetal and adult tissues. *Journal of Biological Chemistry*, **261**, 14539–44.

Maes, M., Maiter, D., Thissen, J-P., Underwood, L.E. & Ketelslegers, J-M. (1991). Contributions of growth hormone receptor and postreceptor defects to growth hormone resistance in malnutrition. *Trends in Endocrinology and Metabolism*, **2**, 92–7.

Mesiano, S., Young, I.R., Hey, A.W., Browne, C.A. & Thorburn, G.D. (1989). Hypophysectomy of the fetal lamb leads to a fall in the plasma concentration of insulin-like growth factor I (IGF-I), but not IGF-II. *Endocrinology*, **124**, 1485–91.

Mirlesse, V., Frankenne, F., Alsat, E., Poncelet, M., Hennen, G. & Evain-Brion, D. (1993). Placental growth hormone levels in normal pregnancy and in pregnancies with intrauterine growth retardation. *Pediatric Research*, **34**, 439–42.

Oliver, M.H., Harding, J.E., Breier, B.H., Evans, P.C. & Gluckman, P.D. (1993). Glucose but not a mixed amino acid infusion regulates plasma insulin-like growth factor (IGF)-I concentrations in fetal sheep. *Pediatric Research*, **34**, 62–5.

Oliver, M.H., Harding, J.E., Breier, B.H. & Gluckman, P.D. (1994). Fetal insulin-like growth factor (IGF)-I and IGF-II are regulated differently by glucose or insulin in the sheep fetus. *Journal of Developmental Physiology*, 'in press'.

Osborn, B.H., Fowlkes, J., Han, V.K.M. & Freemark, M. (1992). Nutritional regulation of insulin-like growth factor-binding protein gene expression in the ovine fetus and pregnant ewe. *Endocrinology*, **131**, 1743–50.

Pintar, J.E., Cerro, J., Streck, R., Wood, T., Rogler, L., Green, B. & Grewal, A. (1994). Expression and function of IGFBPs during rodent development. In *The Insulin-like Growth Factors and Their Regulatory Proteins*, ed. R.C. Baxter, P.D. Gluckman & R.G. Rosenfeld. pp. 253–61. Excerpta Medica, Amsterdam.

Smith, R.M., Garside, W.T., Aghayan, M., Shi, C-Z., Shah, N., Jarett, L. & Heyner, S. (1993). Mouse preimplantation embryos exhibit receptor-mediated binding and transcytosis of maternal insulin-like growth factor I. *Biology of Reproduction*, **49**, 1–12.

Soos, M.A., Field, C.E., Nave, B.T. & Siddle, K. (1994). Hybrid and atypical insulin-like growth factor receptors. In *The Insulin-like Growth Factors and Their Regulatory Proteins*, ed. R.C. Baxter, P.D. Gluckman & R.G. Rosenfeld. pp. 95–106. Excerpta Medica, Amsterdam.

Straus, D.S. & Takemoto, C.D. (1990). Effect of dietary protein deprivation on insulin-like growth factor (IGF)-I and -II, IGF binding protein-2, and serum albumin gene expression in rat. *Endocrinology*, **127**, 1849–60.

Unterman, T.G., Simmons, R.A., Glick, R.P. & Ogata, E.S. (1993). Circulating levels of insulin, insulin-like growth factor-I (IGF-I), IGF-II, and IGF-binding proteins in the small for gestational age fetal rat. *Endocrinology*, **132**, 327–36.

Vileisis, R.A. & D'Ercole, A.J. (1986). Tissue and serum concentrations of somatomedin-C/insulin-like growth factor I in fetal rats made growth retarded by uterine artery ligation. *Pediatric Research*, **20**, 126–30.

Wang, H.S. & Chard, T. (1992). The role of insulin-like growth factor-I and insulin-like growth factor binding protein-1 in the control of human fetal growth. *Journal of Endocrinology*, **132**, 11–19.

Wang, C-Y., Daimon, M., Shen, S-J., Engelmann, G.L. & Ilan, J. (1988). Insulin-like growth factor-I messenger ribonucleic acid in the developing human placenta and in term placenta of diabetics. *Molecular Endocrinology*, **2**, 217–29.

5

Metabolism and growth during neonatal and postnatal development

MICHAEL E. SYMONDS

Introduction

The metabolic adaptations which occur between fetal and neonatal life represent a transition from a quiescent inactive state in which inhibitory stimuli dominate to one of near maximal rates of metabolic activity that are rarely matched during postnatal or adult life. These responses are necessary in order to establish breathing and maintain body temperature after birth, which are both important in determining not only survival but also an individual's ability to thrive. During late gestation, fetal energy demands are small (Power, 1989) and the conservation of energy by the fetus is a prerequisite for ensuring both growth and development (Jansen & Chernick, 1991). A major determinant of fetal development is the maternal metabolic and hormonal environment, which has a large influence on nutrient partitioning and therefore energy supply to the growing fetus (see Symonds & Lomax, 1992). The mother's influence on fetal growth and development is not confined to changes in nutrient supply, as the maternal environment also regulates fetal temperature both throughout the day (Gluckman et al., 1984) and during acute or chronic changes in metabolism (see Symonds et al., 1993).

Low rates of metabolic activity by the fetus are not only necessary to ensure growth but may contribute to periodic episodes of fetal breathing. This point is emphasized by the finding that cold stimulation of cutaneous thermoreceptors not only stimulates metabolism in conjunction with the onset of shivering activity but also results in continuous breathing (Johnston, Gunn & Gluckman, 1988). In contrast, activation of non-shivering thermogenesis in fetal brown adipose tissue is inhibited, which is partly a consequence of placental inhibitory factors such as prostaglandin E_2 (Gunn, Ball & Gluckman, 1993). The ability of brown adipose tissue to generate rapidly large amounts of heat is the result of the electron transport chain becoming uncoupled from ATP synthesis, an effect mediated by a unique mitochondrial uncoupling protein (UCP; see Cannon & Nedergaard, 1985). The ontogeny of brown adipose tissue development in utero is another factor which acts to prevent premature activation since mRNA for UCP remains low during fetal life (Casteilla et al., 1989) as does the amount of UCP (thermogenic capacity) and its thermogenic activity (GDP binding to UCP; Klaus et al., 1991) as illustrated in Fig. 5.1. At the same time, a number of other stimulatory factors that are recruited in order to increase metabolic rate after birth remain at basal levels during fetal life. These include minimal activity of the sympathetic nervous system (Eliot et al., 1981) and low rates of triiodothyronine production, which are the dominant hormonal mechanisms regulating metabolic rate during neonatal life (Symonds, Clarke & Lomax, 1994*a*). One mechanism by which plasma concentrations of triiodothyronine are kept at basal levels during fetal life is the low activity of iodothyronine 5′deiodinase in hepatic and brown adipose tissue (Fig. 5.1) which represent the primary sites of peripheral triiodothyronine synthesis from thyroxine. There is increasing evidence which indicates that changes in sympathetic nervous activity and thyroid status during and following birth can be as important in regulating metabolism and subsequent growth (Symonds et al., 1994*a*) of the neonate, as the effect of removing placental or fetal inhibitory factors.

Birth

Normal parturition at term and concomitant exposure to the cold stimulus of the extrauterine environment are key stimuli for the establishment of both continuous breathing and thermogenesis as metabolic rate rapidly rises. Changes in metabolism by brown adipose tissue and the liver play a primary role in the initiation and maintenance of these responses as a consequence of postpartum increases in thermogenic activity of brown adipose tissue plus type I (Michaelis constant (K_m) in the micromolar range) iodothyronine 5′deiodinase activities in both brown adipose tissue and liver (Fig. 5.1). In contrast, type II (K_m in nanomolar range) iodothyronine 5′deiodinase activity, which is found in brown adipose tissue but not the liver, does not increase after birth in lambs (Fig. 5.1) although high activities have been found in premature infants (Houstek et al., 1993). Sustained iodothyronine 5′deiodinase activity may also be necessary for maintaining fetal brown adipose tissue development since

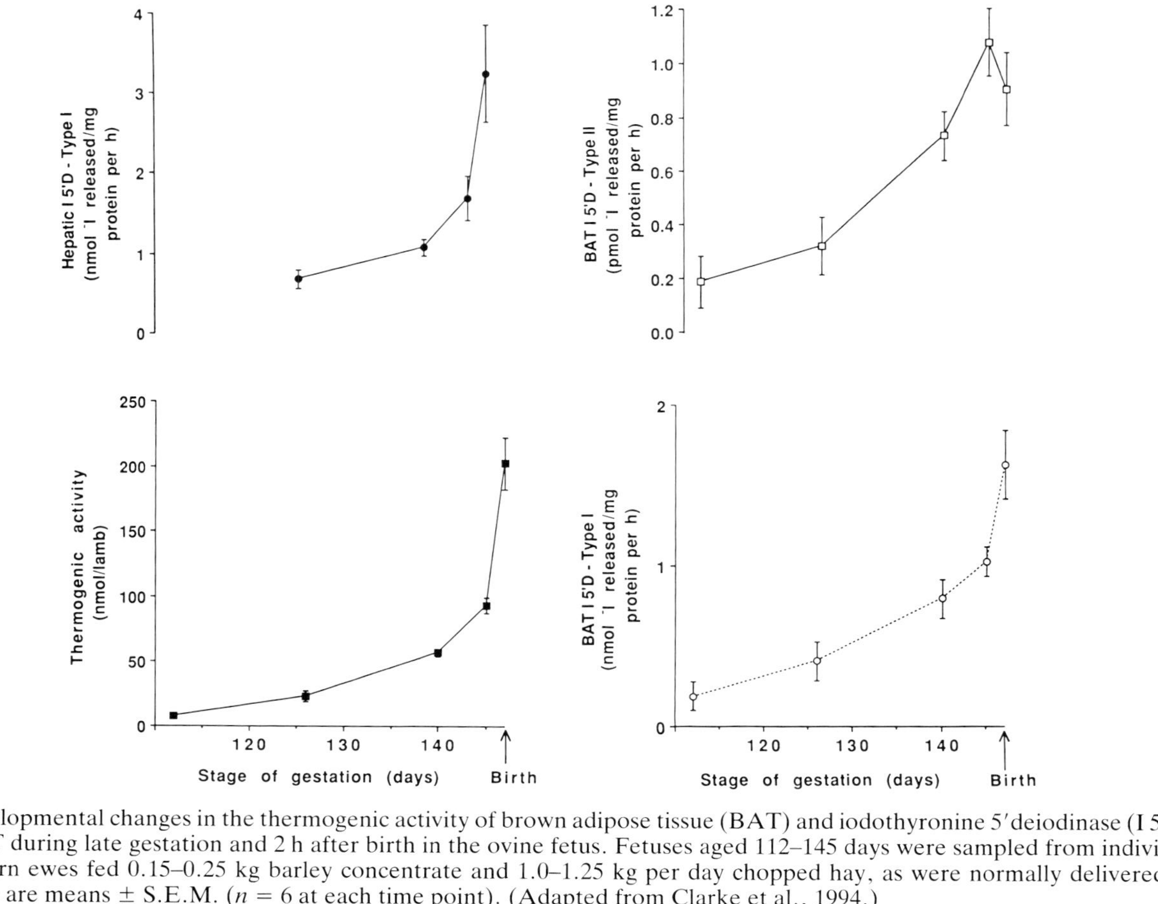

Fig. 5.1. Developmental changes in the thermogenic activity of brown adipose tissue (BAT) and iodothyronine 5′deiodinase (I 5′D) in liver and BAT during late gestation and 2 h after birth in the ovine fetus. Fetuses aged 112–145 days were sampled from individually housed unshorn ewes fed 0.15–0.25 kg barley concentrate and 1.0–1.25 kg per day chopped hay, as were normally delivered term lambs. Values are means ± S.E.M. (n = 6 at each time point). (Adapted from Clarke et al., 1994.)

the postpartum rise in mRNA for UCP is inhibited if iodothyronine 5′deiodinase activity is blocked in utero (Giralt et al., 1990).

After birth, not only is heat production by brown adipose tissue and hepatic triiodothyronine synthesis stimulated, but there is also a transition from net anabolism to catabolism as lipid and glycogen stores are mobilized in order to meet the three- to four-fold increase in metabolic rate (Mellor & Cockburn, 1986). The extent of these adaptations is strongly influenced by the mother's ability to supply glucose to the fetus during late gestation (Symonds & Lomax, 1992). Maternal undernutrition reduces maternal glucose production which results in inhibition of fetal brown adipose tissue and liver development. These effects can be overcome by chronic maternal cold exposure, induced by winter shearing. Lambs which are born from underfed, cold exposed (i.e. shorn) ewes are better adapted to meet the cold challenge of the extrauterine environment. This is a result of these lambs possessing more brown adipose tissue and exhibiting a higher metabolic rate and breathing frequency during non-rapid eye movement sleep (non-REM) over the first day of neonatal life (Symonds et al., 1992, 1993).

Maturity of an individual at birth has a large impact on metabolic adaptation to the extrauterine environment. This effect is particularly noticeable in altricial species such as rodents, which are immature at birth and benefit from the protection of a higher local environment owing to huddling in a nest, than in precocious species, such as lambs, which are mature at birth and do not rely on this behaviour to the same extent. Differences in temperature control are reflected in brown adipose tissue development since this peaks several days after birth in rats (Nedergaard, Connolly & Cannon, 1986) compared with 1–2 h postpartum in sheep (Symonds et al., 1994*b*). Not all mammals possess brown adipose tissue, as this is absent in piglets, which are therefore entirely dependent on shivering thermogenesis in order to increase heat production (Mellor & Cockburn, 1986). This is a comparatively inefficient mechanism by which to maintain body temperature, as it increases air movement around the animal thereby reducing external insulation. Lambs are able to recruit both non-shivering and shivering thermogenesis after birth, although shivering alone is insufficient to maintain body temperature (Symonds & Lomax, 1993) and it only appears to be recruited when heat production by brown adipose tissue is limited (Symonds et al., 1992). Infants are entirely dependent on non-shivering thermogenesis in order to increase metabolic rate at birth (Mellor & Cockburn, 1986) although this process takes several hours to become fully effective (Smales & Kime, 1978)

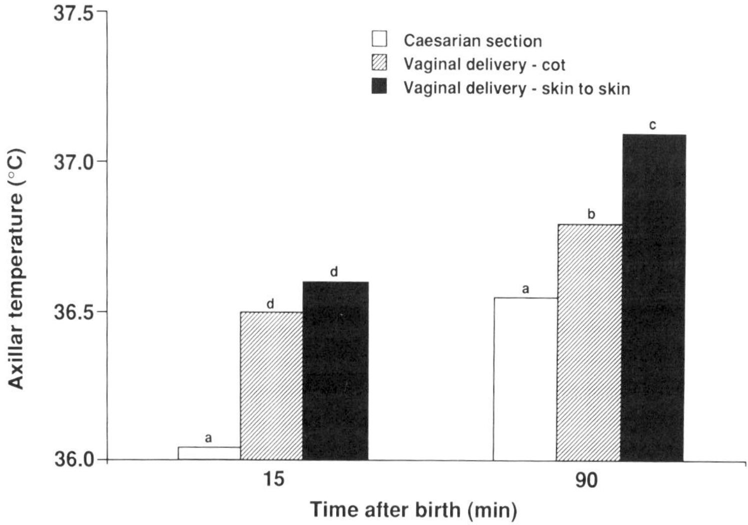

Fig. 5.2. Effect of type of delivery on axillar temperature in newborn infants. Full-term infants were delivered either by Caesarean section or vaginally and placed in a cot or delivered vaginally and placed in direct contact with the mother. Significant differences at each time point are represented by different letters ab $P < 0.05$; ac $P < 0.01$; ad $P < 0.0001$. (Adapted from Christensson et al., 1992, 1993.)

which may explain why body temperature falls appreciably after birth in some cases. The extent to which infants are capable of thermoregulating efficiently after birth is highly influenced by the immediate postpartum environment, since full-term infants which are kept in skin-to-skin contact with the mother have axillary, interscapular and skin temperatures 0.3–1.0 °C above those placed in a cot (Christensson et al., 1992; Fig. 5.2). These differences are partly due to preservation of energy stores but are also a result of skin-to-skin contact promoting metabolic adaptation, thereby indicating altricial characteristics of newborn infants.

An additional factor which has a major impact on metabolic adaptation at birth is the route of delivery since Caesarean section delivery of full-term infants or lambs significantly reduces body temperature (Symonds & Lomax, 1993; Christensson et al., 1993; Fig. 5.2). This response appears to be mediated via a reduction in the thermogenic activity of brown adipose tissue in conjunction with lower plasma concentrations of thyroid hormones (Symonds et al., 1994*a*). Treatment of Caesarean section delivered lambs with a β_3-agonist (Zenecca D7114) does enhance their ability to thermoregulate and restore body temperature, although the sensitivity of brown adipose tissue to β_3-adrenergic stimulation in Caesarean section delivered lambs differs from those delivered vaginally (Symonds et al., 1994*b*). The extent to which thyroid status and thermoregulation is altered following Caesarean section is further influenced by the environmental temperature. Delivery into a cool (15 °C) compared with a warm (30 °C) ambient temperature increases the plasma concentrations of thyroid hormones, which benefits the neonatal lamb by enabling it to produce a greater thermogenic response via shivering thermogenesis (Clarke et al., 1994). These observations are in contrast with the effect of Caesarean section delivery of rat pups at term, in which an increase in mRNA for UCP is observed 6 h after birth when delivered into a warm ambient temperature of 37 °C and this response is doubled when delivered into a cold ambient temperature of 21 °C. However, these adaptations in brown adipose tissue activity are inhibited when rat pups are delivered one day prematurely via Caesarean section (Giralt et al., 1990).

Suckling

Following birth and removal from the placenta the neonate is dependent on an exogenous source of food in order to meet its nutritional requirements. The extent to which a newborn animal can survive without adequate feeding is dependent on maturity at birth and its endogenous energy stores which consist primarily of lipid and glycogen (Mellor & Cockburn, 1986). In altricial species milk is not only a source of nutrition but is essential to ensure gastrointestinal development (Weaver, 1992). The first milk produced is colostrum which is rich in immunoglobulins that provide essential protection against gastrointestinal and respiratory tract infections (Casey, 1989). The immune system of all mammalian species is underdeveloped at birth, and so the neonate is dependent on its mother's milk to provide protection against a variety of potentially pathogenic organisms, including viruses, bacteria, fungi and yeasts (Mepham, 1989). This immuno-protective role is very important in domestic species, such as calves and lambs, in which there is no immune transfer in utero. It could also be important in the establishment of suckling in conjunction with the gradual adaptation to enteral feeding aimed at effective use of milk constituents. However, any additional role that colostrum may have on metabolic and endocrine adaptations after birth has not been fully investigated.

During neonatal development there is a large requirement for fat in order to provide energy, insulation, neural tissue and membrane synthesis (Weaver, 1992). In the full-term individual born from a well-nourished mother, utilization of its own adipose depots, in conjunction with an adequate supply of breast milk, can satisfy this demand. Pigs are not endowed with brown adipose tissue and possess only small amounts of white adipose tissue at birth, so that colostral fat is the primary source for fat oxidation and its supply is essential in maintaining metabolic homeostasis (Herpin, Le Dividich & Van Os, 1992). Milk is composed of an array of substances which have a marked diversity in their functions in addition to meeting the neonate's nutrient requirements (Mepham, 1989). These include protective and trophic factors as well as acting as digestive enzymes (Weaver, 1992). The ability of breast-fed infants to influence milk production directly is not only essential to ensure growth, but can be important during periods of illness when protein catabolism occurs, for which an infant can compensate by increasing protein intake from breast milk (Heinig et al., 1993).

Irrespective of maturity at birth, the ability of offspring to maintain the necessary stimulus for milk production has a large impact on both maternal and neonatal metabolism. This point is illustrated by the finding that milk synthesis is regulated by autocrine factors which appear to be directly influenced by the rate of infant feeding, at least in the short-term (Daly, Owens & Hartmann, 1993). Rates of milk production can therefore vary between breasts and interfeed intervals, which are positively correlated with both the degree to which the breast is emptied and its storage capacity for milk. These findings highlight the importance of entrainment between mother and offspring which is not confined to nutrient supply but extends to more complex neuro-behavioural mechanisms including sleep/wake cycles (McKenna et al., 1990).

An important feature of milk with respect to meeting the high energy demands of the neonate is its high-fat and low-carbohydrate composition. It is essential that hepatic glucose production via gluconeogenesis is maximized in order to ensure that the neonate's obligatory demands for glucose, such as for maintaining brain function, are met. Studies with rats have demonstrated that this is achieved by ensuring a low insulin/glucagon molar ratio which acts to maintain high activities of gluconeogenic enzymes (Girard et al., 1992). This endocrine environment is the result of changes in pancreatic responsiveness to amino acids after birth (Bassett et al., 1982) which are mediated via the postpartum surge in catecholamine secretion (Sperling et al., 1984). Changes in the control of insulin or glucagon release following maternal diabetes or inadequate fetal growth and development can result in hypoglycaemia, because this not only reduces gluconeogenesis but enhances glucose utilization (Girard et al., 1992). However, under normal conditions, fatty acid oxidation and utilization are promoted in order to minimize glucose metabolism, particularly when minimal metabolic rate is high and glucose concentration in plasma is low (Symonds et al., 1989*a*).

The magnitude of metabolic responses to feeding alter with postnatal age, to the extent that there is a rise in growth hormone, insulin and glucose response to feeding, together with a decrease in dietary-induced thermogenesis and plasma concentration of triiodothyronine. These endocrine and metabolic adaptations are important in stimulating and/or facilitating normal growth and development (Symonds et al., 1989*a*).

Weaning

During the suckling and weaning periods metabolism and growth are highly influenced by nutrient supply in the diet. The transition from consuming milk alone, which is characterized with a high-fat/low-carbohydrate composition, to high-carbohydrate/low-fat diet after weaning has a large impact on growth and development. Well-fed neonates have the potential to maximize their growth rate which is reflected in the appreciable quantities of protein and lipid tissue deposited (Whyte & Bayley, 1990). Skeletal muscle growth is characterized by the differentiation and proliferation of satellite cells, but overall growth is far slower than that of adipose tissue in which a marked hyperplasia and hypertrophy of adipose cells occurs (Bell, 1992). After weaning relative growth rate slows, which is reflected in a decreased rate of fractional synthesis and deposition of protein, plus an increased partitioning of nutrients towards lipid tissue. The endocrine and metabolic adaptations, which regulate these processes, are primarily in response to altered fat and carbohydrate intake (Girard et al., 1992). This results in an increased insulin/glucagon molar ratio, plus changes in insulin-like growth factor-I (IGF-I) status which may decrease the influence of growth hormone on nutrient utilization (Bell, 1992). Hepatic metabolism is particularly sensitive to this altered endocrine environment which causes specific changes in enzyme activity, thereby promoting glucose oxidation and reducing fat oxidation. Consequently, rates of glycolysis, glycogen and lipid synthesis are enhanced whilst gluconeogenesis is decreased (Girard et al., 1992). The extent to which these processes may be manipulated during postnatal life is not only determined by dietary factors. For example, thyroid status has a profound influence on postnatal growth as hypothyroidism promotes both lipid and glycogen deposition which could be associated with changes in metabolic rate plus a direct involvement in development of the somatotrophic axis (Symonds et al., 1994*a*).

It should be noted that the ability to maintain adequate or maximal growth in postnatal life may be dependent on the nutritional and endocrine status during fetal and/or neonatal life, since these are critical periods in which cell number is determined. The long-term consequences of nutrient restriction during early life is becoming a key area for current research, as this may provide an explanation for the onset of cardiovascular disease during adult life including ischaemic heart disease, respiratory disease, impaired glucose tolerance, diabetes, obesity and hypertension (Barker, 1992).

Nutrient intake and growth

The growth potential, particularly for protein and lipid, is far greater after birth compared with fetal life (Whyte & Bayley, 1990). Changes in nutrient intake over the first weeks and months of postnatal life predominantly alter adipose tissue and muscle growth, rather than the major organs which tend to grow at a similar rate to the whole body. As with size at birth, it is not only absolute weight which should be taken into consideration, but changes in conformation are equally important when considering growth. This point is particularly relevant when assessing tissue responses to nutritional manipulations such as those observed between breast-fed and formula-fed infants. A perceived benefit of formula feeding is that this doubles protein supply in comparison with breast feeding, thereby enabling recommended dietary allowances to be met (Heinig et al., 1993). Recent results from the DARLING study (Davis Area Research on Lactation, Infant Nutrition and Growth; Heinig et al., 1993) indicate formula feeding is not advantageous as the extra protein consumed is offset by an increase in energy expenditure (White & Bayley, 1990), decreased efficiency of nitrogen utilization, and an increase in fat deposition, as well as imposing a greater metabolic stress on the liver and kidneys (Heinig et al., 1993). This reflects the ability of breast-fed infants to effectively utilize a diet perceived to be protein deficient for growth rather than catabolic processes. It also emphasizes the point that when estimates of nutrient requirements based on metabolic data are made, this should take into account changes in growth characteristics between breast-fed and formula-fed infants (Heinig et al., 1993).

Differences in metabolic adaptation observed between breast-fed and formula-fed infants are mediated in part via altered endocrine responses to feeding. This is linked to the different amino acid contents of these diets which act to stimulate insulin secretion in formula-fed infants, thereby increasing the molar insulin/glucagon ratio (Salmenpera et al., 1988) which results in an enhanced rate of lipid deposition (Girard et al., 1992). Furthermore, although gut regulatory responses to feeding decrease with age, changes in gut regulatory peptides after feeding tend to be greater in formula-fed infants (Salmenpera et al., 1988).

It is not only the composition of milk but quantity consumed which has a large impact on growth and metabolism. This point is illustrated in Fig. 5.3 in which differences in liver and adipose tissue growth between laboratory-reared lambs (i.e. 'formula-fed') at high (320 g milk powder/day) and low (200 g milk powder/day) planes of nutrition are compared with a ewe-reared (i.e. 'breast-fed') group. All lambs were maintained at similar ambient temperatures of 5–15 °C which is well within the operant range for this species, although ewe-reared lambs had the option of selecting a warm environment by contact with the ewe or sibling. It is likely that differences in endocrine status and growth between 'formula-fed' and 'breast-fed' are nutritionally mediated as the lipid and protein content of milk replacer is less than half that of mature ewe's milk. Ewe-reared lambs attained the maximum growth rate which was associated with accelerated liver maturation and higher hepatic iodothyronine 5′deiodinase activity which could explain the high plasma concentrations of triiodothyronine in this group. But, despite this higher circulating concentration of triiodothyronine, perirenal adipose tissue had a low thermogenic activity (indicating loss of brown adipose tissue characteristics) and the marked hyperplasia observed was primarily due to lipid deposition (indicating appearance of white adipose tissue). These results suggest that nutritionally mediated effects on adipose tissue development are due to the appearance of white adipocytes being inversely proportional to the retention of brown adipose tissue characteristics. Ewe-reared lambs also had a higher plasma concentration of insulin which supports the proposal that insulin regulates nutritionally mediated changes in growth during neonatal development (Bassett, 1992).

In formula-fed lambs, whole-body, liver and adipose tissue growth and plasma concentration of insulin were all directly influenced by the level of feed intake (Fig. 5.3), but this did not affect hepatic iodothyronine

5′deiodinase activity, or the plasma concentration of triiodothyronine. Similarly, the thermogenic activity of brown adipose tissue was unaffected, but both type I and II iodothyronine 5′deiodinase activities were approximately ten-fold higher in lambs fed at a high level of the formula diet, compared with ewe-reared or restricted-fed laboratory reared groups. Despite these large differences in iodothyronine 5′deiodinase activities, no comparable effects were observed on the plasma concentration of triiodothyronine. These findings indicate that, in contrast to studies involving cold exposed rodents (see Symonds & Lomax, 1992), the activity of iodothyronine 5′deiodinase in adipose tissue has a very limited role in regulating the peripheral triiodothyronine production and in maintaining brown adipose tissue characteristics postnatally. Another consistent difference between lambs fed at a high level of formula diet was the two- to four-fold higher plasma concentration of IGF-I. A high circulating concentration of IGF-I in conjunction with a low plasma concentration of triiodothyronine could have a primary role in determining tissue growth and development in formula-fed neonates. It has been suggested that IGF-I does not act to limit tissue growth (Bassett, 1992) but there is increasing evidence to indicate that interactions between thyroid hormones and IGF-I are as important in regulating nutrient metabolism (Symonds et al., 1994*a*) as pancreatic hormones (Girard et al., 1992).

Environmental influences on metabolism and growth

Changes in ambient temperature represent the major environmental challenge to newborn mammals. An obligatory requirement to respond to warm or cold thermal stimuli in conjunction with the establishment of enteral feeding are potentially the most demanding challenges to metabolic homeostasis during postnatal life. Metabolic adaptation is not completed in the immediate neonatal period but continues over several weeks or months, depending on maturity at birth (Symonds & Lomax, 1992). The time course and extent of this process is linked to behavioural state and is highly influenced by sleep state organization (i.e. slow wave or non-REM sleep compared with rapid eye movement (REM) sleep) in both lambs in which non-REM sleep predominates (Andrews et al., 1990) and infants in which a greater proportion of sleep is REM (Azaz et al., 1992). Metabolic rate does decrease between wakefulness and sleep, although the preferred sleep state is that in which oxygen consumption is highest. Acute exposure to a cool ambient temperature is characterized by an increased amount of time spent in this particular sleep state, although in infants the magnitude of response decreases with age (Azaz et al., 1992).

Over the first two months of life, there is a fall in both the upper (above which panting occurs and is indicative of a heat losing state) and, to a greater extent, lower (below which oxygen consumption increases and is indicative of a heat producing state) critical temperatures bordering thermoneutrality (Symonds et al., 1989*b*). These developmental processes occur over the period in which plasma concentrations of triiodothyronine decrease, and brown adipose tissue adopts the characteristics of white adipose tissue to the extent that shivering rather than non-shivering thermogenesis is the dominant response to acute cold exposure during non-REM sleep (Symonds et al., 1989*b*, 1992). As a consequence of these adaptations there is a widening of the thermoneutral zone, decrease in minimal metabolic rate, improved thermal efficiency and increase in body temperature (Fig. 5.4). The rate at which these developments proceed is dependent on the ambient temperature in which an individual is reared, and can be accelerated by rearing in a warm environment and hypothyroidism (Fig. 5.4). Continuous warm exposure, plus hypothyroidism, has a pronounced inhibitory effect on metabolic rate and body temperature, although these conditions have less influence on the thermogenic activity of brown adipose tissue. There is, however, increasing evidence to indicate that hypothyroidism in warm-reared lambs results in a chronic impairment in metabolism that is symptomatic with a failure to thrive and unexpected death during postnatal life (Symonds, Andrews & Johnson, 1989*b*; Symonds et al., 1994*a*).

Developmental changes in the control of metabolism not only influence the partitioning of nutrients between requirements for thermoregulation and growth but also have a large impact on breathing control.

Fig. 5.3. Comparison of artificial rearing with ewe rearing of lambs on metabolism and growth over the first month of postnatal life. Lambs were either artificially reared at a low (200 g/day, ■, ($n = 7$)) or high level (320 g/day, ▨, ($n = 7$)) of milk replacer (Volac Lamlac, Royston, Herts) or reared with their ewe (□, ($n = 8$)) at similar ambient temperatures (5–15 °C). Jugular venous blood samples were taken at 31 days of age, after which lambs were humanely killed for sampling of liver and perirenal adipose tissue. Values are means ± S.E.M. I 5′D = iodothyronine 5′deiodinase. For perirenal adipose tissue weight, inserted histograms and error bars are for lipid weight, and for I 5′D activity, inserted histograms and error bars are for type II enzyme activity. (Adapted from Darby et al., 1994 and Symonds, unpublished.)

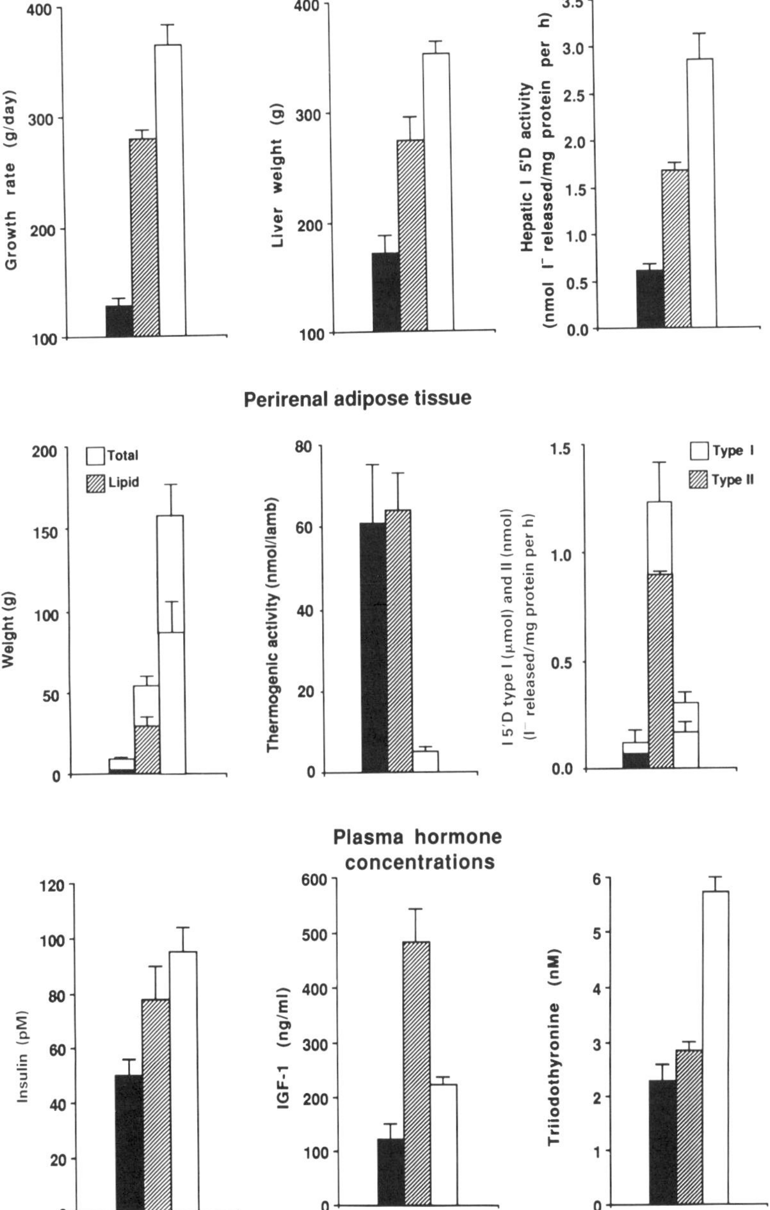
Growth rate (g/day)
Liver weight (g)
Hepatic I 5'D activity
(nmol I⁻ released/mg protein per h)
Perirenal adipose tissue
Total
Lipid
Weight (g)
Thermogenic activity (nmol/lamb)
Type I
Type II
I 5'D type I (μmol) and II (nmol)
(I⁻ released/mg protein per h)
Plasma hormone concentrations
Insulin (pM)
IGF-1 (ng/ml)
Triiodothyronine (nM)

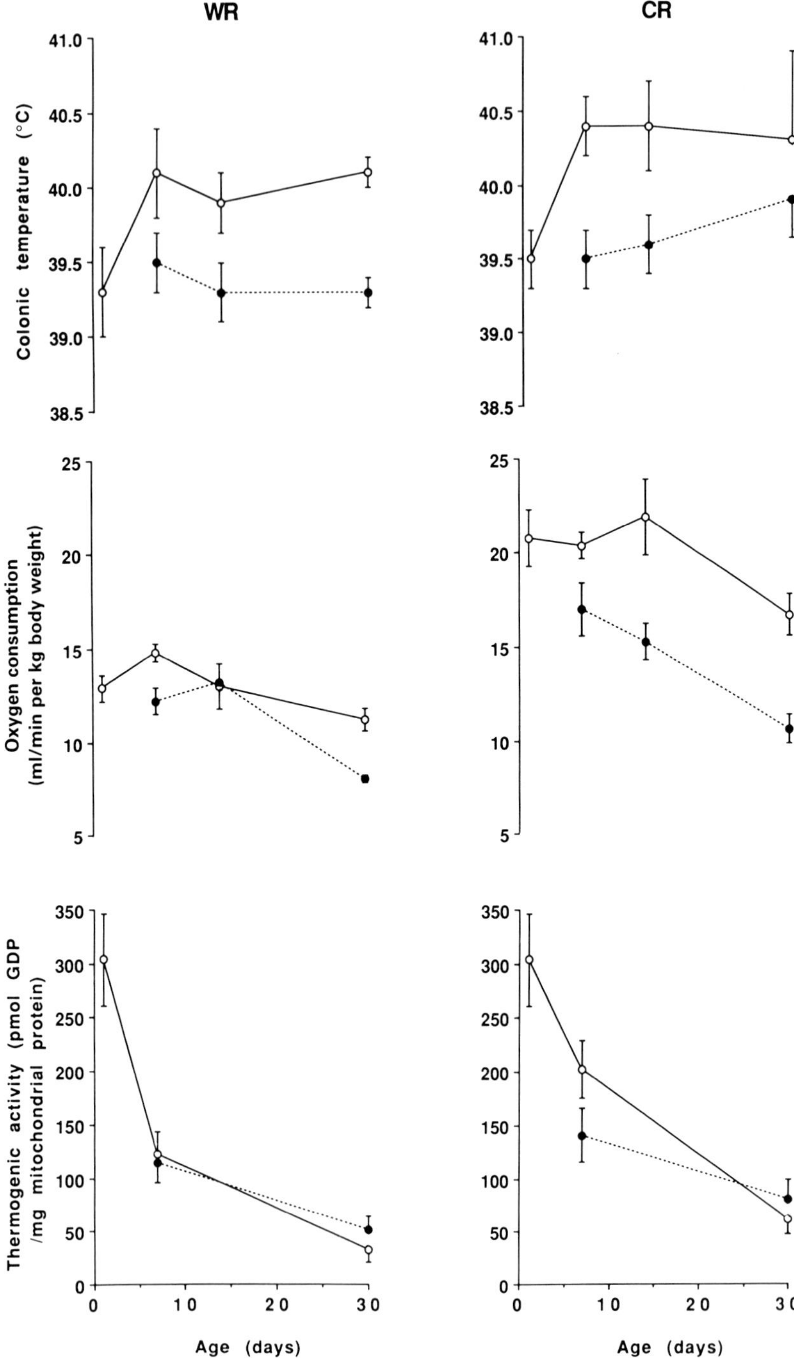
WR
CR
Colonic temperature (°C)
41.0
40.5
40.0
39.5
39.0
38.5
Oxygen consumption
(ml/min per kg body weight)
25
20
15
10
5
Thermogenic activity (pmol GDP
/mg mitochondrial protein)
350
300
250
200
150
100
50
0
0
10
20
30
Age (days)

This is because the decrease in oxygen requirements (per kg body weight) with increasing age and ambient temperature are associated with both a fall in breathing frequency and lengthening of expiratory time (Symonds et al., 1993). It is therefore when metabolic and breathing rates are both minimal that a marked recruitment of laryngeal 'braking' of expiratory airflow occurs. The use of this mechanism is important not only in maximizing oxygen exchange across the lung but also in maintaining breathing rhymicity. There is now strong evidence indicating that development of both thermoregulatory and breathing control mechanisms is not only determined by the postnatal environment, but is highly influenced by the maternal metabolic and hormonal status prenatally (Symonds et al., 1992, 1993). Chronic maternal undernutrition over the final month of gestation can result in a neonate with reduced brown and white adipose tissue stores plus a failure to exhibit the predicted recruitment of laryngeal braking during later life (Symonds et al., 1993).

It must be noted when considering current in vivo research on neonatal metabolism that many studies have been conducted in either anaesthetized or restrained animals and on individuals which are deprived of their mother whilst studies are conducted. These factors are being shown to be of increasing importance when considering neonatal development, because there is strong evidence of entrainment of sleep cycles and therefore of metabolic and breathing control between mother and offspring (McKenna et al., 1990). It must be remembered that the normal practice is for parents and offspring of most mammalian species to feed and sleep together, and it is only in very recent times that infants have been allowed to sleep in isolation. This practice may be of benefit to clinicians and basic scientists but it goes against the evolution of physiological control mechanisms over the past 4 million years (McKenna et al., 1990). In terms of metabolism and growth of an individual in the developed world, there is a strong case that the failure to adhere to the once accepted practices of co-sleeping and breast feeding has resulted in an increased

---

Fig. 5.4. Effect of ambient temperature and hypothyroidism on metabolic adaptation in the developing lamb. Twin lambs were either reared artificially in a warm (25 °C; WR) or cool (days 1–14 15 °C; days 15–30 10 °C; CR) ambient temperature and measurements of oxygen consumption and colonic temperature made during non-rapid eye movement sleep at an ambient temperature close to their rearing temperature. Lambs were either euthyroid controls (○) or made hypothyroid (●) by administration of an oral, daily dose of methimazole (50 mg/kg body weight). Values are means ± S.E.M. (n = 7 at each time point, with exception of hypothyroid lambs reared in the warm when n = 5).

incidence of respiratory disorders, allergic conditions plus the occurrence of sudden infant death syndrome (Mepham, 1989).

Conclusions

The ability of the neonate to adapt effectively to changes in nutrient supply, ambient temperature and parental stimulation has a large impact on metabolism and growth. In recent years many current clinical practices have dramatically increased the number of Caesarean section deliveries, survival of premature babies and the success rate from in vitro fertilization. All these manipulations are likely to result in specific neuroendocrine adaptations which could have long-term consequences on growth and development. It is therefore important that careful consideration of developmental changes in metabolism and tissue growth is taken into account when management strategies aimed at ensuring survival and well-being during neonatal and postnatal life are planned.

Acknowledgements

The author would like to thank the Wellcome Trust, AFRC, MRC and MAFF for their support. A gift of rabbit anti-IGF-I antisera (No. UB3–189) was made by NIDDK, National Institutes of Health and the National Hormone and Pituitary Program, University of Maryland School of Medicine, Baltimore, MD, USA.

References

Andrews, D.C., Ball, N.J., Symonds, M.E., Vojeck, L. & Johnson, P. (1990). The effect of ambient temperature and age on sleep state in developing lambs. In *Sleep*, ed. J. Horne. pp. 115–19. Pentenagel, Bochum.

Azaz, Y., Fleming, P.J., Levine, M., McCabe, R. Stewart, A. & Johnson, P. (1992). The relationship between environmental temperature, metabolic rate, sleep state and evaporative water loss in infants from birth to three months. *Paediatric Research*, **32**, 417–23.

Barker, D.P. (1992). The effect of nutrition of the fetus and neonate on cardiovascular disease in adult life. *Proceedings of the Nutrition Society*, **51**, 135–44.

Bassett, J.M. (1992). The endocrine regulation of growth during early life: a nutritional perspective. In *Neonatal Survival and Growth, Occasional Publication No. 15 – British Society of Animal Production,* ed. M.A. Varley, P.E.V. Williams & T.L.J. Lawrence. pp. 47–62. BSAP, Edinburgh.

Bassett, J.M., Madhill, D., Burks, A.H. & Pinches, R.A. (1982). Glucagon and insulin release in the lamb before and after birth: effects of amino acids in vitro and in vivo. *Journal of Developmental Physiology*, **4**, 379–89.
Bell, A.W. (1992). Foetal growth and its influence on postnatal growth and development. In *The Control of Fat and Lean Deposition*, ed. P.J. Buttery, K.N. Boorman & D.B. Lindsay. pp. 111–27. Butterworth-Heinemann Ltd, Oxford.
Cannon, B. & Nedergaard, J. (1985). The biochemistry of an inefficient tissue: brown adipose tissue. *Essays in Biochemistry*, **20**, 110–64.
Casey, C.E. (1989). The nutritive and metabolic advantages of homologous milk. *Proceedings of the Nutrition Society*, **48**, 271–81.
Casteilla, L., Champigny, O., Bouilland, F., Robelin, J. & Ricquier, D. (1989). Sequential changes in the expression of mitochondrial protein mRNA during the development of brown adipose tissue in bovine and ovine species. *Biochemical Journal*, **257**, 665–71.
Christensson, K., Siles, C., Cabrera, T., Belaustequi, A., Fuente, P. De La, Lagercrantz, H., Puyol, P. & Winberg, J. (1993). Lower body temperatures in infants delivered by Caesarean section than vaginally delivered infants. *Acta Paediatrica*, **82**, 128–31.
Christensson, K., Siles, C., Moreno, L., Fuente, P De La, Lagercrantz, H., Puyol, P. & Winberg, J. (1992). Temperature, metabolic adaptation and crying in healthy full-term newborns cared for skin-to-skin or in a cot. *Acta Paediatrica*, **81**, 488–93.
Clarke, L. (1994). Manipulation and control of thermoregulation in the newborn lamb. PhD Thesis. University of Reading, UK.
Clarke, L., Darby, C.J., Lomax, M.A. & Symonds, M.E. (1994). Effect of ambient temperature during the first day of life on thermoregulation in neonatal lambs delivered by Caesarean section. *Journal of Applied Physiology*, 1481–8.
Daly, S.J., Owens, R.A. & Hartmann, P.E. (1993). The short-term synthesis and infant-regulated removal of milk in lactating women. *Experimental Physiology*, **78**, 209–20.
Darby, C.J., Clarke, L., Lomax, M.A. & Symonds, M.E. (1994). Brown adipose tissue and liver development during early postnatal life in hand-reared and ewe-reared lambs. *Journal of Developmental Physiology* (in press).
Eliot, R.J., Klein, A.H., Glatz, T.H., Nathanielsz, P.W. & Fisher, D.A. (1981). Plasma norepinephrine, epinephrine and dopamine concentrations in maternal and fetal sheep during spontaneous parturition and in premature sheep during cortisol-induced parturition. *Endocrinology*, **108**, 1678–82.
Giralt, M., Martin, J., Iglesias, R., Vinars, O., Villarroya, F. & Mampel, T. (1990). Ontogeny and perinatal modulation of gene expression in rat brown adipose tissue. *European Journal of Biochemistry*, **193**, 297–302.
Girard, J., Ferre, P., Pegorier, J.P. and Duee, P.H. (1992). Adaptations of glucose and fatty acid metabolism during perinatal period and suckling–weaning transition. *Physiological Reviews*, **72**, 507–62.
Gluckman, P.D., Gunn, T.R., Johnston, B.M. & Quinn, J.P. (1984). Manipulation of the temperature of the fetal lamb in utero. In *Animal Models in Fetal Medicine*, ed. P.W. Nathanielsz. pp. 37–56. Perinatology Press, New York.
Gunn, T.R., Ball, K.T. & Gluckman, P.D. (1993). Withdrawal of placental

prostaglandins permits thermogenic responses in fetal sheep brown adipose tissue. *Journal of Applied Physiology*, **74**, 998–1004.

Heinig, M.J., Nommsen, L.A., Peerson, J.M., Lonnerdal, B. & Davey, K.G. (1993). Energy and protein intakes of breast-fed and formula-fed infants during the first year of life and their association with growth velocity: the DARLING study. *American Journal of Clinical Nutrition*, **58**, 152–61.

Herpin, P., Le Dividich, J. & Van Os, M. (1992). Contribution of colostral fat to thermogenesis and glucose homeostasis in the newborn pig. *Journal of Developmental Physiology*, **17**, 131–41.

Houstek, J., Vizek, K., Pavelka, S., Kopecky, J., Krejcova, E., Hermanska, J. & Cermakova, M. (1993). Type II iodothyronine 5′-deiodinase and uncoupling protein in brown adipose tissue of human newborns. *Journal of Clinical Endocrinology and Metabolism*, **77**, 382–7.

Jansen, A.H. & Chernick, V. (1991). Fetal breathing and development of control of breathing. *Journal of Applied Physiology*, **70**, 1431–46.

Johnston, B.M., Gunn, T.R. & Gluckman, P.D. (1988). Surface cooling rapidly induces coordinated activity in the upper and lower airway muscles of the fetal lamb in utero. *Pediatric Research*, **23**, 257–61.

Klaus, S., Casteilla, L., Bouilland, F. & Ricquier, D. (1991). The uncoupling protein UCP: a membraneous mitochondrial ion carrier exclusively expressed in brown adipose tissue. *International Journal of Biochemistry*, **23**, 791–801.

McKenna, J.J., Mosko, S., Dungy, C. & McAninch, J. (1990). Sleep and arousal patterns of co-sleeping human mother/infant pairs: a preliminary physiological study with implications for the study of sudden infant death syndrome (SIDS). *American Journal of Physical Anthropology*, **83**, 331–47.

Mellor, D.J. & Cockburn, F. (1986). A comparison of energy metabolism in the new-born infant, piglet and lamb. *Quarterly Journal of Experimental Physiology*, **71**, 361–79.

Mepham, T.B. (1989). Science and the politics of breastfeeding: birthright or birth rite? *Science and Public Policy*, **16**, 181–91.

Nedergaard, J., Connolly, E. & Cannon, B. (1986). Brown adipose tissue in the mammalian neonate. In *Brown Adipose Tissue*, ed. P. Trayhurn. pp. 152–213. Edward Arnold, London.

Power, G.G. (1989). Biology of temperature: the mammalian fetus. *Journal of Developmental Physiology*, **12**, 295–304.

Salmenpera, L. Perheentupa, J., Silmes, M.A., Adrian, T.E., Bloom, S.R. & Aynsley-Green, A. (1988). Effects of feeding regimen on blood glucose levels and plasma concentrations of pancreatic hormones and gut regulatory peptides at 9 months of age: comparison between infants fed with milk formula and infants exclusively breast-fed from birth. *Journal of Pediatric Gastroenterology and Nutrition*, **7**, 651–6.

Smales, O.R.C. & Kime, R. (1978). Thermoregulation in babies immediately after birth. *Archives of Diseases in Childhood*, **53**, 58–61.

Sperling, M.A., Ganguli, S., Leslie, N. & Landt, K. (1984). Fetal–perinatal catecholamine secretion: role in perinatal glucose homeostasis. *American Journal of Physiology*, **247**, E69–74.

Symonds, M.E., Andrews, D.C. & Johnson, P. (1989*a*). The endocrine and metabolic response to feeding in the developing lamb. *Journal of Endocrinology*, **123**, 295–302.

Symonds, M.E., Andrews, D.C. & Johnson, P. (1989*b*). The control of thermoregulation in the developing lamb during slow wave sleep. *Journal of Developmental Physiology*, **11**, 289–98.

Symonds, M.E., Bird, J.A., Clarke, L., Darby, C.J., Gate, J.J. & Lomax, M.A. (1994*c*). Nutrition, temperature and homeostasis during perinatal development. *Journal of Developmental Physiology* (in press).

Symonds, M.E., Bird, J.A., Clarke, L., Darby, C.J., Gate, J.J. & Lomax, M.A. (1994*b*). Manipulation of brown adipose tissue development in neonatal and postnatal lambs. In *Temperature Regulation*, ed. A.S. Milton. pp. 309–314. Birkhauser, Switzerland.

Symonds, M.E., Bryant, M.J., Clarke, L., Darby, C.J. & Lomax, M.A. (1992). Effect of maternal cold exposure on brown adipose tissue and thermogenesis in the neonatal lamb. *Journal of Physiology*, **455**, 487–502.

Symonds, M.E., Clarke, L., & Lomax, M.A. (1994*a*). The regulation of neonatal metabolism and growth. In *Early Fetal Growth and Development, Proceedings of the Twenty-seventh Study Group of the Royal College of Obstetricians and Gynaecologists*, ed. D. Donnai, S.K. Smith & R.H.T. Ward. pp. 407–19. RCOG, London.

Symonds, M.E. & Lomax, M.A. (1992). Maternal and environmental influences on thermoregulation in the neonate. *Proceedings of the Nutrition Society*, **51**, 165–72.

Symonds, M.E. & Lomax, M.A. (1993). Brown adipose tissue and the control of thermoregulation in the developing infant during sleep. In *Proceedings of the Second Sudden Infant Death Syndrome Family International Conference*, ed. A.M. Walker, C. McMillen, D. Barnes, K. Fitzgerald & M. Willinger. pp. 208–11. Perinatology Press, USA.

Symonds, M.E. Lomax, M.A., Kenward, M.G., Andrews, D.C. & Johnson, P. (1993). Effect of the prenatal maternal environment on the control of breathing during non-rapid eye movement sleep in the developing lamb. *Journal of Developmental Physiology*, **19**, 43–50.

Weaver, L.T. (1992). Breast and gut: the relationship between lactating mammary function and neonatal gastrointestinal function. *Proceedings of the Nutrition Society*, **51**, 155–63.

Whyte, R.K. & Bayley, H.S. (1990). Energy metabolism of the newborn infant. In *Advances in Nutritional Research, Vol. 8*. ed. H.H. Draper. pp. 79–108. Plenum Press, New York.

Part Two

Pathophysiology

6

Experimental restriction of fetal growth

JULIE A. OWENS, P.C. OWENS and
JEFFREY S. ROBINSON

Introduction

Restricted fetal growth is common in human pregnancy and is associated with increased perinatal morbidity and mortality and an increased risk of adverse outcomes in later life. Similarly, restricted fetal growth in domestic animals results in poor perinatal outcome and reduced productivity. The term 'restricted fetal growth' is used increasingly in preference to 'intrauterine growth retardation', since the latter has unfortunate connotations for consumers of health services. To prevent, diagnose and treat restricted fetal growth successfully, greater understanding of its origins and consequences, as well as careful evaluation of potential therapeutic strategies, is needed. The study of experimental restriction of fetal growth in animals is an essential element in obtaining this knowledge.

Experimentally, the approaches used to restrict fetal growth in animals reflect the different questions being asked. Some are devised to mimic known or suspected causes of naturally occurring fetal growth restriction, to determine if such factors are involved causatively by imposing them for varying periods at different stages of development. Some perturbations can be produced chronically, and are used to examine the consequences for the individual in the medium to long term. Yet others are designed to identify/delineate the specific physiological, cellular and molecular mechanisms by which perturbations restrict growth and alter development of key fetal organs and tissues.

This chapter will document these varied approaches and put them into the context of our current understanding of human and animal fetal growth restriction. The consequences of experimental restriction of fetal growth and their relevance to the human condition have been reviewed previously and referenced in detail (Owens, Owens & Robinson, 1989*b*; Owens, 1991; Thorburn & Harding, 1994; Robinson, Owens & Owens,

1994). This chapter summarizes that information and extends to new questions to be addressed by the study of experimental fetal growth restriction – i.e. the long-term consequences for the adult of intrauterine perturbation, which include an increased risk of certain adult onset diseases (Barker, 1994), and the consequences of perturbation of the early embryonic environment for subsequent development.

Restricted fetal growth in the human: origins, phenotypes and outcomes

Origins

Many conditions are associated with human fetal growth restriction (Table 6.1). Some are intrinsic, that is, originating or acting from within the fetus, while others are extrinsic and include different aspects of the maternal environment and the state of the mother herself or of the placenta (Table 6.1). Many of these extrinsic conditions are characterized by physiological or pathophysiological changes, consistent with reduced delivery of essential substrates to the fetus, either as a result of their reduced abundance within the mother or due to impaired placental development and function (Table 6.2). The major substrates for fetal growth and development are oxygen, glucose, lactate and amino acids in all mammalian species studied so far (Fowden, 1994). Other substances are required but in lesser amounts, including lipids and ketone bodies and a variety of micronutrients. Fetal growth and development are largely determined by the interaction between genome and the availability of these substrates, which are essential for growth. The placenta, in turn, is a major determinant of substrate availability within the fetus, because of (a) its substrate transfer functions, (b) its high metabolic rate, which makes it a significant competitor with the fetus for those substrates, (c) its modification of nutrients and (d) cycling of substrates with the fetus (Hay & Wilkening, 1994). In addition, the placenta elaborates a variety of hormones and factors into the fetus and mother, to coordinate and influence their metabolic and physiological adaptation during pregnancy. In human fetal growth restriction, even apparently diverse extrinsic conditions may act by a final common mechanism: restriction of the delivery of essential substrates to the fetus. Intrinsic factors may act by limiting the ability of fetal cells and tissues to utilize substrates, even when provided in sufficient abundance.

Table 6.1. *Conditions associated with human fetal growth restriction*

Intrinsic			
Fetal factors:			
Intrauterine infections			
Chromosomal mosaicism			
Chromosomal anomalies			
Congenital malformations			
Inborn errors of metabolism			
Anaemia (Rh disease)			
Extrinsic			
Environmental factors:	Maternal factors:	Placental factors:	Other factors:
High altitude	Undernutrition (including anorexia)	Abnormalities:	Reproductive technologies
Variable nutrition	Low maternal weight gain	Chromosomal mosaicism	
Pollution	Maternal age 16<	Infarcts, focal lesions	
Hyperthermia	Drug use	Abnormal placentation	
Irradiation	Smoking		
	Alcohol		
	Illicit drugs		
	Low socio-economic status		
	Medical complications:		
	Acute or chronic hypertension		
	Antepartum haemorrhage		
	Severe chronic infections		
	Anaemia		
	Disseminated lupus erythematosus		
	Lupus obstetric syndrome		
	Malignancy		
	Abnormalities of the uterus		
	Uterine fibroids		

Table 6.2. *Human fetal growth restriction: Initiating causes, sites of action, short- and long-term consequences*

INITIATING CAUSES **Sites of Action**	CONSEQUENCES FOR THE PLACENTA: **Growth and Functional Development**	CONSEQUENCES FOR THE FETUS: **Metabolism and Endocrinology**	 **Growth and Development**
Maternal: Reduced substrate availability: oxygen calorie deficiency protein-calorie deficiency micronutient deficiency mineral deficiency (iron, iodine)	Reduced delivery of substrates to the placenta Altered placental development (including placentomegaly)	***In utero*:** Hypoxaemia, hypercapnia, hypoglycaemia, acidosis, hypoaminoacidaemia, (essential amino acids); increased blood alanine, lactate, triglycerides Reduced plasma insulin, thyroid hormones, IGF-I, ACTH; increased plasma cortisol, IGFBP-1 **Perinatal:** Asphyxia, acidosis, hypoglycaemia	***In utero*:** Normal then arrested growth velocity, normal or low birthweight, low ponderal index (< 10 percentile), soft tissue wasting **Perinatal:** Increased morbidity and mortality, catch-up growth **Adult:** Increased risk of cardiovascular disease, hypertension, hyperlipidaemia, non-insulin-dependent diabetes
Placental Defective placentation Placental damage	Reduced placental volume, weight Reduced surface area for exchange of bood solutes Reduced uterine and/or umbilical blood flows Reduced placental clearance of solutes Increased resistance in umbilical and uterine circulations Early maturation or slowing of growth Failure of normal ontogenic changes in perfusion, resistance, surface area		
Fetal Chromosomal mosaicism Reduced cell proliferation Reduced cardiac output Absence of glands/ organs providing anabolic drive to growth	Reduced substrate acquisition and delivery to fetal tissues	***In utero*:** Increased inhibitory/ decreased stimulatory drive to growth?	***In utero*:** Low growth velocity, low birthweight (<10 percentile), normal ponderal index, reduced cell numbers in tissues **Perinatal:** No catch-up growth

Phenotype and outcomes

Human fetal growth has been characterized using a range of anthropometric measures, including birthweight, length, head circumference and body proportions, as indicated by ponderal index (weight (g) × 100/length^3) or birthweight to length ratio. The consequences of perturbation in utero for the human have usually been described as varying in terms of phenotype and outcome, with two main patterns apparent: primary and secondary intrauterine growth restriction (Fay & Ellwood, 1993). These types of altered fetal growth have been distinguished on the basis of birthweight and body proportions and described as differing in terms of their short- and long-term outcomes and as to whether they originate from perturbation within the fetus or outside it or in the timing of the perturbation (Fay & Ellwood, 1993; Robinson et al., 1994). Primary growth restriction has been defined by a low birthweight for gestational age (<10th percentile), but a normal ponderal index, reflecting a uniform or symmetrical reduction in growth. Secondary growth restriction is characterized by reduced birthweight and low ponderal index (<10th percentile) or asymmetric growth restriction. However, the limitations of data supporting this long held view have led to a re-examination of the patterns of human fetal growth. In one recent study of a large cohort of infants, for whom gestational age was independently and accurately determined, no evidence for the existence of two distinct subtypes of fetal growth restriction could be found (Kramer et al., 1989). Rather, fetal growth restriction was usually found to be disproportionate with increased length and head circumference for weight and increased variability in body proportions. Disproportionality was just as evident at earlier gestational ages as at term and post term, and increased with severity of fetal growth restriction (Kramer *et al.*, 1990). Thus, human fetal growth restriction may well be largely disproportionate, regardless of timing of onset.

Infants described as being symmetrically growth restricted appear well nourished and rarely show evidence of asphyxia (Fay & Ellwood, 1993). This suggests that the cause is constitutive or inherent to the fetus. Many such infants may, in fact, be normally grown with a genetically low drive to growth, or in some cases, incorrectly dated in terms of gestational age. Some may also result from either genetic or metabolic abnormality or the direct action on the fetus of an external agent, such as infection, without the involvement of pathology in other systems such as the mother or placenta. Many of these factors will exert their influence from early in gestation. These infants have normal rates of perinatal morbidity and mortality, unless chromosomal abnormalities are present, but have significantly lower than normal scores on parameters of mental development. Limited data available suggest that these infants are at greater risk of spastic cerebral palsy. Such infants commonly fail to undergo catch-up growth and remain smaller and lighter, with smaller head circumferences, for up to at least four years of age, which is also consistent with a low drive to growth. Further studies, particularly in populations exposed to chronically adverse environments, are needed to determine if human fetal growth restriction can be symmetrical or uniform as well as disproportionate and if so, the factors responsible (Kramer et al., 1990).

Asymmetrically growth-restricted infants have relative sparing of brain growth while liver and lymphoid tissues are disproportionately reduced in size (Naeye, 1965; Brooke, Wood & Butters, 1984). They appear thin or wasted and are relatively long for their weights, as indicated by their anthropometric measurements. Infants with this type of fetal growth restriction have a higher incidence of perinatal morbidity and mortality, including asphyxia during labour and acidosis, hypoglycaemia and hypothermia after birth (Fay & Ellwood, 1993). In addition, small size and disproportionate growth at birth are associated with increased risk of death from cardiovascular diseases and of non-insulin dependent diabetes, hypertension and hyperlipidaemia (Barker, 1994). However, such infants often undergo catch-up growth postnatally, with rates of growth in the first month or months of life that are greater than those of infants who are symmetrically small and, in some studies, greater than those of normally grown infants. Catch-up growth reduces the risk of neurological handicap and the later onset in the adult of the diseases described above.

Disproportionate fetal growth restriction appears to result from the arrest of normal growth at any stage of pregnancy, although it is often described as being of late onset. Because the infants appear malnourished, the primary cause is presumed to be restriction of the supply of essential substrates, particularly nutrients. In the large study referred to previously (Kramer et al., 1990), fetuses with tall mothers or pregnancy-related hypertension and male fetuses tended to be disproportionately grown, but these factors could account for only a small proportion of the variation in growth pattern. The influence of placental size on fetal growth or growth pattern was not evaluated. However, in other large studies, placental weight was highly correlated with birthweight and birth length (Karlberg, Albertsson-Wikland & Lawrence, 1994). In smaller studies, disproportionate fetal growth restriction was often associated with an abnormal or a small placenta, often with signs of ischaemia and infarction.

Normally, major reductions in the placental barrier to diffusion of oxygen, and presumably of other substances, between maternal and fetal blood occur in the human and other species with advancing gestation (Mayhew, Jackson & Boyd, 1993). The harmonic mean thicknesses of membranes, which these substances must traverse from maternal to fetal blood, decrease, and the areas of surfaces responsible for exchange (syncytiotrophoblast, fetal endothelium) and vascular space volumes increase, particularly in the second half of gestation. The rates of umbilical and uterine blood flow increase greatly throughout gestation, paralleling these vascular changes. Placental glucose transport capacity increases substantially during the second half of pregnancy, owing to an increase in transporter protein number rather than affinity, and may be accounted for largely by the increase in surface area of villi that occurs concomitantly (Hay & Wilkening, 1994). Failure of such ontogenic structural and physiological changes to occur may contribute to fetal growth restriction.

Reduced placental weight, volume, exchange surface area, perfusion and clearance have been found in association with secondary or disproportionate fetal growth restriction (Owens et al., 1989*b*). Transport of mannitol and of the branched chain amino acids, leucine and glycine, across the placenta of growth-restricted fetuses in vivo is reduced (Konje et al., 1994). Reduced transport of a non-metabolizable amino acid analogue, methylaminoisobutyric acid, occurs in vitro in vesicles of microvillous membranes prepared from placentae associated with fetal growth restriction (Dicke & Henderson, 1988; Mahendran et al., 1991). Abnormal maternal vasculature supplying the placenta also occurs, with and without pre-eclampsia. Defective second wave trophoblastic invasion resulting in failure of these vessels, the spiral arteries, to dilate is consistently found in pre-eclampsia (Khong et al., 1986) and is increasingly implicated in intrauterine growth restriction (Sheppard & Bonnar, 1988). While pre-eclampsia is associated with secondary fetal growth restriction, uncomplicated maternal hypertension in women does not reduce fetal growth and may even increase the surface area for exchange within the placenta. However, maternal conditions, such as pre-eclampsia and complicated hypertension (e.g. renal disease), are associated with poor prenatal growth and may exacerbate pre-existing placental damage or inadequacy.

Cordocentesis has enabled direct characterization of the metabolic and endocrine state of growth-restricted fetuses and their relationship to other parameters (Table 6.2) (Montemagno & Soothill, 1994, see chapter 8). However, a major confounding factor in studies utilizing this procedure may be that it perturbs the metabolic and endocrine parameters under study. A heterogeneous group characterized by a reduced abdominal circumference or birthweight, rather than body proportions, has been investigated in many studies utilizing cordocentesis. Nevertheless, various metabolic indices determined in this way indicate that deficient substrate supply occurs in fetal growth restriction and correlates with decreased blood flow velocity in the fetal descending aorta or increased resistance in umbilical and uterine arteries (Montemagno & Soothill, 1994). Fetal hypoxia and acidosis (often a mixed acidosis characterized by hypercapnia and lactic acidosis) are associated with increased resistance in uterine arteries or in the fetoplacental circulation. Some small fetuses are also hypoglycaemic, while their plasma concentrations of triglycerides are increased. Plasma levels of essential amino acids, particularly the branched chain amino acids, leucine, isoleucine and valine, as well as those of others, including serine, tyrosine, taurine and ornithine, are reduced in some small fetuses. Normally, the margin between placental delivery of leucine and phenylalanine and fetal utilization of these amino acids is small in the term human fetus, suggesting that any reduction in their supply will impact adversely on fetal protein accretion and growth, as well as fetal oxidative metabolism (Chien et al., 1993). The reduced circulating levels of these amino acids in small fetuses suggest that impaired supply of essential amino acids may have a role in the aetiology of restricted fetal growth. In contrast, levels of other non-essential amino acids, glycine and alanine are increased, but generally the picture resembles that of chronically undernourished protein-calorie-deprived children. Moreover, at term, measurement of the amino acid flux across the umbilical circulation, by cordocentesis at Caesarean delivery of human infants, shows a reversal of the normal pattern of uptake of amino acids in the growth-retarded fetus with, instead, a net loss of mainly the non-essential amino acids (Cetin et al., 1988; Hayashi et al., 1978).

These metabolic disturbances in small human fetuses are accompanied by a variety of endocrine changes with a reduction in the abundance of anabolic factors and an increase in the abundance of inhibitory or catabolic factors (Table 6.2) (Montemagno & Soothill, 1994). Fetal hypoinsulinaemia occurs, and to a greater extent than expected from the degree of hypoglycaemia present. Reduced concentrations of insulin-like growth factor-I (IGF-I; a major growth-promoting factor in the fetus)

(Lassarre et al., 1991) and increased concentrations of IGF-binding protein-1 (IGFBP-1; a binding protein which inhibits the stimulatory actions of IGF-I on glucose utilization) (Wang et al., 1991) also occur in the small fetus. Cortisol is increased, as is noradrenaline in small hypoxic fetuses. In some small fetuses, TSH is increased and thyroid hormones are decreased and are related to the extent of fetal hypoxaemia and acidaemia.

Since dispoportionate fetal growth restriction is characterized by perinatal hypoxaemia and hypoglycaemia, those small fetuses shown to have metabolic and endocrine disturbances in utero are thought to be suffering from growth restriction rather than being genetically small, but this requires further study. This also suggests that inadequate placentation, with consequently impaired placental function and reduced substrate supply to the fetus, causes fetal growth restriction. However, other extrinsic factors may also alter fetal growth through similar final mechanisms, such as maternal anaemia, altitude, and maternal undernutrition. By reducing the availability within the mother of substrates for transfer to the fetus by the placenta, all these conditions will cause deficits in oxygen or nutrients within the conceptus, whether or not they also impair placental functional development.

Other origins of fetal growth restriction

Recent studies suggest that external perturbation of the early or peri-implantation environment of the developing individual can alter fetal growth rate substantially for the remainder of gestation. Reproductive technology is associated with reduced birthweight in singleton human infants (Wang et al., 1994*a*), suggesting that disturbance of the early embryonic environment, either in vitro or as influenced by the hormonal manipulation of the mother, or in the population of women requiring such treatment, is adverse and results in restricted fetal growth. To date, much of the work on the importance of the early environment of the oocyte, zygote and developing embryo has focused on embryo survival as an outcome, rather than on longer-term growth and development.

Experimental restriction of fetal growth

Experimental interventions which influence or restrict fetal growth indirectly via maternal or placental manipulation are extrinsic to the fetus in nature (Table 6.3). These can be classified further according to the

Table 6.3. *Experimental restriction of fetal growth: interventions and sites of action*

Site of intervention	Species
Maternal	
Altered maternal substrate availability	
Maternal undernutrition:	Sheep, pig, rat, mouse
Protein-calorie deficiency	
Selected nutrient deficiency	
Micronutrient deficiency	
Maternal hypoxaemia:	Sheep, rat, guinea pig
altitude	
hypobaric hpoxaemia	
normobaric hypoxaemia	
reduced maternal fractional inspired oxygen content	
intratracheal nitrogen	
carbon monoxide	
anaemia	
methhaemoglobinaemia	
Maternal hypertension	Baboon, sheep, rat
Placental	
Reduction/restriction of placental growth	Sheep
Reduction in number of implantation sites (uterine/endometrial caruncles) prior to pregnancy by hemihysterectomy or carunclectomy	
Maternal hyperthermia	
Separation of placentomes during pregnancy	

Interference with uteroplacental vasculature	Sheep, monkey, guinea pig, rabbit, rat
Partial occlusion of uterine artery	
Embolization of uteroplacental circulation	
Ligation of interplacental vessels	
Ligation of uterine artery	
Interference with fetoplacental circulation	Sheep
Embolization via umbilical artery	
Fetal	
Viral infection	Mouse
Organ/gland ablation	Sheep, monkey
Hypophysectomy, hypothalamic-pituitary disconnection	
Thyroidectomy, radioactive iodine	
Pancreatectomy (surgical, chemical: streptozotocin)	
Nephrectomy	
Other:	Sheep
Banding ascending aorta	
Fistula	
Gene deletion:	Mouse
Insulin-like growth factor axis:	
IGF-I, IGF-II, type 1 receptor, type 2 receptor, IGFBPs	
c-jun	

basis of the initial insult employed: altered maternal substrate availability, interference with vasculature in either the uteroplacental or fetoplacental circulations and restriction or restraint of placental growth and development (Owens et al., 1989*b*). While the initial targets and nature of these interventions vary, their long-term consequences for fetal growth and outcome develop many common elements.

Practical limitations have meant that the majority of techniques used to restrict fetal growth experimentally in animals are extrinsic. Increasing application of molecular biology, particularly of transgenesis and null mutations, has meant that the types of intrinsic interventions possible have expanded, as has our ability to examine the role of specific elements in the mechanisms by which fetal growth is restricted. Various species have been used in the study of fetal growth restriction, each offering different advantages, as well as disadvantages. The sheep has been extensively utilized, by virtue of its size, docility and tolerance of chronic instrumentation, which allows invasive access to the fetus in the absence of anaesthesia and with minimal stress, and hence it will be the focus here. While many elements of reproduction are common to most mammalian species, important differences in maternal adaptation to pregnancy, in the developmental patterns of key systems and in placentation, do exist. These differences, or the potential for them, must be understood in comparative studies of early development.

Substrate delivery and growth: responses to experimental intervention

The ontogeny of fetal growth and development differs from that of the placenta (Fig. 6.1). In terms of mass, placental growth occurs largely in the first half of gestation, whereas most fetal growth takes place in the last third of gestation. Extensive placental structural remodelling and development, which occur during the second half of gestation, enhance placental substrate transfer function to meet the increasing demands of the much larger fetus (Hay & Wilkening, 1994). Unsurprisingly, the responses of the fetus and placenta to perturbation vary with the stage of gestation at which it is imposed. The consequences for specific tissues will depend in part on the developmental stage and processes active when perturbation is experienced – morphogenesis, growth (hyperplasia and hypertrophy) or maturation/ differentiation.

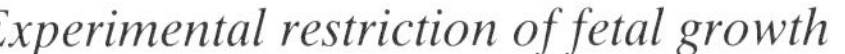

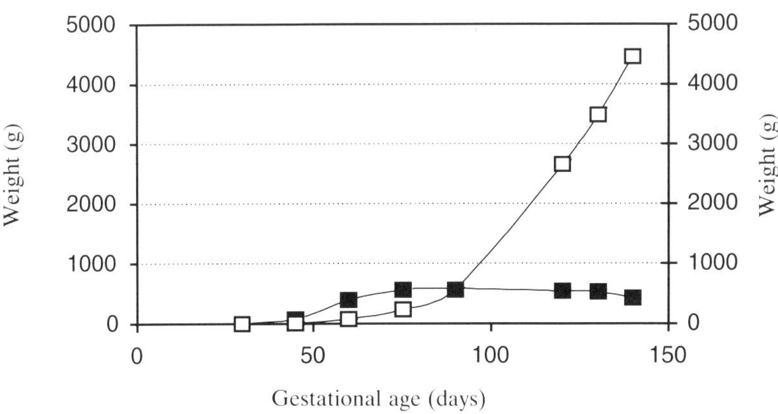

Fig. 6.1. Ontogeny of placental and fetal growth in sheep. Placental (■) and fetal (□) weight between days 30 and 140 of gestation (Owens, DeBarro & Robinson, unpublished data).

Intervention in the mother

Maternal substrate deprivation reduces the rate of delivery of substrates to the uterus for transfer by the placenta to the fetus, by lowering their concentrations in maternal blood. Either chronic maternal hypoglycaemia or hypoxaemia alone can reduce fetal growth or birthweight in most species examined (Owens et al., 1989*b*). In sheep, moderate maternal undernutrition for most of gestation (maternal arterial glucose ~70% control), which reduces availability of the major fetal substrate, glucose, reduces fetal growth by approximately 30% (Mellor, 1983), while a comparable decrease in maternal oxygenation (chronic maternal hypobaric hypoxaemia) reduces fetal weight in late gestation by slightly less (Jacobs et al., 1988*c*). In sheep, placental weight is also reduced by chronic maternal hypoglycaemia or by chronic maternal hypoxaemia, but more variably. In other species, maternal undernutrition and hypoxaemia also reduce fetal growth and often placental growth (Winnick & Noble, 1966; Tapanainen et al., 1994). When undernutrition or hypobaric hypoxaemia are imposed only in the last third of gestation in sheep, fetal growth is restricted to almost the same degree as when limitations are imposed for most of pregnancy (Mellor, 1983; Jacobs et al., 1988*c*). In contrast, placental weight is less affected by perturbation in late gestation. Thus the fetus and placenta appear most susceptible to reduced substrate availability during periods of their most rapid growth in terms of mass: the first half of gestation for the placenta and late gestation for the fetus. However, the limitations of weight as an indicator of growth and development should be noted, both for the fetus as well as the placenta, where substantial changes in connective tissue content of fetal villi and weight (which occur with gestation and in response to perturbation), may obscure changes in other structural characteristics more directly related to function.

More specific deprivation of the mother of particular macro- and micronutrients has been imposed in other species, particularly the rat, where protein deprivation of the mother from before pregnancy reduces fetal weight and birthweight (Langley & Jackson, 1994). Interestingly, placental weight is usually increased by maternal protein deprivation and the resulting growth-restricted offspring with a large placenta goes on to develop hypertension postnatally (Langley & Jackson, 1994), as does this phenotype in human populations.

The spontaneously hypertensive rat (SHR) has reduced uteroplacental blood flow and delivers offspring which are small at birth and have large placentae (Erkadius et al., 1994*a*). Between mid- and late gestation, fetal and placental weight are reduced in SHR, suggesting that the restriction of fetal growth in this strain is a consequence of early impairment of placental development and function (Erkadius, Morgan & Nicolantonio, 1994*b*). Just before term, placental weight increases to above normal in the pregnant SHR. The mechanism by which late onset placentomegaly occurs in the pregnant SHR and its impact on placental function and subsequent development of the fetus are not known. Similarly, the extent to which genetic factors, as opposed to maternal influences via the uterine environment, are responsible for the development of hypertension in the offspring of SHR rats requires further study. Prolonged blockade of nitric oxide synthesis in pregnant rats, by continuous infusion with L-nitro-arginine, also produces chronic maternal hypertension and substantial fetal growth retardation (Molnar et al., 1994).

Reduced progesterone abundance, following ovulation in mice, retards subsequent embryonic growth (McRae, 1994). Conversely, excess progesterone in the first few days of pregnancy in sheep increases fetal weight (Kleeman, Walker & Seamark, 1995). Progesterone supplementation reduces embryo mortality and increases birthweight in overfed pigs, which have lower than normal peripheral progesterone levels (Parr et al., 1994). In vitro culture of sheep and cattle embryos (for longer periods than commonly used in human reproductive technology) increases fetal weight, birthweight and gestational length, compared to in vivo culture of embryos (Walker et al., 1992). In addition, growth of the viscera is enhanced disproportionately relative to skeletal growth in the fetus, following in vitro culture of ruminant embryos (Farin, Farin & Yang, 1994). Whether the mechanisms involved operate by reprogramming of subsequent growth and development at the embryonic stage or by some other pathway is not clear. In both cases, the selection or operative mechanism may be a mismatching of the zygote with its tubal or uterine environment. The potential contribution of perturbation of the early embryonic environment to fetal growth restriction, and the phenotype produced, needs further investigation.

Intervention in the placenta

Placental growth can be restricted from early in pregnancy in sheep by reducing the number of sites available for implantation prior to pregnancy (Robinson et al., 1979) or by subjecting the ewe to heat stress throughout mid-gestation (Bell, Wilkening & Meschia, 1987). When placental growth is restrained to less than half of normal in terms of weight in the sheep, fetal growth is reduced in late gestation and to a greater extent than is achieved by either chronic maternal oxygen or nutritional deprivation alone. Placentally restricted fetal sheep are chronically hypoxaemic and hypoglycaemic in late gestation (Robinson et al., 1979; Owens, Falconer & Robinson, 1987*a*, *b*). Restriction of placental growth reduces placental weight and various functional characteristics including the rates of umbilical and uterine blood flows and flow determined clearance of antipyrine or ethanol (Fig. 6.2) (Bell et al., 1987; Owens, Falconer & Robinson, 1986, 1987*c*). Restricted implantation also reduces the surface area of the exchange epithelia in the ovine placenta by late gestation (Chidzanja, Robinson & Owens, 1993). Placental transfer of antipyrine (blood flow determined), methyl-glucose (a non-metabolizable analogue of glucose) and of urea (a measure of permeablity) decreases with placental weight following restricted implantation and reduced placental delivery of both oxygen and glucose to the conceptus and fetus results (Fig. 6.3) (Owens et al., 1987*a*,*b*). When placental growth is restricted, consumption of these substrates by the gravid uterus and fetus decreases, but to a lesser extent than does their delivery, due to increased extraction (Fig. 6.3). While this compensatory response helps to maintain consumption by the conceptus and fetus, the margin of safety, between delivery and consumption or the demand for oxygen and glucose, is reduced as a consequence. Any increase in fetal

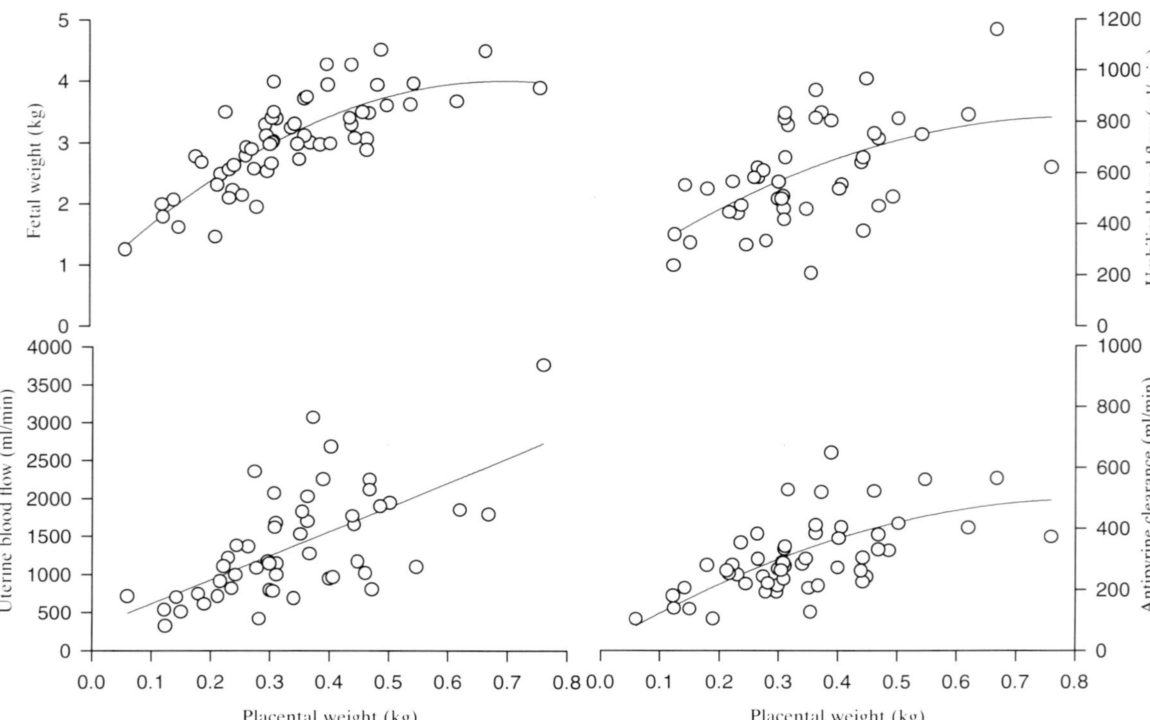

Fig. 6.2. Relationship between function and growth in the sheep placenta in late gestation. Some sheep were subjected to restriction of implantation by surgical removal of most placental implantation sites from the uterus prior to pregnancy. (Adapted from Owens et al., 1989*a*.)

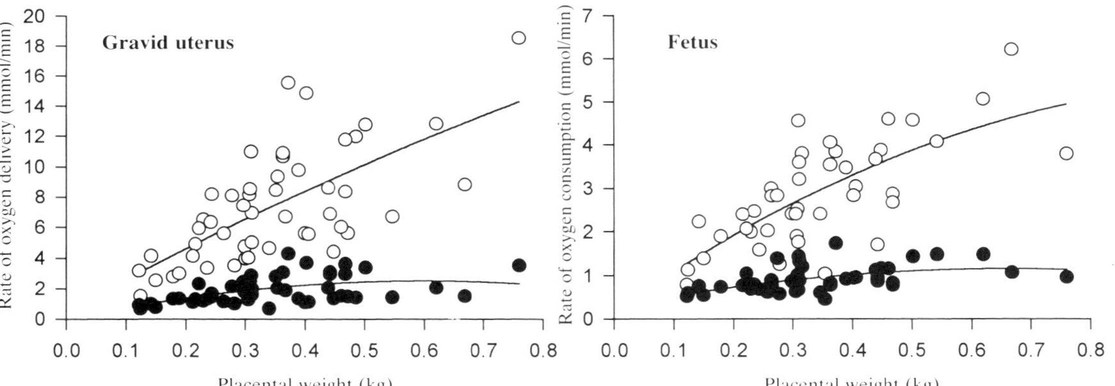

Fig. 6.3. Effect of restricting placental growth on oxygen delivery to (○) and consumption by (●) the gravid uterus and fetus in sheep in late gestation. Placental growth was restricted as described in Fig. 6.2. (Adapted from Owens et al., 1989*a*.)

demand, for example with fetal activity or change in fetal sleep state, or a decrease in delivery, such as reduced placental perfusion during contractions, may cause the reduced margin of safety to be exceeded. Continuous monitoring of oxygen saturation in placentally restricted and growth-retarded fetal sheep shows transient further reductions in oxygen saturation associated with fetal activity or uterine contractions (Robinson, Falconer & Owens, 1985). The consequences may be further altered development of, or damage to, key organs, or even fetal death.

Uteroplacental blood flow can be reduced chronically in sheep in late gestation by repetitive embolization of the uteroplacental circulation with microspheres (Charlton & Johengen, 1987). Maternal hyperthermia in late gestation also reduces maternal placental blood flow (Bell et al., 1987). These perturbations produce fetal hypoxaemia and hypoglycaemia, presumably by reducing uteroplacental perfusion initially and reducing placental size and functionality and, in turn, fetal growth eventually. In other species, such as rodents and primates, ligation of uterine arteries, spiral arterioles or interplacental vessels also reduces placental and fetal growth, usually in association with fetal hypoxaemia and hypoglycaemia (Owens et al., 1989*b*). Reduced placental transfer of oxygen, glucose and amino acid analogues is also found following uterine artery ligation in rats and guinea pigs, and results in fetal hypoxaemia, hypoglycaemia and fetal growth restriction (Jansson & Persson, 1990). Mechanical occlusion of a maternal iliac artery in the pregnant sheep in late gestation reduces uteroplacental blood flow and produces fetal hypoxaemia in the short term (Clark, Durnwald & Austin, 1982). In the longer term, mechanical reduction of uteroplacental perfusion in sheep retards fetal growth, but in the apparent absence of fetal hypoxaemia or hypoglycaemia. The mechanism by which this intervention restricts fetal growth is therefore unknown, but adverse effects on amino acid supply or placental production of growth-inhibitory substances have been proposed and are under investigation.

Embolization of the feto-placental circulation in sheep by repetitive administration of microspheres for ten days in late gestation increases resistance and reduces umbilical blood flow, but only in some studies does it reduce fetal weight (Trudinger et al., 1987; Gagnon et al., 1994). Fetal hypoxaemia and marginal hypoglycaemia develop, but their magnitude and the length of treatment may be too short to reduce growth consistently or substantially. In contrast, ligation of one umbilical artery in the fetal sheep, in mid-gestation, reduces fetal growth substantially, and in late gestation, can result in fetal death (Emmanoulides, Townsend

& Bauer, 1968). The difference in outcome for fetal growth and viability between these procedures may reflect differences in the magnitude of any resultant increase in resistance and reduction in umbilical blood flow, as well as the much more rapid time of onset of such changes in the latter intervention.

Intervention in the fetus

Congenital failure of growth and development of some fetal endocrine glands and organs is associated with reduced fetal growth in humans. Similarly, ablation of some tissues, but not others, in fetal sheep alters and restricts growth. In contrast to postnatal life, growth before birth appears to be largely growth hormone independent, but is clearly dependent on thyroid hormones and insulin which, in part, mediate the influence of oxygen and nutrient supply (Fowden, 1989). Removal of the pituitary of the fetal sheep in mid-gestation restricts growth of both somatic and skeletal tissues, particularly that of fetal thyroid, adrenals, heart and lungs, but not that of the brain and liver (Deayton, Young & Thorburn, 1993). Growth of the thyroid is reduced disproportionately, while that of the brain, liver and kidneys is relatively maintained. In contrast, hypophysectomy of fetal sheep in late gestation has little effect apart from a reduction in skeletal growth, retardation of skeletal maturation and an increase in fat deposition (Stevens & Alexander, 1986; Mesiano et al., 1987). Supplementation of hypophysectomized fetal sheep with a growth hormone extract prevented this accumulation of subcutaneous fat (Stevens & Alexander, 1986). This suggests that the hypothalamo-pituitary axis strongly influences early, but not late, fetal growth. Thyroidectomy in mid-gestation produces a similar pattern of fetal growth restriction to hypophysectomy (Hopkins & Thorburn, 1972), suggesting that the actions of the pituitary on fetal development may be mediated substantially through the thyroid hormone axis. Pancreatectomy of fetal sheep in late gestation causes proportionate restriction of fetal growth, except for relative maintenance of brain growth and disproportionate reduction in the growth of the spleen and thymus (Fowden, 1989). Generally, soft tissue growth is reduced to a greater extent than that of skeletal tissues by pancreatectomy. In contrast to these endocrine gland ablations, adrenalectomy has no obvious effect on fetal growth, although the adrenal and cortisol are clearly critical in maturation of fetal tissues and in the onset of parturition. Studies in which excess hormone has been delivered chronically to fetuses have generally found little evidence that thyroid hormone or growth hormone can accelerate fetal growth, while insulin supplementation does increase fat deposition and size of the liver, which appears to reflect accumulation of glycogen.

The insulin-like growth factor (IGF) family, IGF-I and IGF-II are polypeptide mitogens, are among the major growth factors controlling mammalian growth (Cohick & Clemmons, 1993). They differ from most other growth factors, in that they are able to act both locally and in an endocrine fashion. The actions of the IGFs are in turn, modulated by a family of six specific binding proteins (IGFBPs), which usually inhibit, but can also facilitate, their anabolic, mitogenic and differentiative activities on a wide variety of cell types and tissues. Both IGF-I and -II exert many of their actions via the type 1 receptor, while IGF-II can also bind to the type 2 receptor, the cation-independent mannose-6-phosphate lysosomal enzyme receptor. The IGFs are produced at multiple sites, although the liver has the highest abundance of IGF-I mRNA postnatally, and has been proposed as the major source of circulating IGF-I (Pell, Saunders & Gilmour, 1993). In fetal life, many extrahepatic tissues have a similar or greater abundance of IGF-I mRNA, and certainly of IGF-II mRNA, than the liver (Dickson, Saunders & Gilmour, 1991; O'Mahoney, Brandon & Adams, 1991). High concentrations of IGFs are found in fetal blood from early gestation, consistent with IGFs having endocrine actions in the fetus (Carr et al., 1995). Glucose availability controls IGF-I and -II levels in fetal blood, in the former case probably via insulin (Oliver et al., 1993). Less is known of the influence of oxygenation on IGFs in the fetus, but acute hypoxia also reduces circulating IGF-I in fetal sheep, while the impact on IGF-II is not known. Fetal hypophysectomy reduces circulating IGF-I, but not IGF-II, in fetal sheep in late gestation (Mesiano et al., 1989). Thyroid hormone replacement partially restored fetal plasma IGF-I levels in hypophysectomized fetal sheep, suggesting that pituitary-dependent factors, including thyroid hormone, regulate IGF-I in the fetus.

Determining the role of polypeptide growth factors in fetal growth has been more difficult owing to their production by multiple tissues, and has been made possible only by the use of gene deletion and identification of natural mutations. Surprisingly, the absence of many growth factors is associated with an apparently normal phenotype, presumably due to maternal rescue or redundancy (Ferguson, 1994). Exposure of such animals to perturbation may also be necessary for expression of any consequent abnormality. However, deletion of either or both of the genes for IGF-I and IGF-II, or the type 1 receptor, which mediates many of their actions, restricts fetal growth substantially (Liu et al., 1993; Baker et al., 1993). Retarded skeletal maturation and poor development of muscle, including the diaphragm, are also seen following deletion of the IGF-I gene in mice. Chronic IGF-I supplementation of fetal sheep in late gestation promotes growth of many organs and endocrine glands and accelerates maturation of skeletal tissues (Lok et al., 1993). Maternal inheritance of an inactivated type 2 receptor gene, which binds IGF-II and mannose-6-phosphate-containing ligands and which is maternally imprinted (paternal allele is silenced), increases fetal weight by 30%, but causes fetal death at term (Wang et al., 1994*a*). These responses are probably the result of excess IGF-II in the second half of gestation. Consistent with this is the finding that these mutant mice could be rescued by concomitant deletion of the IGF-II gene. In addition, these findings support the hypothesis of fetal growth being determined by the balance between maternal constraint of growth and paternal drive to growth through imprinting of the type 2 receptor and the IGF-II genes, respectively, at least in mice (Haig & Graham, 1991). Thus, both IGF-I and -II are needed for normal fetal growth and development, and may partly mediate the influence of substrate availability on growth. These responses to intervention within the fetus not only delineate the origins of very specific types of fetal growth restriction, but help to identify the molecular and cellular mechanisms or pathways by which extrinsic interventions and conditions alter fetal growth.

Naturally occurring mutations and gene targeting experiments in mice have identified factors and genes which are essential for appropriate placental growth and development (Cross, Werb & Fisher, 1994). Most of these are lethal, in that the absence of the factor or functional gene blocks a major event in placentation, from blastocyst formation and implantation, through to chorioallantoic development (Cross et al., 1994). Less extreme variations in the abundance of these critical factors, due either to genetic influences or extrinsic perturbations, may impair placental functional development and contribute to fetal growth restriction. Deletion of the gene for IGF-II is not lethal, but substantially reduces placental weight in mice from day 13 onwards (Baker et al., 1993). This contrasts with the lack of effect of the absence of IGF-I on placental growth and, together with other experimental deletions and natural mutations, suggests that IGF-II influences placental growth via an unknown receptor (Baker et al., 1993). However, the impact of IGF gene deletion on placental structural and functional characteristics needs to be much more closely examined.

Viral infection reduces fetal growth in many species. Where fetal growth has been characterized in sufficient detail, the type of fetal growth restriction produced is assymetrical with reduced growth and function of the lymphoid tissues in the neonate.

Functional outcome for fetus and placenta

The consequence of most extrinsic interventions is asymmetrical fetal growth restriction, with body weight being reduced to a greater extent than crown–rump length (Owens et al., 1989*b*). Commonly, brain weight is maintained relative to body weight, while that of the liver and lymphoid tissues are disproportionately reduced. Other organs are generally reduced in proportion to body weight. Endocrine glands, such as the adrenal and thyroid, may actually maintain or even increase their growth, and consequently are often increased in size relative to body weight.

Regardless of the impact of perturbation on their size, all those organs studied so far show altered structural development consistent with altered and impaired function. For the majority, delayed maturation or immaturity is found in fetal growth restriction. Restriction of implantation in sheep, or uterine artery ligation in guinea pigs, to restrict placental and fetal growth, alters development of the brain (Rees, Bocking & Harding, 1988; Jones, 1989). In the growth-restricted fetal sheep, growth of neuropil in the cerebellum, motor and visual cortices and the hippocampal formation is reduced as is that of granule cell dendrites and the Purkinje cell dendritic tree, suggesting that neuronal connectivity and function may be adversely affected. Reduced rates of myelin formation are seen in brain of the growth-restricted fetal guinea pig. While gut weight is reduced to a similar extent to body weight in placentally restricted fetal sheep, small intestine weight as a fraction of gut is disproportionately reduced (Avila et al., 1989). Along with this disproportionate reduction in weight, thinning of the small intestinal wall, a reduction in its surface area, reduced epithelial regenerative capacity and retardation of epithelial maturation are also apparent. The fetal lung is usually reduced in weight to the same extent as body weight by placental restriction, but development of the mucosal and submucosal layers of the fetal airways alters, with a reduction in the ciliated border on epithelial cells in the latter and a reduction in the extent of folding (Rees et al., 1991). In addition, the volume of lung liquid is reduced relative to lung weight, as is phospholipid content of lung liquid. Growth and maturation of skeletal tissues is retarded in the growth-restricted fetal guinea pig, while ultrastructural changes in skeletal muscle suggest immaturity as well as restricted growth (Jones, 1989). These changes in organs and tissues, which are essential in adaptation to postnatal life, indicate that altered functional capacity in experimental fetal growth restriction partly underlies the associated increase in morbidity and mortality observed in the perinatal period. The functional consequences of the changes in size of various endocrine glands in fetal growth restriction have been examined to a limited extent and evidence for altered endocrine function is detailed later. Other recent reviews have focused on changes in functional capacities of various organs and tissues in experimental and human fetal growth restriction, which could explain the longer-term consequences of fetal growth restriction in adult life (Barker, 1994).

Experimental perturbations which act on the placenta often evoke a compensatory response. In sheep, these may include overgrowth or regrowth of individual cotyledons or placentomes or structural remodelling of the placenta, which enhance function (Robinson et al., 1979; Owens et al., 1987*c*). Restriction of implantation in sheep increases the relative abundance and surface area of the epithelial cell layers responsible for exchange, fetal trophectoderm and feto-maternal syncytium (Chidzanja, Robinson & Owens, 1993). Placental compensation is particularly marked if intervention takes place in the first half of gestation, when placental growth is maximal, and is observed in many species. The initial stimuli and the mechanisms responsible are unknown but, once delineated, may offer new approaches to treating placental insufficiency.

Feto-placental metabolic and endocrine responses to experimental intervention: mechanisms leading to altered growth and development

The impact of experimental interventions on feto-placental metabolism is determined by their effect on substrate abundance in the mother, the functional transport capacity of the placenta and, additionally, by the outcome for placental competition for and modification of substrates to be delivered to the fetus. The metabolic adaptations of the fetus and placenta to intervention is accompanied by endocrine changes, which will partly mediate their impact on fetal growth and development.

Substrate availability within the conceptus

Experimental interventions in the mother, which reduce the availablity of a specific substrate, e.g. oxygen or glucose, generally induce a deficit in the same substance within the conceptus. Depending on the stage of gestation at which the limitation is imposed, any subsequent impairment of placental functional development may lead to deficits in other substrates in the longer term. Experimental restriction of placental capacity to deliver substrates to the fetus, due to either intervention in the placenta or the mother, generally results in fetal hypoglycaemia and hypoxaemia in late gestation (Owens et al., 1989*b*). Restriction of placental supply of substrates by uterine artery ligation in guinea pigs in early gestation produces fetal hypoglycaemia and evidence of hypoxaemia as early as mid-gestation (Jones et al., 1990). Fetal hypoxaemia is accompanied by the development of elevated lactate concentrations in late gestation, whether or not fetal hypoglycaemia is also present (Owens et al., 1987*b*; Jacobs et al., 1988*b*; Jones et al., 1990).

The impact of experimental restriction of fetal growth on the levels of individual amino acids in fetal blood appears to depend on what other deficits in major substrates are produced. Where fetal hypoglycaemia is present, with or without hypoxaemia, the concentrations of amino acids in fetal blood generally increase, particularly those of the branched chain amino acids (Lemons & Schreiner, 1984). Thus glucose deficit appears to limit the ability of the fetus to utilize amino acids, resulting in their accumulation in fetal blood. If placental transfer of amino acids has been affected also, either by hypoglycaemia or concomitant hypoxaemia, it is not evident from the net outcome for amino acid availability in the fetus. Studies using non-metabolizable analogues of amino acids have shown reduced placental transfer of such analogues following experimental restriction of placental function by uterine artery ligation in rats and guinea pigs (Jansson & Persson, 1990). Interventions which produce fetal hypoxaemia alone reduce the concentrations of amino acids in fetal blood, particularly those of the branched chain amino acids in fetal sheep (Owens, Falconer & Robinson, 1989*a*). An exception is alanine, concentrations of which increase in parallel with circulating lactate concentrations in hypoxaemic fetal sheep (Jacobs et al., 1988*b*).

The effect of experimental perturbation on lipid metabolism shows species differences, since placental transport of fatty acids varies considerably between species, and appears to be a major determinant of the fat content of the developing fetus. In species with substantial placental transfer of fatty acids, such as the guinea pig and human, maternal free fatty acid levels are an important determinant of transfer. Ligation of the uterine artery in guinea pigs reduces free fatty acid levels in fetal blood, presumably due to reduced placental transfer, whereas maternal starvation increases their concentrations, paralleling the concomitant increase in maternal free fatty acids (Jones et al., 1990). In contrast to these species, the epitheliochorial placenta of the sheep is relatively impermeable to fatty acids, and placental restriction does not alter concentrations of free fatty acids in fetal blood, or those of acetate and ketone bodies. Placental and fetal synthesis of fatty acids or placental production from maternally derived triacylglycerols, lipoproteins and phospholipids occurs, but the impact of restriction of fetal growth on these processes has been little studied. Reduced fat deposition is a common characteristic of the growth-restricted fetus in the guinea pig and human, but whether reduced delivery or production of precursors or reduced utilization of these is responsible is not known.

Partition of substrates between fetus and placenta

The placenta is a highly metabolically active organ and competes with the fetus for major substrates, even in late gestation, when fetal size far exceeds that of the placenta (Hay & Wilkening, 1994). Normally, the placenta consumes half of the oxygen and two-thirds of the glucose taken up from the mother by the gravid uterus in sheep (Fig. 6.4). Utero-placental glucose uptake is regulated by, and varies considerably with, the concentrations of glucose in fetal and maternal blood in late gestation (Aldoretta et al., 1994). In contrast, uteroplacental oxygen consumption (on a weight-specific basis) generally varies little with acute and chronic variations in glucose suppply to, and uptake by, the placenta (Aldoretta et al., 1994). A significant fraction of the glucose consumed by the placenta is converted to lactate, which is released into both the umbilical and uterine circulations (Fig. 6.4). The placenta is far less permeable to lactate than to glucose and this may represent a mechanism for 'trapping' carbohydrate within the fetal circulation for utilization, occurring in all species studied. Placental lactate production normally varies in parallel with utero-placental glucose uptake (Aldoretta et al., 1994). The placenta also releases ammonia into both the fetal and uterine circulations (Hay & Wilkening, 1994).

When implantation and hence subsequent placental growth are chronically restricted in sheep, oxygen and glucose are redistributed from the placenta to the fetus in late gestation (Fig. 6.4) (Owens et al., 1987*a*,*b*). This is accounted for in part by the relative maintenance of fetal compared to placental growth following restriction. However, a decrease in placental consumption of oxygen and glucose on a weight-specific basis also occurs. At the same time, uteroplacental production of lactate increases, particularly that released into the umbilical circulation,

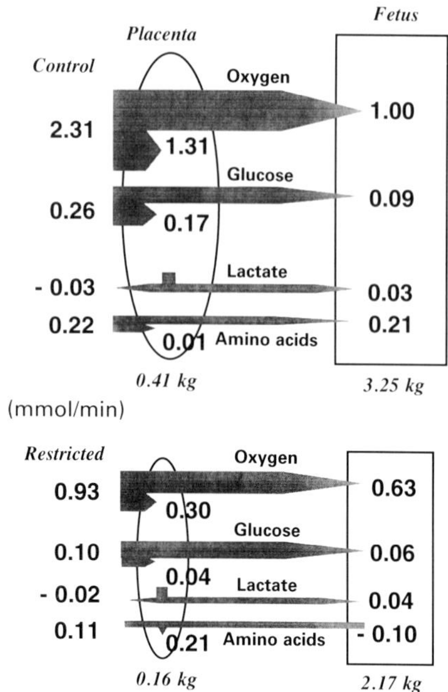

Fig. 6.4. Partitioning of substrates between placenta and fetus: effect of restriction of placental and fetal growth. Rates of flux of substrates in mmol/min between mother, placenta and fetus in control sheep and in sheep with restricted placental and fetal growth in late gestation. Placental growth was restricted as described in Fig. 6.2. Mean placental and fetal weights are shown in italics. (Adapted from Owens et al., 1989*a*.)

thereby increasing the availability of this substrate to the growth restricted fetus. The impact of restriction of placental and fetal growth on ammonia production by the placenta has not been determined, but increased concentrations of ammonia are seen in the blood of growth-restricted fetuses in several species (Owens et al., 1989*b*).

Most of the amino acids taken up from the mother by the placenta in late gestation are transferred to the fetus (Fig. 6.4). However, selective cycling of certain amino acids between the placenta and fetus occurs, in some cases involving the fetal liver (Hay & Wilkening, 1994). The fetus, largely the fetal liver, takes up glutamine and glycine from the placenta and, in turn, releases their metabolic products, glutamate and serine respectively, back to the placenta for uptake. A similar reciprocal exchange involving feto-hepatic uptake of asparagine from, and release of aspartate to, the placenta has also been observed in vivo in sheep. The placenta in the human and sheep contains very high concentrations and activities of the branched chain amino acid aminotransferases. Consistent with this, net placental uptake of the branched chain amino acids and their transamination to the corresponding keto-acid for release largely into the fetal circulation occurs in sheep in late gestation (Smeaton et al., 1989). The importance and role of these cycles in fetal and placental metabolism and growth remain to be determined.

Restriction of placental growth in sheep alters the exchange of amino acids across the placenta in late gestation. The growth-restricted fetal sheep releases many, mainly non-essential, amino acids back to the placenta, suggesting that fetal growth restriction may result not only from slower growth but also from net loss of nitrogen, possibly protein, and hence 'wasting' in late gestation (Owens et al., 1989*b*). This could provide an explanation for the 'wasting' of growth-restricted human fetuses observed using ultrasound (Divon et al., 1986). As a consequence of this reversal of the flux of amino acids from fetus to placenta, uteroplacental consumption of amino acids such as alanine and the branched chain amino acids greatly increases, and may provide alternative substrates to sustain placental oxidative metabolism and the concomitant increases in lactate production, while placental glucose consumption is reduced (Owens et al., 1987*a*). This increase in consumption of the branched chain amino acids is not accompanied by an increase in placental production of their corresponding 2-keto acids (Smeaton et al., 1989), suggesting they may be utilized largely within the small placenta, and may be important in its adaptation to restriction. Similar changes in the exchange of amino acids between fetus and placenta are seen in pregnant sheep subjected to undernutrition or fasting.

As in the growth-restricted human fetus, placentally restricted fetal sheep consume glucose and oxygen at lower than normal absolute rates in late gestation (Owens et al., 1987*a*). With the exception of restriction produced by chronic maternal undernutrition in the sheep in late gestation, weight-specific rates of uptake of oxygen and glucose by the restricted fetus are largely normal, as is the glucose/oxygen quotient. Thus fetal growth appears to proceed at a rate consistent with the availability of glucose and oxygen at least in the longer term. The rate of fetal glucose utilization on a weight-specific basis actually increases, as fetal weight decreases, following placental restriction in sheep (Owens et al., 1989*a*). This may, in part, reflect the relative maintenance of brain growth, and hence increase in glucose demand. Fetal glucose utilization is maintained in part by increased endogenous production of glucose and partly by reduced loss of glucose back to the placenta. The latter may partly explain the reduction in placental glucose uptake which occurs following restriction. Despite the increase in lactate availability in the growth-restricted fetal sheep, fetal uptake does not increase consistently, while the rate of fetal lactate utilization has not been investigated under these circumstances. In the human and sheep fetus, amino acids are used extensively for oxidation as well as for accretion in protein and hence growth (Fowden, 1994). Amino acids provide even more energy (40%) for the fetus than glucose (30%). The impact of chronic restriction of substrate supply in utero upon these processes has not been determined. However, maternal undernutrition or fasting in sheep increases fetal leucine oxidation and urea production (Fowden, 1994). This increased fetal amino acid catabolism in reponse to maternal nutritional deprivation is accompanied by reduced rates of fetal protein synthesis and accretion in sheep and rats and reduced uptake or increased release of various amino acids by the skeletal muscle of fetal hindlimb. The effect of chronic hypoxia alone on fetal metabolism is unknown; however, acute hypoxaemia in sheep reduces protein synthesis by about 70%, suggesting that substantial reductions in protein accretion and growth will ensue (Milley, 1987). However, chronic maternal hypobaric hypoxaemia has a much more modest impact on fetal growth in sheep (Jacobs et al., 1988*c*), suggesting that adaptations occur to ameliorate the effect of oxygen deficit on nitrogen metabolism within the conceptus.

Endocrine responses and relationship to substrate supply

A wide range of endocrine changes occur in the growth-restricted fetus (Robinson et al., 1980; Harding, Jones & Robinson, 1985; Jones, 1989). Because the placenta is impermeable to many hormones, particularly polypeptide hormones, the fetus is substantially autonomous in its endocrinology. In consequence, the hormonal changes observed in fetal growth restriction substantially reflect the fetal response to perturbation of its environment, specifically, changes in the supply of essential substrates, with subsequent changes in fetal metabolism and growth.

The origin of many of the endocrine changes in fetal growth restriction appears to be the associated deficits in substrate availability, particularly of oxygen or glucose or both. The placentally restricted fetus, which is chronically hypoxaemic and hypoglycaemic, has higher basal and stimulated cortisol concentrations in blood (Robinson et al., 1980). This greater rise in cortisol appears to be due to oxygen deficit, since it occurs and is accelerated with chronic fetal hypoxaemia (Jacobs et al., 1988*a*), but not with hypoglycaemia alone. Enhanced adrenal growth, either in absolute or relative terms, occurs concomitantly. The adrenal cortex of the growth-restricted fetal sheep responds to repeated episodes of acute hypoxia with a larger than normal increase in cortisol (Robinson, Jones & Kingston, 1983). This accelerated maturation of the fetal adrenal cortex may enhance development of other cortisol-dependent systems in the fetus. In contrast, maturation of the fetal adrenal medulla appears to be delayed. The higher concentrations of catecholamines in plasma of growth-restricted fetal sheep are accompanied by a delay in the ontogenic fall in the ratio of noradrenaline to adrenaline (Jones & Robinson, 1983).

The placentally restricted hypoxaemic and hypoglycaemic fetal sheep also has reduced plasma concentrations of T3 and T4 in late gestation (Robinson et al., 1980; Harding et al., 1985). Chronic hypoxaemia delays the rise in plasma T3 levels in the fetus in late gestation, while T4 levels are only reduced transiently (Jacobs *et al.*, 1988a). In both perturbations, the relative size of the thyroids increases, but the structural and functional consequences of this are unknown. Fetal plasma insulin concentrations are reduced in fetal growth restriction produced by restriction of placental growth and by maternal undernutrition (Robinson et al., 1980; Harding et al., 1985), but not in that resulting from hypoxaemia alone (Jacobs et al., 1988*a*). While both glucose and amino acids can stimulate insulin release by the fetal pancreas, only glucose is reduced consistently along with fetal growth in these perturbations, suggesting that glucose deficit is responsible for hypoinsulinaemia in fetal growth restriction. The high concentrations of adrenaline in the growth-restricted fetus may also inhibit insulin secretion. The concentrations of IGF-I are reduced consistently in fetal growth restriction characterized by chronic fetal hypoglycaemia in rodents as well as sheep (Straus et al., 1991; Owens et al., 1994), while chronic fetal hypoxaemia in rats has no effect (Tapanainen et al., 1994). IGF-I mRNA and protein are reduced in the liver, but not lung, of growth-restricted fetal rats (Straus et al., 1991). In placentally restricted fetal sheep, IGF-I mRNA is reduced in fetal skeletal muscle, lung and kidney and correlates with fetal blood concentrations of IGF-I protein (Kind et al., 1995). Thus production of IGF-I is reduced at multiple sites in association with reduced circulating levels, implying both local and endocrine activities will be reduced. In addition, the size of both kidney and liver correlated with local abundance of IGF-I mRNA and with circulating IGF-I, suggesting both local and endocrine control of their growth are possible. In these restricted fetal sheep, hepatic IGF-I mRNA correlated with insulin and fetal blood PO_2, but not glucose, suggesting that reduced substrate availability is affecting IGF-I production, in part via other hormonal mediators. In contrast, concentrations of IGF-II are generally unchanged or increase in fetal growth restriction, until very late in gestation, when they are reduced in very growth-restricted hypoxaemic and hypoglycaemic fetal sheep (Owens et al., 1994). This reduction in circulating IGF-II in placentally restricted fetal sheep, coincides with, and may be due to, their accelerated rise in cortisol, a factor known to inhibit hepatic IGF-II gene expression in fetal sheep in late gestation (Li et al., 1993). Moreover, chronically hypoxaemic fetal rats have increased concentrations of IGF-II in plasma (Tapanainen et al., 1994). This suggests that reduced availability of IGF-II does not contribute to restriction of fetal growth until near term, and then only in severe restriction of substrate supply and growth. Increased production of IGFBP-1 and -2 also occurs in chronically hypoxic fetal rats, while increased IGFBP-2 occurs in placentally restricted fetal sheep, even before fetal hypoxia and significant restriction of fetal weight can be detected (Carr, Owens & Wallace, 1994). Thus fetal growth restriction characterized by hypoxaemia and /or hypoglycaemia is characterized by an increased abundance of factors generally inhibitory to the actions of IGFs, as well as a reduced abundance of the IGFs themselves.

Conclusions

Studies of experimental restriction of fetal growth have revealed much about the origins of altered growth before birth but have, until recently, focused mainly on the consequences of perturbation in the second half of gestation. The importance of the peri-implantation period and the first half of gestation is now being recognized in considering the aetiology of altered fetal growth and development. In addition, the functional outcomes of restriction for many fetal systems have been described in only limited terms so far. Both the short and particularly the long-term consequences of fetal growth restriction for the individual need to be investigated in far greater detail, as do the physiological, cellular and molecular mechanisms responsible. Those long-term consequences include new and previously unsuspected links between growth before birth and risk of developing major adult-onset diseases. Finally, the use of experimental restriction of fetal growth continues to offer an efficient and the most appropriate approach to developing and testing new approaches to the diagnosis and treatment of fetal growth restriction and its long-term sequelae effectively.

References

Aldoretta, P.W., Carter, T.D. & Hay, W.W.(1994). Ovine uteroplacental glucose and oxygen metabolism in relation to chronic changes in maternal and fetal glucose concentrations. *Placenta*, **15**, 753–64.

Avila, C.G., Harding, R., Rees, S. & Robinson, P.M. (1989). Small intestinal development in growth retarded fetal sheep. *Journal of Pediatric Gastroenterology and Nutrition*, **8**, 507–15.

Baker, J., Liu, J.-P., Robertson, E.J. & Efstratiadis, A. (1993). Role of insulin-like growth factors in embryonic and post-natal growth. *Cell*, **75**, 73–82.

Barker, D.J.P. (1994). *Mothers, Babies and Disease in Later Life*. BMJ Publishing Group, London.

Bell, A.W., Wilkening, R.B. & Meschia, G. (1987). Some aspects of placental function in chronically heat-stressed ewes. *Journal of Developmental Physiology*, **9**, 17–29.

Brooke, O.G., Wood, C. & Butters, F. (1984). The body proportions for small-for-dates infants. *Early Human Development*, **10**, 85–94.

Carr, J.M., Owens, J.A., Grant, P.A., Walton, P.E., Owens, P.C. & Wallace, J.C. (1995). Circulating insulin-like growth factors (IGFs) IGF-binding proteins (IGFBPs) and tissue mRNA levels of IGFBP-2 and IGFBP-4 in the ovine fetus. *Journal of Endocrinology*, In Press.

Carr, J.M., Owens, J.A. & Wallace, J.C. (1994). Altered ontogeny of insulin-like growth factor binding proteins in the growth retarded fetal sheep. In *Proceedings of the Australian Society for Medical Research*, **33**, Oral 4–5.

Cetin, I., Marconi, A.M., Bozzetti, P., Sereni, L.P., Corbetta, C., Pardi, G. & Battaglia, F.C. (1988). Umbilical amino acid concentrations in appropriate and small-for-gestational age infants: a biochemical difference present in utero. *American Journal of Obstetrics and Gynecology*, **158**, 120–6.

Charlton, V. & Johengen, M. (1987). Fetal intravenous nutritional supplementation ameliorates the development of embolization-induced growth retardation in the sheep. *Pediatric Research*, **22**, 55–61.

Chidzanja, S.C., Robinson, J.S. & Owens, J.A. (1993). Compensatory placental growth occurs by mid gestation following restricted implantation in sheep. In *Proceedings of the Australian Society for Medical Research*, **32**, 40.

Chien, P.F.W., Smith, K., Watt, P.W., Scrimgeour, C.M., Taylor, D.J. & Rennie, M.J. (1993). Protein turnover in the human fetus studied at term using stable isotope tracer amino acids. *American Journal of Physiology*, **265**, E31–5.

Clark, K.E., Durnwald, M. & Austin, J.E. (1982). A model for studying chronic reduction in uterine blood flow in pregnant sheep. *American Journal of Physiology*, **242**, H297–301.

Cohick, W.S. & Clemmons, D.R. (1993). The insulin-like growth factors. *Annual Reviews of Physiology*, **55**, 131–53.

Cross, J.C., Werb, Z. & Fisher, S.J. (1994). Implantation and the placenta: Key pieces of the development puzzle. *Science*, **266**, 1508–18.

Deayton, J.M., Young, I.R. & Thorburn, G.D. (1993). Early hypophysectomy of sheep fetuses: effects on growth, placental steroidogenesis and prostaglandin production. *Journal of Reproduction and Fertility*, **97**, 513–20.

Dicke, J.M. & Henderson, G.I. (1988). Placental amino acid uptake in normal and complicated pregnancies. *American Journal of Medical Sciences*, **295**, 223–7.

Dickson, M.C., Saunders, J.C. & Gilmour, R.S. (1991). The ovine insulin-like growth factor-I gene: characterisation, expression and identification of a putative promoter. *Journal of Molecular Endocrinology*, **6**, 17–31.

Divon, M.Y., Chamberlain, P.F., Sipos, L., Manning, F. & Platt, L.D. (1986). Identification of the small-for-gestational age fetus with the use of gestational age independent indices of fetal growth. *American Journal of Obstetrics and Gynecology*, **155**, 1197–201.

Emmanoulides, G.C., Townsend, D.E. & Bauer, R.A. (1968). Effects of single umbilical artery ligation in the lamb fetus. *Pediatrics*, **42**, 919–27.

Erkadius, Di Iulio, J., Lucente, F., Brannich, C., Morgan, T. & Nicolantonio, R.D. (1994*a*). Role of uterine factors in the development of hypertension in SHR. *Clinical and Experimental Pharmacology and Physiology*, **21**, 239–42.

Erkadius, Morgan, T.O. & Nicolantonio, R.D. (1994*b*). Role of the uterine environment in the development of hypertension in the spontaneously hypotensive rat. *Placenta*, **15**, A16.

Farin, P.W., Farin, C.E. & Yang, L. (1994). In vitro production of bovine embryos is associated with altered fetal development. *Theriogenology*, **41**, 193.

Fay, R.A. & Ellwood, D.A. (1993). Categories of intrauterine growth retardation. *Fetal and Maternal Medicine Review*, **5**, 203–12.

Ferguson, M.W.J. (1994). Overviews of mechanisms in embryogenesis. In *Early Fetal Growth and Development*, ed. R.H.T. Ward, S.K. Smith & D. Donnai, pp. 1–19. RCOG Press, London.

Fowden, A.L. (1989). The endocrine regulation of fetal metabolism and growth. In *Advances in Fetal Physiology, Research in Perinatology*, vol. 8, ed. P.D. Gluckman, B.M. Johnston & P.W. Nathanielz, pp. 229–243. Perinatology Press, Ithaca, NY.

Fowden, A.L. (1994). Fetal metabolism and energy balance. In *Textbook of Fetal Physiology*, ed. G.D. Thorburn & R. Harding, pp. 70–82. Oxford University Press, Oxford.

Gagnon, R., Challis, J., Johnston, L. & Fraher, L. (1994). Fetal endocrine responses to chronic placental embolization in the late-gestation ovine fetus. *American Journal of Obstetrics and Gynecology*, **170**, 929–38.

Haig, D. & Graham, C. (1991). Genomic imprinting and the strange case of the insulin-like growth factor II receptor. *Cell*, **64**, 1045–6.

Harding, J.E., Jones, C.T. & Robinson, J.S. (1985). Studies on experimental growth retardation in sheep. The effects of a small placenta in restricting fetal growth. *Journal of Developmental Physiology*, **7**, 427–42.

Hay, W.W. & Wilkening, R.B. (1994). Metabolic activity of the placenta. In *Textbook of Fetal Physiology*, ed. G.D. Thorburn & R. Harding, pp. 30–47. Oxford University Press, Oxford.

Hayashi, S., Sareda, K., Sagawa, N., Yamoda, W. & Kido, K. (1978). Umbilical vein-artery differences of plasma amino acids in the last trimester of human pregnancy. *Biology of the Neonate*, **34**, 11–18.

Hopkins, P.S. & Thorburn, G.D. (1972). The effects of fetal thyroidectomy on the development of the ovine fetus. *Journal of Endocrinology*, **54**, 55–6.

Jacobs, R., Owens, P.C., Falconer, J. & Robinson, J.S. (1988*a*). Effect of chronic hypoxia on hormone concentrations in fetal sheep. In *Proceedings of the Society for Gynecological Investigation*, A252.

Jacobs, R., Owens, J.A., Falconer, J., Webster, M.E.D. & Robinson, J.S. (1988*b*). Changes in metabolite concentrations in fetal sheep subjected to prolonged hypobaric hypoxia. *Journal of Developmental Physiology*, **10**, 113–21.

Jacobs, R., Robinson, J.S. Owens, J.A., Falconer, J. & Webster, M.E.D. (1988*c*). The effect of prolonged hypobaric hypoxia on growth of fetal sheep. *Journal of Developmental Physiology*, **10**, 97–112.

Jansson, T. & Persson, E. (1990). Placental transfer of glucose and amino acids in intrauterine growth retardation: Studies with substrate analogs in the awake guinea pig. *Pediatric Research*, **28**, 203–8.

Jones, C.T. (1989). Observations on the control of prenatal growth in the guinea pig. In *Advances in Fetal Physiology, Research in Perinatal Medicine*, vol. 8, ed. P.D. Gluckman, B.M. Johnston & P.W. Nathanielz, pp. 287–302. Perinatology Press, Ithaca, NY.

Jones, C.T., Lafeber, H.N., Rolph, T.P. & Parer, J.T. (1990). Studies on the growth of the fetal guinea pig. The effects of nutritional manipulation on prenatal growth and plasma somatomedin activity and insulin-like growth factor concentrations. *Journal of Developmental Physiology*, **13**, 189–97.

Jones, C.T. & Robinson, J.S. (1983). Studies on experimental growth retardation in sheep. Plasma catecholamines in fetuses with small placentae. *Journal of Developmental Physiolgy*, **5**, 77–87.

Karlberg, J., Albertsson-Wikland, K. & Lawrence, C. (1994). Birth size related to placental weight and maternal height. In *Proceedings, 14th International Symposium on Growth and Growth Disorders*.

Khong, T.Y., DeWolf, F., Robertson, W.B. & Brosen, I. (1986). Inadequate maternal vascular response to placentation in pregnancies complicated by pre-eclampsia and by small-for-gestational age infants. *British Journal of Obstetrics and Gynaecology*, **93**, 1049–59.

Kind, K.L., Owens, J.A., Robinson, J.S., Quinn, K.J., Grant, P.A., Walton, P.E., Gilmour, R.S. & Owens, P.C. (1995). Effect of restriction of placental growth on expression of insulin-like growth factors in fetal sheep: relationship to fetal growth, circulating insulin-like growth factors and binding proteins. *Journal of Endocrinology*, In Press.

Kleeman, D.O., Walker, S.K. & Seamark, R.F. (1995). Enhanced fetal growth in sheep administered progesterone during the first three days of pregnancy. *Journal of Reproduction and Fertility*, In press.

Konje, J.C., Smith, K., Downie, S., Taylor, D.J. & Rennie, M.J. (1994). Mannitol transfer across the human placenta: evidence for diminished rates of carrier-mediated transfer in small-for-gestational age pregnancy. *Journal of Physiology*, in Press.

Kramer, M.S., McLean, F.A., Olivier, M., Willis, D.M. & Usher, R.H. (1989) Body proportionality and head-length 'sparing' in growth-retarded neonates: a critical reappraisal. *Pediatrics*, **84**, 717–23.

Kramer, M.S., Olivier, M., McLean, F.H., Dougherty, G.E., Willis, D.M. & Usher, R.D. (1990). Determinants of fetal growth and body proportionality. *Pediatrics*, **86**, 18–26.

Langley, S.C. & Jackson, A.A. (1994) Increased systolic blood pressure in adult rats induced by fetal exposure to maternal low protein diets. *Clinical Science*, **86**, 217–22.

Lassarre, C., Hardovin, S., Daffos, F., Forestier, F., Frankienne, F. & Binoux, M. (1991). Serum insulin-like growth factors and insulin-like growth factor binding proteins in the human fetus. Relationships with growth in normal subjects and subjects with intrauterine growth retardation. *Pediatric Research*, **29**, 219–25.

Lemons, J.A. & Schreiner, R.L. (1984). Metabolic balance of the ovine fetus during the fed and fasted states. *Annals of Nutrition and Metabolism*, **28**, 268–80.

Li, J., Saunders, J.C., Gilmour, R.S., Silver, M. & Fowden, A.L. (1993). Insulin-like growth factor-II mRNA expression in fetal tissues of the sheep during late gestation: effects of cortisol. *Endocrinology*, **132**, 2083–9.

Liu, J.-P., Baker, J., Perkins, A.S., Robertson, E.J. & Efstratiadis, A. (1993). Mice carrying null mutations of the genes encoding insulin-like growth factor I (Igf-I) and type-1 IGF receptor (Igfr). *Cell*, **75**, 59–72.

Lok, F., Owens, J.A., Mundy, L., Owens, P.C. & Robinson, J.S. (1993). Insulin-like growth factor-I promotes growth selectively in fetal sheep. In *The Proceedings of The Endocrine Society of Australia,* **36 (A7)**, p. 68.

McRae, A.C. (1994). Effects of the anti-progestin and anti-glucocorticoid steroid RU486 on cell proliferation in oviductal embryos of lactating mice. *Journal of Reproduction and Fertility,* **100**, 307–13.

Mahendran, D., Donnai, D.P, D'Souza, S., Glazier, J.D., Boyd, R.D.H. & Silby, C.P. (1991). Na+/H+ exchange and sodium dependent methylamino-isobutyric acid (Me AIB) transport in the placentae of small for gestational age rats (IUGR). *Placenta*, **12**, 415–6.

Mayhew, T.M., Jackson, M.R. & Boyd, P.A. (1993). Changes in oxygen diffusive conductances of human placentae during gestation (10–41 weeks) are commensurate with the gain in fetal weight. *Placenta*, **14**, 51–61.

Mellor, D. (1983). Nutritional and placental determinants of foetal growth rate in sheep and consequences for the newborn lamb. *British Veterinary Journal,* **139**, 307–24.

Mesiano, S., Young, I.R., Baxter, R.C., Hintz, R.L., Browne, C.A. & Thorburn, G.D. (1987). Effect of hypophysectomy with and without thyroxine replacement on growth and circulating concentrations of IGF-I and IGF-II in the fetal lamb. *Endocrinology*, **120**, 1821–30.

Mesiano, S., Young, I.R., Hey, A.W., Browne, C.A. & Thorburn, G.D. (1989). Hypophysectomy of the fetal lamb leads to a fall in the plasma concentration of insulin-like growth factor I, but not IGF-II. *Endocrinology*, **124**, 1485–91.

Milley, J.R. (1987). Protein synthesis during hypoxia in fetal lambs. *American Journal of Physiology,* **252**, E519–24.

Molnar, M., Suto, T., Toth, T. & Hertelendy, F. (1994). Prolonged blockade of nitric oxide synthesis in gravid rats produces sustained hypertension, proteinuria, thrombocytopenia and intrauterine growth retardation. *American Journal of Obstetrics and Gynecology*, **170**, 1458–66.

Montemagno, R. & Soothill, P.W. (1994). The biochemistry of small for gestational age fetuses. In *Early Fetal Growth and Development*, ed. R.H.T. Ward, S.K. Smith & D. Donnai, pp. 391–405. RCOG Press, London.

Naeye, R.L. (1965). Malnutrition: probably cause of fetal growth retardation. *Archives Pathology*, **79**, 284–91.
O'Mahoney, J.V., Brandon, M.R. & Adams, T.E. (1991). Developmental and tissue specific regulation of ovine insulin-like growth factor-II (IGF-II) mRNA expression. *Molecular and Cellular Endocrinology*, **78**, 87–96.
Oliver, M.H., Harding, J.E., Brier, B.H., Evans, P.C. & Gluckman, P.D. (1993). Glucose but not mixed amino acid infusion regulates plasma insulin-like growth factor-I concentrations in fetal sheep. *Pediatric Research*, **34**, 62–5.
Owens, J.A. (1991). Endocrine and substrate control of fetal growth: placental and maternal influences and insulin-like growth factors. *Reproduction, Fertility and Development*, **3**, 501–17.
Owens, J.A., Falconer, J. & Robinson, J.S. (1986). Effect of restriction of placental growth on umbilical and uterine blood flows. *American Journal of Physiology*, **250**, R427–34.
Owens, J.A., Falconer, J.& Robinson, J.S. (1987*a*). Effect of restriction of placental growth on fetal and utero-placental metabolism. *Journal of Developmental Physiology*, **9**, 225–38.
Owens, J.A., Falconer, J. & Robinson, J.S. (1987*b*). Restriction of placental growth on oxygen delivery to and comsumption by the pregnant uterus and fetus. *Journal of Developmental Physiology*, **9**, 137–50.
Owens, J.A., Falconer, J. & Robinson, J.S. (1987*c*). Restriction of placental size in sheep enhances the efficiency of placental transfer of antipyrine, 3-0-methyl-D-glucose but not of urea. *Journal of Developmental Physiology*, **9**, 457–64.
Owens, J.A., Falconer, J. & Robinson, J.S. (1989*a*). Glucose metabolism in pregnant sheep when placental growth is restricted. *American Journal of Physiology*, **257**, R350–7.
Owens, J.A., Kind, K.L., Carbone, F., Robinson, J.S. & Owens, P.C. (1994). Circulating insulin-like growth factors-I and -II and substrates in fetal sheep following restriction of placental growth. *Journal of Endocrinology*, **1540**, 5–13.
Owens, J.A., Owens, P.C. & Robinson, J.S. (1989*b*). Experimental fetal growth retardation: metabolic and endocrine aspects. In *Advances in Fetal Physiology, Research in Perinatology, vol. 8*, ed. P.D. Gluckman, B.M. Johnston & P.W. Nathanielz, pp. 263–286. Perinatology Press, Ithaca, NY.
Parr, R.A., Miles, M.A., Cash, M.P. & Waters, J.M. (1994). Timing of progesterone and embryonic survival in overfed gilts. In *Proceedings of the Australian Society for Reproductive Biology*, 78.
Pell, J.M., Saunders, J.C. & Gilmour, R.S. (1993). Differential regulation of transcription initiation from insulin-like growth factor-I (IGF-I) leader exons and of tissue IGF-I expression in response to changed growth hormone and nutritional status in sheep. *Endocrinology*, **132**, 1797–807.
Rees, S., Bocking, A.D. & Harding, R. (1988). Structure of the fetal sheep brain in experimental growth retardation. *Journal of Developmental Physiology*, **100**, 211–24.
Rees, S., Ng, J., Dickson, K., Nicholas, T. & Harding, R. (1991). Growth retardation and the development of the respiratory system in fetal sheep. *Early Human Development*, **26**, 13–27.
Robinson, J.S., Hart, I.C., Kingston, E.J., Jones, C.T. & Thorburn, G.D. (1980). Studies on the growth of the fetal sheep. The effects of reduction

of placental size on hormone concentration in fetal plasma. *Journal of Developmental Physiology*, **2**, 239–48.

Robinson, J.S., Falconer, J. & Owens, J.A. (1985). Intrauterine growth retardation: clinical and experimental. *Acta Paediatrica Scandinavica*, Suppl **319**, 135–40.

Robinson, J.S., Jones, C.T. & Kingston, E.J. (1983). Studies on experimental growth retardation in sheep. The effects of maternal hypoxaemia. *Journal of Developmental Physiology*, **5**, 89–100.

Robinson, J.S., Kingston, E.J., Jones, C.T. & Thorburn, G.D. (1979). Studies on experimental growth retardation in sheep. The effect of removal of endometrial caruncles on fetal size and metabolism. *Journal of Developmental Physiology*, **1**, 379–98.

Robinson, J.S., Owens, J.A. & Owens, P.C. (1994). Fetal growth and growth retardation. In *Textbook of Fetal Physiology*, ed. G.D. Thorburn & R. Harding, pp. 83–94. Oxford University Press, Oxford.

Sheppard, B.L. & Bonnar, J. (1988). The maternal blood supply to the placenta in pregnancy complicated by intrauterine fetal growth retardation. *Trophoblast Research,* **3**, 69–81.

Smeaton, T.C., Owens, J.A., Kind, K.L. & Robinson, J.S. (1989). The placenta releases branched-chain keto acids into the umbilical and uterine circulations in the pregnant sheep. *Journal of Developmental Physiology*, **12**, 95–9.

Straus, D.S., Ooi, G.T., Orlowski, C.C. & Rechler, M.M. (1991). Expression of the genes for insulin-like growth factor-I (IGF-I), IGF-II, and IGF-binding proteins 1 and 2 in fetal rat under conditions of intrauterine growth retardation caused by maternal fasting. *Endocrinology*, **128**, 518–25.

Stevens, D. & Alexander, G. (1986). Lipid deposition after hypophysectomy and growth hormone treatment in the sheep fetus. *Journal of Developmental Physiology*, **8**, 139–45.

Tapanainen, P.J., Borg, P., Wilson, K., Unterman, T.G., Vreman, H.J. & Rosenfeld, R.G. (1994). Maternal hypoxia as a model for intrauterine growth retardation: effects on insulin-like growth factors and their binding proteins. *Pediatric Research*, **36**, 152–8.

Thorburn, G.D. & Harding, R. (1994). *Textbook of Fetal Physiology*. Oxford University Press, Oxford.

Trudinger, B.J., Stevens, D., Connelly, A., Hales, J.R.S., Alexander, G., Bradley, L., Fawcett, A. & Thompson, R. (1987). Umbilical artery flow velocity waveforms and placental resistance: the effects of embolization of the umbilical circulation. *American Journal of Obstetrics and Gynecology*, **157**, 1443–8.

Walker, S.K., Heard, T.M., Bee, C.A., Frensham, A.B., Warnes, D.M. & Seamark, R.F. (1992). Culture of embryos of farm animals. In *Development and Manipulation in Animal Production*, ed. A. Lauria & F. Gandolfi, pp. 77–92. Portland Press, London.

Wang, J.X., Clark, A.M., Kirby, C.A., Philipson, G., Petrucco, O., Aderson, G. & Matthews, C.D. (1994*a*). The obstetric outcome of singleton pregnancies following in vitro fetilization/gamete intra-fallopian transfer. *Human Reproduction*, **9**, 141–6.

Wang, Z.Q., Fung, M.R., Barlow, D.P. & Wagner, E.F. (1994*b*). Regulation of embryonic growth and lysosomal targeting by the imprinted Igf 2/Mpr gene. *Nature*, **372**, 464–7.

Wang, H.S., Lim, J., English, J., Irvine, L. & Chard, T. (1991). The concentration of insulin-like growth factor-I and insulin-like growth factor-binding protein-1 in human umbilical cord serum at delivery: relation to fetal weight. *Journal of Endocrinology,* **129**, 459–64.

Winnick, M. & Noble, A. (1966). Cellular response in rats during malnutrition at various ages. *Journal of Nutrition*, **89**, 300–12.

7

Placental changes in fetal growth retardation

T.Y. KHONG

Introduction

Many factors, which may be maternal, fetal or maternal–fetal, may contribute, either singly or synchronously, to intrauterine fetal growth retardation (IUGR). Pathophysiological studies have concentrated on pre-eclampsia, with which IUGR is commonly associated. It is now apparent that 'idiopathic' IUGR, not associated with pre-eclampsia, shares much of the pathophysiology of pre-eclampsia, with hypoperfusion of the intervillous space as a feature. The underlying pathology has often been ascribed to 'placental insufficiency' or, more correctly, uteroplacental insufficiency. It is necessary, therefore, to review the morphological features of the maternal blood supply to the placenta in normal pregnancy before describing the features in pre-eclampsia and IUGR. It is useful also to understand the techniques that have been used for obtaining the maternal tissue and their limitations to underscore these studies. Finally, the pathology of the placenta in pre-eclampsia and in IUGR is described.

Sampling the uteroplacental vasculature

Placental bed biopsy

Early morphological studies of human placentation were based on the delivered placenta, on sporadic specimens from hysterectomy during pregnancy and on specimens obtained at autopsy following maternal death. Examination of the delivered placenta provided only an incomplete picture of the maternal side of the blood supply. The autopsy material was, thankfully, rare and often suffered from postmortem artefacts. Much use was therefore made of the Caesarean hysterectomy specimens, including specimens removed with the placenta in situ so as to preserve the relationship between the placenta and the placental bed. Studies in early and late pregnancy were conducted on these tissues. However, it was only after a method of sampling the placental bed at Caesarean section was described (Dixon & Robertson, 1958) that systematic studies on the maternal blood supply to the placenta and fetus could be achieved by allowing large numbers of cases to be studied by a larger group of researchers.

In coining the term 'placental bed', Dixon and Robertson wished to focus attention on the area where the genetically dissimilar maternal tissue and fetal trophoblast intermingled most intimately and, as importantly, where the spiral arteries destined to supply the placenta and fetus were localized. They emphasized, therefore, that the placental bed included decidua basalis and the subjacent myometrium.

Tissue from the pregnant uterus can be obtained either at Caesarean section or vaginally immediately postpartum. The latter method, using a cervical punch biopsy or specially adapted ovum or other forceps, is generally less reliable even though the precise location of the placenta may have been determined by ultrasound during pregnancy. The potential risks of perforation and an inability to visualize any excessive bleeding at the biopsy site detracts from a biopsy via the vagina. On the other hand, the method clearly facilitates study of large numbers of cases and also allows the placental bed from cases that are clinically not severe enough to be subjected to a Caesarean section to be studied. Finally, the vaginal approach has been used successfully to study the placental bed in miscarriages, although a sharp curette would yield more tissue of the uterus, both placental and non-placental bed (Khong, Liddell & Robertson, 1987*a*).

Biopsies of the placental bed are best taken under direct visualization of the placental site at Caesarean section or at hysterotomy in early pregnancy. Two methods are available. In the first, the true centre of the placenta and not the site of insertion of the umbilical cord is identified digitally by the assistant after delivery of the baby (Dixon & Robertson, 1958; Robertson et al., 1986). After the placenta is peeled away, the placental site can be seen. This appears to be depressed, focally disrupted and friable when compared to the smoother decidua parietalis. Biopsies can then be taken with a curved scissors, although this may potentially yield crushing artefacts, or by blunt dissection using a non-toothed forceps and scalpel. The biopsies do not need to be deep as the superficial few millimetres of myometrium will contain the myometrial segments of the spiral arteries. Placental bed biopsies of approximately 10 mm in length and width and 7 mm in depth will yield good material for study. There usually is no need to secure haemostasis although use of absorbable sutures has been recommended if thought necessary. A second method to ensure that a biopsy comes from the placental site is to thrust a cervical punch biopsy or other forceps through the placenta before peripheral separation is complete (Dixon & Robertson, 1958). One disadvantage of this method is the uncertainty of the depth to which the forceps needs to be thrust before the biopsy is taken as a superficial biopsy will yield potentially only tissue from the basal zone of the placenta.

The true placental bed can be sampled in over 70% of cases in experienced hands. Blind biopsies with adapted cutting forceps generally result in inadequate material from outside the placental site while direct visualization using the two methods described earlier improves the rate. Accordingly, it is not surprising that biopsies of the placental bed from the antero-fundal area can be unsatisfactory. This can be overcome, to some extent, by exteriorization of the uterus with eversion of the anterior lip of the lower segment incision thus giving good access to the placental site, although the procedure may be uncomfortable to the woman under regional anaesthesia.

The subsequent handling of the biopsy will depend on the interests of the investigator, and these were reviewed recently (Robertson et al., 1986). In so far as morphology of the placental bed is concerned, it is essential that the specimen is properly oriented as there is no defined junction to separate the decidua from the myometrium (Fig. 7.1).

Placental basal plate

Full thickness blocks of the placenta extending from the chorionic plate on the fetal surface to the basal plate on the maternal surface are routinely taken when placentas are submitted for histopathological assessment. Because the uteroplacental arteries terminate in the basal plate at their openings into the intervillous space, sections from these blocks will on occasion contain these terminal segments of the uteroplacental arteries for examination. Distinguishing between uteroplacental arteries and veins can be difficult and care must be exercised (Khong, Sawyer & Heryet, 1992). Generally, the fibrinoid matrix of the walls of the uteroplacental arteries were more clearly demarcated from Nitabuch's fibrinoid layer of the basal plate than that of the veins which merged imperceptibly with Nitabuch's layer. They could also be dis-

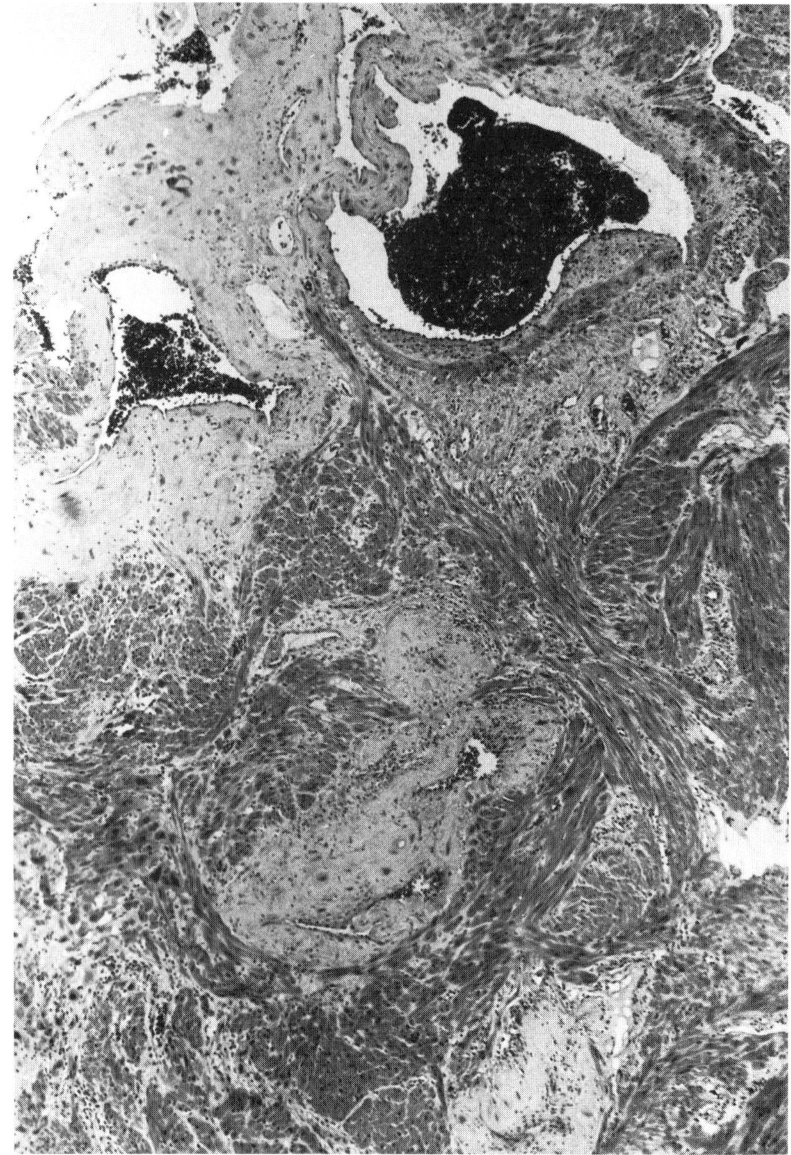

Fig. 7.1. Photomicrograph of a histological section taken from a well-orientated placental bed biopsy showing decidua at the top and myometrium in the lower half. (Haematoxylin and eosin ×50). (Reproduced from Robertson et al., 1986.)

tinguished by the occasional finding of placental villi dipping into the orifices of the veins, but not the arteries, at the intervillous space.

Another method of sampling the placenta is to take en face blocks of the basal plate by shaving the maternal surface and embedding this surface 'face on' (Khong & Chambers, 1992). This would comprise a larger surface area and, accordingly, have a greater chance of including a spiral artery for assessment. A potential pitfall of this unconventional method of sampling is the possible confusion between the thick muscular arteries of mainstem villi and unconverted spiral arteries retaining their musculo-elastic tissue within their walls (see below). However, mainstem villi are invested by a layer of syncytiotrophoblast and surrounding fetal mesenchyme while maternal arteries are surrounded by decidua or extravillous trophoblast of the residual cytotrophoblastic shell embedded within Nitabuch's layer.

A limitation of the basal plate block, whether en face or full thickness, in so far as examination of the uteroplacental vasculature is concerned, is the failure to provide any information regarding the status of the maternal blood supply more proximally in the deeper decidua basalis and myometrium. Nevertheless, it is a valuable source of information in pregnancies where placental bed biopsies are unavailable for whatever reason. Furthermore, it supplements studies based on examination of only placental bed biopsies since it allows study of milder cases of pre-eclampsia or intrauterine growth retardation that are not subjected to Caesarean section (Khong et al., 1986).

Uteroplacental circulation

Normal development

The phenomenon of migratory extravillous trophoblast is common to all species, including the human, with haemochorial placentation where the villous trophoblast of the fetal placenta is bathed in maternal blood. Nidation of the blastocyst is followed soon after by infiltration of the decidua basalis by extravillous trophoblast derived initially from the cytotrophoblastic shell and, at a later stage, from the tips of anchoring chorionic villi. Two subsets of extravillous trophoblast are identified on the basis of their topography. Interstitial trophoblast invades the decidual stroma and by the tenth week of gestation will have penetrated into the superficial myometrium. These interstitial trophoblastic cells tend to cluster around the spiral arteries. The second subset, the endovascular trophoblast, migrates retrogradely into the lumina of the spiral arteries

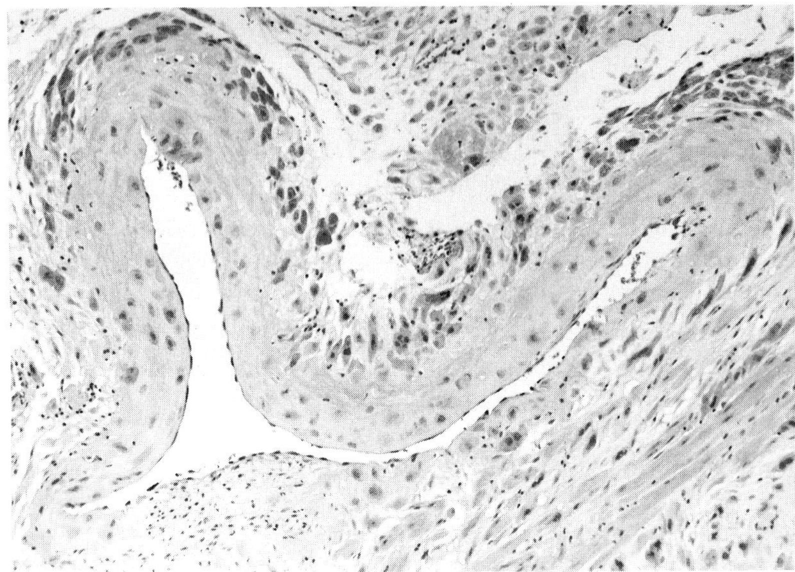

Fig. 7.2. Fully developed physiological changes in the myometrial segment of a uteroplacental artery that is artefactually collapsed ex vivo. The wall is replaced by a prominent fibrinoid matrix in which trophoblastic cells are embedded. Note also the plentiful surrounding perivascular interstitial trophoblast. (Haematoxylin and eosin ×125.)

and invades the arterial wall. This migration is assumed to commence with the trapping of the spiral arteries by the expanding cytotrophoblastic shell from about 4–6 weeks gestation and continues until the end of the first trimester by which time all the decidual segments are affected. There is then a pause until about 15–16 weeks gestation when there is a renewed wave of endovascular trophoblast migration extending beyond the deciduo-myometrial junction into the myometrial segments of the spiral arteries (Pijnenborg et al., 1983).

The actual mechanisms involved are not known but the interaction between extravillous trophoblast, in particular the endovascular trophoblast, and maternal tissue results in transformation of the normally small calibre spiral arteries into flaccid distended tubes (Fig. 7.2). The spiral arteries which supply the endometrium in the non-pregnant uterus are terminal branches of the radial arteries that traverse the uterus after originating from the arcuate arteries in the outer third of the uterus and are similar to other medium-sized arteries in the body with a normal complement of muscular and elastic tissue in their walls. The muscular and elastic components of the arterial wall are replaced by amorphous 'fibrinoid' material embedded within which are endovascular trophoblast. These changes take place in two stages, corresponding to the two waves of endovascular trophoblast migration, affecting decidual and myometrial segments, respectively, and are normally completed by 22–24 weeks gestation (Pijnenborg et al., 1983; Robertson et al., 1986). The changes in the myometrial segments of the spiral arteries may be variable with residual fragments of elastic and muscular tissue present. This is hardly surprising given that there is a greater amount of musculoelastic tissue in the more proximal myometrial segments than in the decidual segments. Most authors found that the morphological changes in normal pregnancies always involved the decidual and myometrial segments of the spiral arteries (Brosens, Robertson & Dixon, 1972; Hustin, Foidart & Lambotte, 1983; Björk et al., 1984; Khong et al., 1986) or even reached the distal portions of the radial arteries (Robertson, Brosens & Dixon, 1975). Other workers found that these changes did not always extend to the myometrial segments (Brosens, Dixon & Robertson 1977; Sheppard & Bonnar, 1981; Gerretsen, Huisjes & Elema, 1981; Frusca et al., 1989; Pijnenborg et al., 1991); between them, these five groups of workers found 6 out of 77 uncomplicated pregnancies without the morphological changes in the myometrial segments of the spiral arteries. It must be emphasized that these dissenting studies examined placental bed biopsies which may be subject to sampling error (see below). Thus, it is safe to conclude that in normal pregnancy virtually all 100–150 spiral arteries, in their entirety, in the placental bed are converted to uteroplacental arteries by the end of the second trimester at the latest. These transformed uteroplacental arteries undergo passive distension resulting in a series of dilated and tortuous channels that open into the intervillous space.

The fully developed uteroplacental arteries apparently lose their ability to respond to vasomotor influences because of the loss of musculoelastic tissue. It is assumed that there is also denervation of the autonomic nerves (Thorbert et al., 1979) attendant with the loss of muscular and elastic tissue from the spiral arteries during their transformation to uteroplacental arteries, although this is as yet unproved (Zuspan et al., 1981). These changes result in a significant drop in peripheral resistance and allow a greater conductance and an almost ten-fold increase in blood flow through these arteries into and through the intervillous space. Thus, despite the marked lack of resemblance of the uteroplacental arteries to the spiral arteries in the non-pregnant state, these changes have been termed physiological changes (Brosens, Robertson & Dixon, 1967) since they allow for the necessary increase in blood flow as pregnancy progresses.

An important consideration in studies of placental bed vascular pathology is that, during the establishment and development of placentation in the first and second trimesters, there is a centrifugal 'fading' of extravillous trophoblast migration from the original nidation site. This has been described analogously as the ripples created by a stone dropped into a still pool of water (Pijnenborg et al., 1981). This means that trophoblast-induced physiological vascular changes in the peripheral zones of the placental bed may be incomplete. Studies of the placental basal plate, where the location of the spiral arteries in relation to the centre of the placental bed can be established firmly, confirm that unaltered decidual segments of spiral arteries may be seen in blocks taken from the margin of the placenta (Khong et al., 1986). Failure to appreciate this feature of trophoblast migration and its effect on physiological changes can lead to misinterpretation, particularly in relation to pathological pregnancies. Hence, the emphasis on ascertaining the true centre of the placenta when obtaining a placental bed biopsy or the taking of basal plate blocks away from the periphery cannot be overstated (Robertson et al., 1986).

Uteroplacental pathology in pre-eclampsia and intrauterine growth retardation

Vascular changes

In the majority of cases, pre-eclampsia manifests as rising blood pressure, proteinuria and oedema in the third trimester of pregnancy. However, evidence is accumulating that in women who are destined to develop pre-eclampsia various biochemical and haematological parameters may be abnormal at an early stage of pregnancy. It has been known for a long time that there is a reduction in blood flow into the intervillous space in cases of pre-eclampsia before clinical signs become apparent and this may be present as early as the second trimester of pregnancy, as shown by uteroplacental Doppler blood flow studies (Bewley, Cooper & Campbell, 1991). It is not surprising, therefore, to discover that these clinical abnormalities are reflected in perturbations in the early stages of placentation.

In 1972, Brosens, Robertson and Dixon showed that in pre-eclampsia, whether arising de novo or superimposed on pre-existing essential or

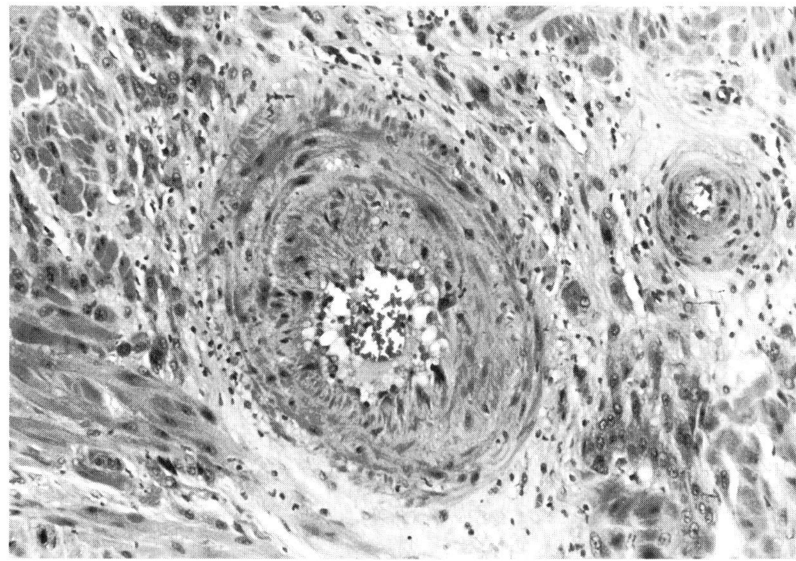

Fig. 7.3. Absence of physiological changes in myometrial segment of spiral artery in the placental bed from a case of pre-eclampsia. Numerous surrounding interstitial trophoblastic cells are present. Compare the luminal diameter with uteroplacental artery in Fig. 7.2. (Haematoxylin and eosin ×150.) (Reproduced from Khong & Sawyer, 1991.)

renal hypertension, the myometrial segments of the spiral arteries did not undergo these physiological changes, leaving them resembling the small calibre vessels in the non-pregnant state (Fig. 7.3). They observed that only the decidual segments underwent the transformation, implying a defect in, or absence of, the second wave of endovascular trophoblast invasion. Although physiological changes have been reported in myometrial segments in pre-eclampsia by some workers (in 20 out of 159 cases) (Sheppard & Bonnar, 1981; Gerretsen et al., 1981; Hustin et al., 1983; Pijnenborg et al., 1991), the general consensus is that there is a maladaptation of the myometrial segments in pre-eclampsia.

Indeed, this deficit is more extensive than originally thought. In pre-eclampsia, physiological changes are lacking in the decidual segments of a proportion, about one third to one half, of spiral arteries in the placental bed (Fig. 7.4) (Khong et al., 1986) in addition to the restriction of physiological changes to decidual segments in the remaining spiral arteries. In effect, not only are there fewer uteroplacental arteries formed in pre-eclampsia with absence of transformation of the spiral arteries throughout their entire length but those that are, are only partially

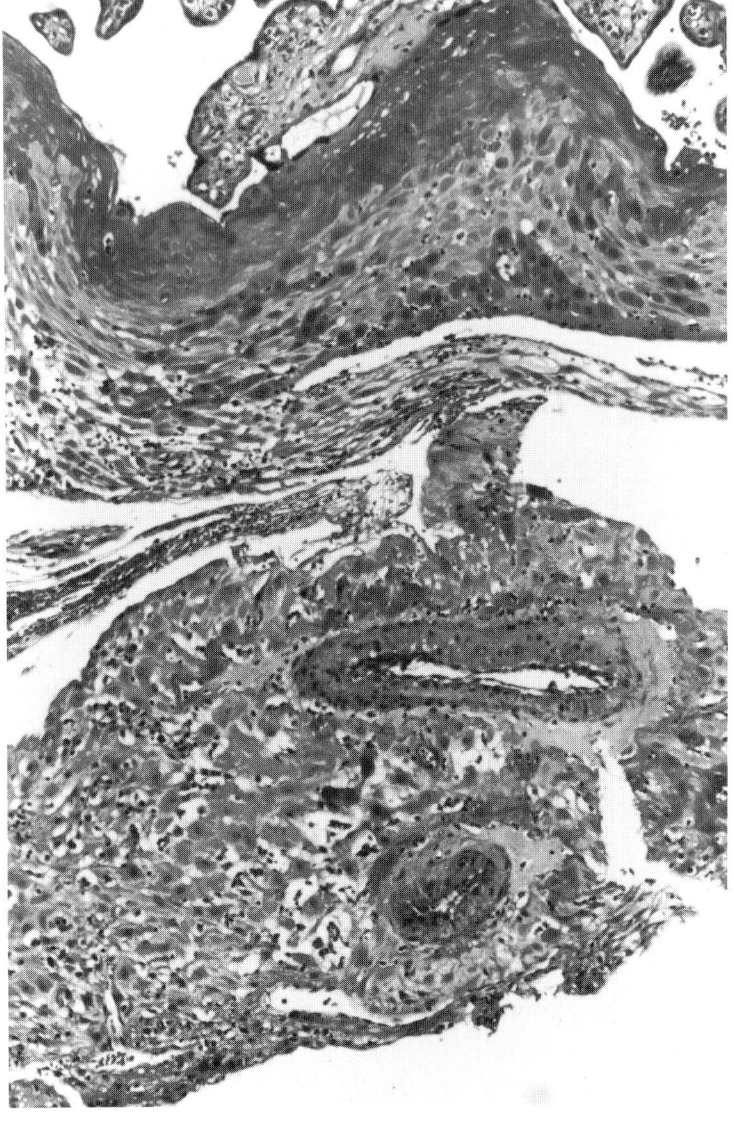

Fig. 7.4. Spiral artery in the basal plate showing absence of physiological changes. (Haematoxylin and eosin ×100.) (Reproduced from Khong, 1993.)

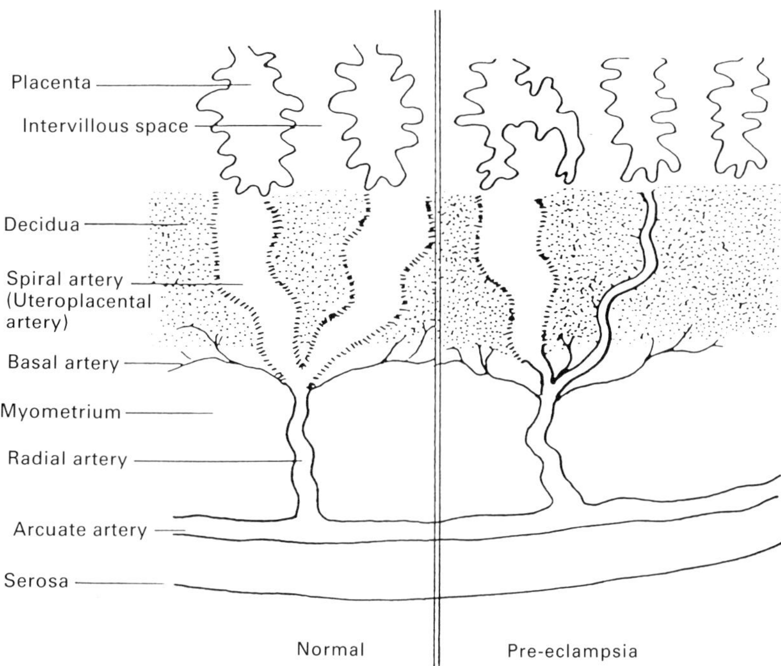

Fig. 7.5. Diagram of the blood supply to the placenta. Note the physiological conversion (hatched) of the spiral arteries throughout their entire length in normal pregnancy (*left*). This is contrasted with physiological changes in some decidual segments (hatched) but absence of such changes in other decidual and myometrial segments in pre-eclampsia (*right*). (Adapted from Khong et al., 1986.)

transformed in the decidual segments (Fig. 7.5). This observation was derived from pregnancy hysterectomy specimens and has been confirmed in placental bed biopsies. It is now clear that some arteries show partial transformation with physiological changes affecting only part of their circumferences (Khong et al., 1986; Pijnenborg et al., 1991), but how they relate to the haemodynamics of uteroplacental blood flow is unclear.

It will be apparent from the foregoing that the finding of uteroplacental arteries showing physiological changes in placental basal plate blocks may not be a reliable indication of normality since the myometrial segments of these vessels may be devoid of physiological changes. The absence of physiological changes in spiral arteries in the basal plate is a diagnostically useful finding as it was seen in 57% of placentas derived from abnormal pregnancies but was not observed in placentas from normal pregnancies (Khong et al., 1986).

When pre-eclampsia develops in a woman with established hypertension, whether essential or renal, the myometrial segments of the spiral arteries which have not undergone physiological changes develop a severe hyperplastic proliferative change to produce a picture of true advanced arteriosclerosis. The degree of arteriosclerotic change is very exaggerated, akin to that seen in other arterial systems in humans when the hypertension is severe and long–standing (Robertson, Brosens & Dixon, 1967).

The vascular changes seen in IUGR appear to be more complex than those seen in pre-eclampsia. Generally, a range from complete physiological changes in decidual and myometrial segments, through changes confined to decidual segments, to absence of changes in decidual and myometrial segments, may be encountered (Khong et al., 1986). Thus, the universal absence of physiological changes in myometrial segments apparently seen in pre-eclampsia is not a feature of IUGR. These studies have not been based on pregnancy hysterectomy specimens and the morphological picture is a composite one derived from studies of placental bed biopsies.

The suggestion that absence of physiological changes may be a result of the various forms of hypertension in pregnancy (Pijnenborg et al., 1991) is untenable since similar defects in placentation are seen in IUGR in normotensive pregnancies. The failure of decidual and myometrial segments of spiral arteries to undergo physiological changes offers a plausible explanation for the reduction in uteroplacental blood flow seen in these pregnancy disorders. It is known that not all pre-eclamptic pregnancies are complicated by IUGR; thus, the depth of restriction of vascular changes may be of less importance in determining whether IUGR will ensue than is whether the number of uteroplacental arteries formed is reduced. While the suggestion that maternal blood pressure is elevated as a compensatory mechanism in maintaining adequate blood supply in pre-eclampsia (Gerretsen et al., 1981) cannot be proven, it is clear that the interaction of blood pressure, morphological features of the placental bed and other factors in determining blood flow are complex.

Abnormalities of trophoblast

When Brosens and colleagues noted that the myometrial segments did not undergo physiological changes in pre-eclampsia, eclampsia and a proportion of IUGR, the implication was that there was a failure of the second wave of endovascular trophoblast migration (Robertson et al.,

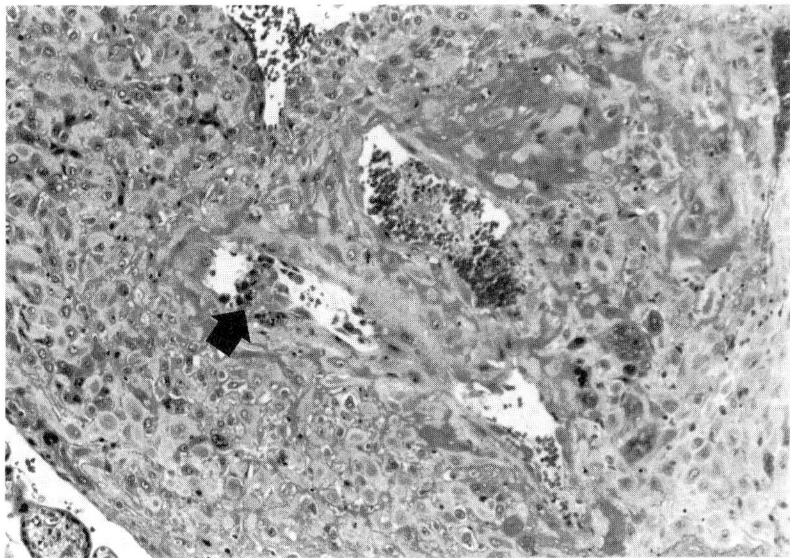

Fig. 7.6. Intraluminal endovascular trophoblast (arrow) in the third trimester of a pregnancy complicated by intrauterine growth retardation. (Haematoxylin and eosin ×140). (Reproduced from Khong & Chambers 1992.)

1975). The finding of a similar defect in decidual segments in these pregnancy disorders suggests that the first wave of endovascular trophoblast migration may be lacking also. This is supported by the observation that in a proportion of miscarriages, physiological changes are absent in the decidual segments at the gestational age when they would be expected to be present (Khong et al., 1987*a*).

Another morphological indicator of defective placentation is the finding of intraluminal endovascular trophoblast in the third trimester in uteroplacental (spiral) arteries in pregnancies complicated by pre-eclampsia and IUGR (Fig. 7.6) (Khong et al., 1986, 1992). Endovascular trophoblast migration is thought to be completed by 24 weeks gestation, and intraluminal endovascular trophoblast is not seen beyond the second trimester in normal pregnancies. Teleologically, we have argued that this may represent a belated response by the fetally derived trophoblast in infiltrating the spiral arteries, in an attempt to transform them into physiologically altered vessels to provide the necessary increase in blood flow (Khong & Robertson, 1992).

Several workers have noted clustering of interstitial trophoblast around physiologically unconverted spiral arteries in abnormal pregnancies (Gerretsen et al., 1983; Pijnenborg et al., 1991), but this needs to be confirmed in hysterectomy specimens to exclude a possible selection bias of placental bed biopsy material as an explanation. Where spiral arteries do not show physiological changes, the only guide as to whether a biopsy has originated from the true centre of the placental bed and not from the margin is the finding of plentiful interstitial trophoblast. Therefore, the clustering of interstitial trophoblast may be a selection bias on the part of the pathologist to confirm its origin from the centre of the placental bed. An alternative explanation is likely also. It will be recalled that in early pregnancy there is clustering of interstitial trophoblast around the spiral arteries and that this is present even prior to their transformation into uteroplacental arteries. It is believed that one action of interstitial trophoblast is to prime the spiral arteries for their subsequent interaction with endovascular trophoblast (Pijnenborg et al., 1983). It is possible therefore that the clustering of interstitial trophoblast around spiral arteries in the third trimester may be a delayed response (teleologically) to attempts to bring about this priming effect on the unconverted arteries, analogous to intraluminal endovascular trophoblast in the third trimester. Parenthetically, interstitial trophoblast migration is disturbed also in miscarriages (Khong et al., 1987*a*). All these features of disturbed extravillous trophoblast migration suggest that there is a temporal window when migration of interstitial and endovascular trophoblast and their interaction with maternal tissue must occur, outside which defective placentation will result (Khong & Robertson, 1992).

Acute atherosis

A distinctive arteriopathy, called acute atherosis, was first described in the uterus in 'hypertensive albuminuric toxemia' of pregnancy. This lesion is characterized by fibrinoid necrosis of the arterial wall, a perivascular lymphocytic infiltrate and, at a later stage, the presence of lipid-laden cells in the damaged wall (Fig. 7.7). Since then, there have been numerous studies of the arteriopathy and it has been described in pre-eclampsia, IUGR and systemic lupus erythematosus (Labarrere, 1988; Khong, 1991*a*). The incidence of acute atherosis ranges from 41–48% in series examining placental and placental bed biopsy material (Khong, Pearce & Robertson, 1987*b*).

It has been described only in vessels inside the uterus in autopsies of women dying from pre-eclampsia or eclampsia (Zeek & Assali, 1950), despite evidence that the pregnancy disorder affects multiple systems.

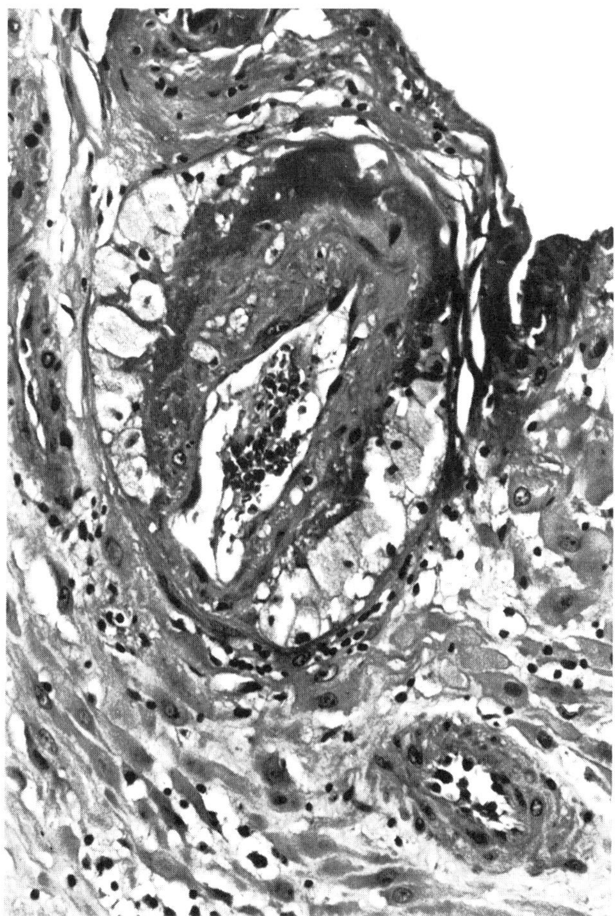

Fig. 7.7. Acute atherosis in a decidual vessel in the decidua parietalis showing fibrinoid necrosis, infiltration by lipophages and a perivascular mononuclear cellular infiltrate. (Haematoxylin and eosin ×200). (Reproduced from Khong et al., 1987*b*.)

Only vessels that have not undergone the physiological changes are affected. Thus, it may be seen in the basal arteries, myometrial and decidual segments of spiral arteries in the placental bed and in the non-placental bed, although it is not seen in the decidua parietalis in IUGR (Khong, 1991*a*). There is extensive luminal obstruction by lipophages, endothelial damage and thrombosis associated with acute atherosis (Khong & Mott, 1993). These further compromise the maternal blood supply to the placenta and fetus which is already limited by the absence of physiological vascular changes in these vessels. These lesions offer the best explanation for decidual necrosis and subsequent abruptio placentae, antepartum haemorrhage and for maternal vascular thrombosis leading to placental infarction.

Although some workers have found an inverse relation between the presence of acute atherosis and birthweight (Maqueo, Azuela & de la Vega, 1964; McFadyen, Price & Geirsson, 1986), this is not supported by critical statistical analysis and, furthermore, there are methodological problems with those studies. No statistically significant relation between acute atherosis and fetal outcome, including birthweight, degree of proteinuria, severity or duration of hypertension was found (Khong et al., 1987*b*).

Analysis of the maternal factors associated with acute atherosis does not support the concept that hypertension in itself causes the lesion (Khong et al., 1987*b*). Much has been made of the similarity of acute atherosis to the arteriopathy seen in allograft rejection reactions, such as cardiac, hepatic and renal transplants. Immunoglobulin (IgM) and complement (C3) deposition in acute atherosis, similar to that seen in acute atherosis-like lesions in cardiac and renal allograft rejections, has been described (Labarrere, 1988). However, as the lesion is seen in maternal vessels, one has to speculate that it is the fetal rejection of the maternal uterus rather than the often- stated rejection of the fetal allograft (Khong & Robertson, 1992). A direct immune attack on fetal tissue is also an unlikely explanation as the lesion is seen best in small arteries relatively remote from trophoblast (Robertson & Khong, 1987). It may be that an inappropriate immune reaction acting in synergy with the haemodynamic disturbances engendered by the hypertension results in the formation of the lesion.

Placental lesions in pre-eclampsia and intrauterine growth retardation

Infarction

The placental lesion most commonly associated with pre-eclampsia is the placental infarct. A placental infarct is a localized area of ischaemic villous necrosis secondary to lesions in the maternal uteroplacental blood supply. An infarct should never be diagnosed without slicing of the placenta, as perivillous fibrin deposition and intraplacental haematomas may simulate the lesion on cursory examination of the maternal surface. Others go further and advocate histological confirmation but, with experience, an infarct can be recognized grossly. A fresh infarct seen in the cut surface of the placenta is dark red and is firmer than healthy villous tissue on palpation. As the infarct ages, it appears brownish, then yellow and finally white and becomes progressively firmer. Histologically, the infarct is characterized by villous crowding, narrowing of the intervillous space, congestion of the fetal vessels and pyknosis of the syncytiotrophoblastic nuclei. As the infarct ages, the villi undergo necrosis and an old infarct consists of 'ghost' villi (Fig. 7.8) (Fox, 1978).

Infarcts are more commonly seen in the periphery of the placenta where they are of no clinical significance to the fetus. However, central infarction may compromise adequate fetoplacental exchange and is clinically significant. It is generally agreed that infarcts occupying less than 10% of the parenchyma are insignificant and that the placenta has a significant functional reserve capacity, being able to withstand the loss of 15–20% of its villous tissue as a result of ischaemic necrosis (Fox, 1978). The extent of placental infarction consistent with fetal survival depends on the integrity of the maternal uteroplacental blood supply. Thus, infarction in itself would be of little or no significance if it occurred in a placenta with an adequate and healthy maternal uteroplacental vasculature. On the other hand, an infarction of one or two placental cotyledons would be devastating to a growth-retarded fetus where there is generalized abnormal maternal uteroplacental vasculature and compromised uteroplacental blood supply. Indeed, the true significance of an infarct is that it is a visible marker of underlying disease of the maternal uteroplacental vasculature. Brosens and Renaer (1972) showed that the spiral arteries underlying infarcts lacked physiological changes or trophoblastic invasion and that there was occlusive thrombosis; this was confirmed by Wallenburg, Stolte and Janssens (1973) who also showed that no significant changes could be seen in the fetal stem vessels.

Placental abruption

Placental abruption or premature separation of the placenta prior to the onset of labour or delivery results in accumulation of blood beneath the placenta and retroplacental haematoma formation. If the placental separation takes place over a long period of time, in stages, the fetus may survive but suffers from deprivation of its maternal blood supply. This prolonged sequence of events often results in retroplacental haematoma that may be organized and firmly attached to the basal plate of the

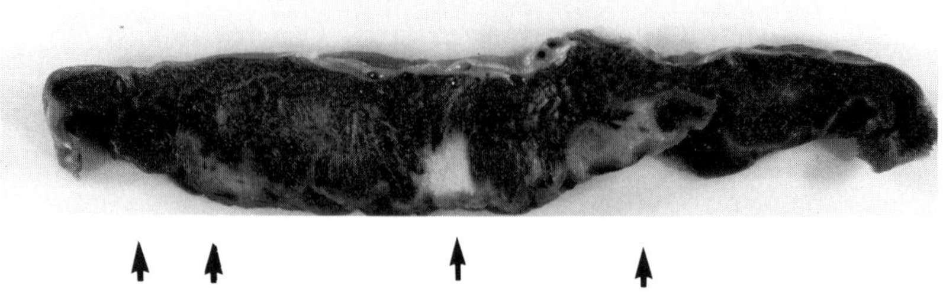

Fig. 7.8*a*. Placental slice showing infarcts of varying ages (arrows).

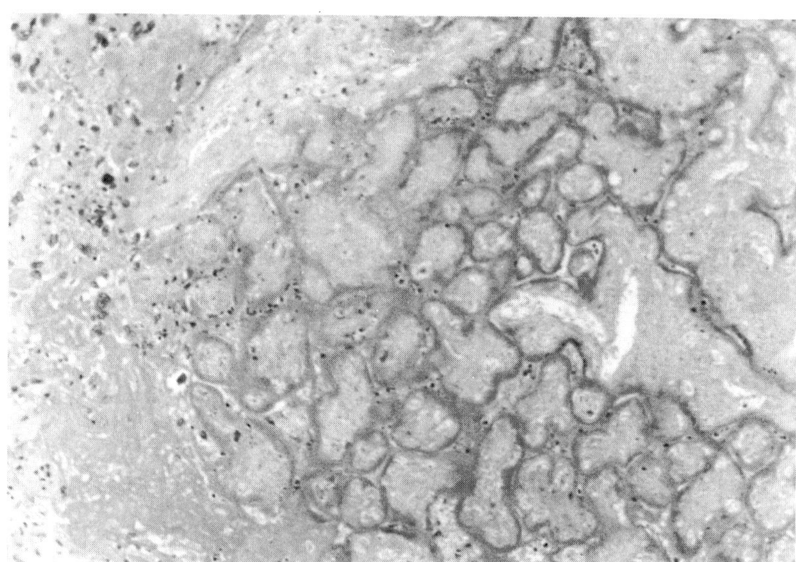

Fig. 7.8*b*. An old placental infarct. The villi have a ghost outline and the villous trophoblast has undergone complete necrosis and is represented by a rim of eosinophilic material. (Haematoxylin and eosin ×140.)

placenta, often indenting into the placental parenchyma with ensuing infarcts. The acute placental abruption, on the other hand, occurring immediately prior to delivery or causing sufficient fetal distress as to warrant emergency delivery may not be recognized reliably by the pathologist, as macroscopic evidence may be absent; there may be no adherent blood clot or indentation of the placental parenchyma. However, there may be histological evidence with intense congestion and dilatation of the fetal vessels of the affected area.

Retroplacental haematoma and placental abruption is often discussed in the context of maternal hypertensive disorders but only about 30% of women with placental abruption have hypertension. Fox (1978) demonstrated that women with pre-eclampsia had a three-fold increase in incidence, while women with chronic hypertension had no increase in incidence.

The bleeding is primarily intradecidual and intramyometrial. Extravasation towards the decidual surface leads to dissection of the decidua and myometrium and placental abruption while extravasation towards the serosal surface produces the typical ecchymoses of the Couvelaire uterus. It is unlikely that the primary source of bleeding is venous as the pressure would be insufficient to cause the extravasation seen in placental abruption. Whether the haemorrhages are due to primary uteroplacental vascular pathology or are preceded by local decidual necrosis, or both, is not certain. Acute atherotic lesions offer a plausible explanation, with their association with thrombosis and subsequent haemorrhage through the weakened vessel walls, but they do not explain the majority of cases which occur in normotensive pregnancies. Thrombosis of the decidual arteries may lead to decidual necrosis and venous haemorrhage. Dommisse and Tiltman (1992) showed that the intramyometrial segments of the spiral arteries lacked physiological changes in about 60% of placental abruption cases, both hypertensive and normotensive patients. Uteroplacental arteries showed intimal or subintimal thickening. Abnormal vessels, not clearly identifiable as arteries or as veins, were seen deep in the myometrium and these showed subintimal fibrosis and thrombosis. The possibilities of arteriovenous malformation or aneurysmal formation were suggested but could not be confirmed.

Villitis

Intravillous inflammation is seen often. When specific aetiological factors, such as rubella, toxoplasmosis, cytomegalovirus, etc., have been

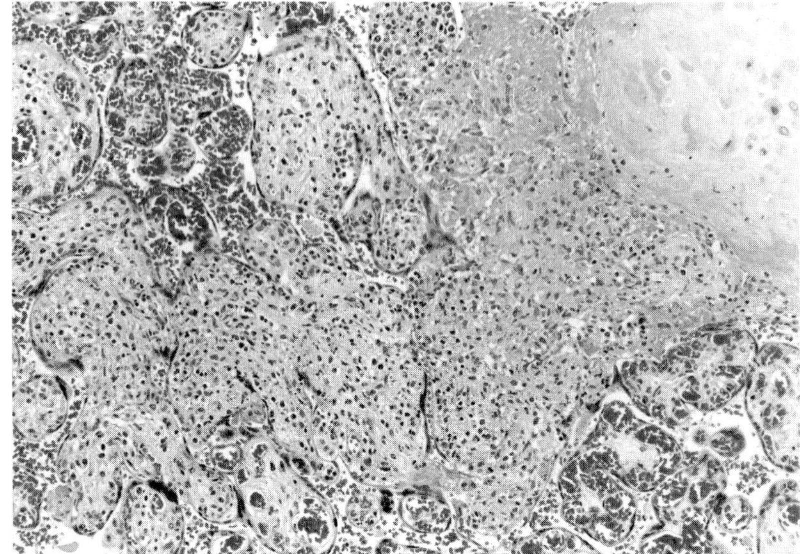

Fig. 7.9. Villitis of unknown aetiology. The hypercellular inflamed villi are contrasted with adjacent normal villi (lower right). (Haematoxylin and eosin ×150.)

eliminated, a large number of cases of villitis are of unknown aetiology. The incidence of villitis of unknown aetiology is influenced by various factors, such as the number of cases studied, the number of placental blocks examined, definition of the lesion, possible population differences and observer reliability (Khong et al., 1993). Be that as it may, the reported incidence ranges from 6% (United States of America) to 34% (Argentina).

Villitis of unknown aetiology is significantly associated with IUGR and pre-eclampsia and may recur in successive pregnancies with similar associations (Redline & Abramowsky, 1985).

The histological aspects of villitis have been well documented, the sine qua non being an intravillous inflammatory infiltrate (Fig. 7.9) (Russell, 1980). The cells participating in the inflammatory process are lymphocytes and macrophages and these usually form a mixed infiltrate. The distribution of the lesion is not uniform throughout the placenta and may be confined to the parabasal and anchoring villi near the basal plate. Similarly, the extent of the villous inflammation may be confined to one or two foci in each of which only a very few villi may be involved, or be extensive in which large areas of most sections are inflamed.

As defined, the aetiology of villitis of unknown aetiology is unclear although infective causes, probably haematogenous, have been proposed. However, attempts to identify an infective agent have been unsuccessful and serological evidence of infection has been singularly negative. Labarrere, Althabe and Telenta (1982) have suggested that villitis may represent a morphological expression of a maternal immune attack against placental tissues and this is corroborated by their finding of villitis in apparently normal pregnancies (Labarrere, McIntyre & Faulk, 1990). However, the fact that most of the inflammatory cells are intravillous, and hence presumably fetal in origin, argues that if an immunopathological process were causative, it would be a graft-versus-host reaction rather than a host-versus-graft reaction (Knox & Fox, 1984).

Most studies report a relation between the degree of villitis present and the severity of IUGR. Cases of widespread, diffuse and necrotizing villitis are exceptional. Most cases of villitis are focal and the degree of villous damage is unlikely to impair placental function on an anatomical basis, given the large functional reserve capacity of the placenta. Until we understand the cause of villitis, we can only speculate that the presence of the lesion serves as a marker for something more widespread, such as an infection or a physiological immunological reaction.

Summary

A range of pregnancy disorders, such as pre-eclampsia, IUGR, miscarriage and placenta accreta, may ensue when there is defective placentation. It may also contribute to preterm delivery (Arias et al., 1993). Recent observations of pregnancy outcomes in a variety of clinical disorders have shown interesting support for the hypothesis that failure to establish an adequate sustaining uteroplacental blood supply could have growth impairing effects on the fetus (Khong, 1991*b*). Although the morphological features and events described in the placental bed in late pregnancy provide a powerful explanation for the hypoperfusion of the intervillous space, the mould is cast in the early stages of pregnancy. This is when the factors that facilitate the interactions between fetal and maternal tissues occur, and when the pivotal influences on promotion or restraint of trophoblast migration are activated. Until these mechanisms are elucidated, any possible therapeutic manipulation of uteroplacental vascular development must remain purely conjectural.

References

Arias, F., Rodriquez, L., Rayne, S.C. & Kraus, F.T. (1993). Maternal placental vasculopathy and infection: two distinct subgroups among patients with preterm labor and preterm ruptured membranes. *American Journal of Obstetrics and Gynecology*, **168**, 585–91.

Bewley, S., Cooper, D. & Campbell, S. (1991). Doppler investigation of uteroplacental blood flow resistance in the second trimester: a screening study for pre-eclampsia and intrauterine growth retardation. *British Journal of Obstetrics and Gynaecology*, **98**, 871–9.

Björk, O., Persson, B., Stangenberg, M. & Václavínková, V. (1984). Spiral artery lesions in relation to metabolic control in diabetes mellitus. *Acta Obstetrica et Gynecologica Scandinavica*, **63**, 123–7.

Brosens, I., Dixon, H.G. & Robertson, W.B. (1977). Fetal growth retardation and the arteries of the placental bed. *British Journal of Obstetrics and Gynaecology*, **84**, 656–63.

Brosens, I. & Renaer, M. (1972). On the pathogenesis of placental infarcts in pre-eclampsia. *Journal of Obstetrics and Gynaecology of the British Commonwealth*, **79**, 794–9.

Brosens, I., Robertson, W.B. & Dixon, H.G. (1967). The physiological response of the vessels of the placental bed to normal pregnancy. *Journal of Pathology and Bacteriology*, **93**, 569–79.

Brosens, I., Robertson, W.B. & Dixon, H.G. (1972). The role of the spiral arteries in the pathogenesis of pre-eclampsia. *Obstetrics and Gynecology Annual*, **1**, 177–91.

Dixon, H.G. & Robertson, W.B. (1958). A study of the vessels of the placental bed in normotensive and hypertensive women. *Journal of Obstetrics and Gynaecology of the British Empire*, **65**, 803–9.

Dommisse, J. & Tiltman, A.J. (1992). Placental bed biopsies in placental abruption. *British Journal of Obstetrics and Gynaecology*, **99**, 651–4.

Fox, H. (1978). *Pathology of the Placenta*. W.B. Saunders, London.

Frusca, T., Morassi, L., Pecorelli, S., Grigolato, P. & Gastaldi, A. (1989). Histological features of uteroplacental vessels in normal and hypertensive patients in relation to birthweight. *British Journal of Obstetrics and Gynaecology*, **96**, 835–9.

Gerretsen, G., Huisjes, H.J. & Elema, J.D. (1981). Morphological changes of the spiral arteries in the placental bed in relation to pre-eclampsia and fetal growth retardation. *British Journal of Obstetrics and Gynaecology*, **88**, 876–81.

Gerretsen, G., Huisjes, H.J., Hardonk, M.J. & Elema, J.D. (1983). Trophoblast alterations in the placental bed in relation to physiological changes in spiral arteries. *British Journal of Obstetrics and Gynaecology*, **90**, 34–9.

Hustin, J., Foidart, J.M. & Lambotte, R. (1983). Maternal vascular lesions in pre-eclampsia and intrauterine growth retardation: light microscopy and immunofluorescence. *Placenta*, **4**, 489–98.

Khong, T.Y. (1991*a*). Acute atherosis in pregnancies complicated by hypertension, by small for gestational age infants, and by diabetes mellitus. *Archives of Pathology and Laboratory Medicine*, **115**, 722–5.

Khong, T.Y. (1991*b*). The Robertson–Brosens–Dixon hypothesis: evidence for the role of haemochorial placentation in pregnancy success. *British Journal of Obstetrics and Gynaecology*, **98**, 1195–9.

Khong, T.Y. (1993). Placenta and umbilical cord and the immunology of pregnancy. In *Fetal and Neonatal Pathology*, ed. J.W. Keeling. Springer-Verlag, London.

Khong, T.Y. & Chambers, H.M. (1992). Alternative method of sampling placentas for the assessment of uteroplacental vasculature. *Journal of Clinical Pathology*, **45**, 925–7.

Khong, T.Y., De Wolf, F., Robertson, W.B. & Brosens I. (1986). Inadequate vascular response to placentation in pregnancies complicated by pre-eclampsia and by small-for-gestational age infants. *British Journal of Obstetrics and Gynaecology*, **93**, 1049–59.

Khong, T.Y., Liddell, H.S. & Robertson, W.B. (1987*a*). Defective haemochorial placentation as a cause of miscarriage: a preliminary study. *British Journal of Obstetrics and Gynaecology*, **94**, 649–55.

Khong, T.Y. & Mott, C. (1993). Immunohistologic demonstration of endothelial disruption in acute atherosis in pre-eclampsia. *European Journal of Obstetrics, Gynecology and Reproductive Biology*, **51**, 193–7.

Khong, T.Y., Pearce, J.M. & Robertson, W.B. (1987*b*). Acute atherosis in pre-eclampsia: Maternal determinants and fetal outcome in the presence of the lesion. *American Journal of Obstetrics and Gynecology*, **157**, 360–3.

Khong, T.Y. & Robertson, W.B. (1992). Spiral artery disease. In *Immunological Obstetrics*, ed. C.B. Coulam, W.P. Faulk & J.A. McIntyre. pp. 492–501. W.W. Norton, New York.

Khong, T.Y. & Sawyer, I.H. (1991). The human placental bed in health and disease. *Reproduction, Fertility and Development*, **3**, 373–7.

Khong, T.Y., Sawyer, I.H. & Heryet, A.R. (1992). An immunohistologic study of endothelialization of uteroplacental vessels in human pregnancy – Evidence that endothelium is focally disrupted by trophoblast in pre-eclampsia. *American Journal of Obstetrics and Gynecology*, **167**, 751–6.

Khong, T.Y., Staples, A., Moore, L. & Byard, R.W. (1993). Observer reliability in assessing villitis of unknown aetiology. *Journal of Clinical Pathology*, **46**, 208–10.

Knox, W.F. & Fox, H. (1984). Villitis of unknown aetiology: Its incidence and significance in placentae from a British population. *Placenta*, **5**, 395–402.

Labarrere, C.A. (1988). Acute atherosis – a histological hallmark of immune aggression? *Placenta*, **9**, 95–108.

Labarrere, C.A., Althabe, O. & Telenta, M. (1982). Chronic villitis of unknown aetiology in placentae of idiopathic small for gestational age infants. *Placenta*, **3**, 309–18.

Labarrere, C.A., McIntyre, J.A. & Faulk, W.P. (1990). Immunohistologic evidence that villitis in human normal term placentas is an immunologic lesion. *American Journal of Obstetrics and Gynecology*, **162**, 515–22.

McFadyen, I.R., Price, A.B. & Geirsson, R.T. (1986). The relation of birthweight to histological appearances in vessels of the placental bed. *British Journal of Obstetrics and Gynaecology*, **93**, 476–81.

Maqueo, M., Azuela, C.J. & de la Vega, M.D. (1964). Placental pathology in eclampsia and pre-eclampsia. *Obstetrics and Gynecology*, 350–6.

Pijnenborg, R., Anthony, J., Davey, D.A., Rees, A., Tiltman, A., Vercruysse, L. & Van Assche, A. (1991). Placental bed spiral arteries in the hypertensive disorders of pregnancy. *British Journal of Obstetrics and Gynaecology*, **98**, 648–55.

Pijnenborg, R., Bland, J.M., Robertson, W.B. & Brosens, I. (1983). Uteroplacental arterial changes related to interstitial trophoblast migration in early human pregnancy. *Placenta*, **4**, 397–414.

Pijnenborg, R., Bland, J.M., Robertson, W.B., Dixon, G. & Brosens, I. (1981). The pattern of interstitial trophoblastic invasion of the myometrium in early human pregnancy. *Placenta*, **2**, 303–16.

Pijnenborg, R., Dixon, G., Robertson, W.B. & Brosens, I. (1980). Trophoblastic invasion of human decidua from 8 – 18 weeks of pregnancy. *Placenta*, **1**, 3–19.

Redline, R.W. & Abramowsky, C.R. (1985). Clinical and pathologic aspects of recurrent placental villitis. *Human Pathology*, **16**, 727–31.

Robertson, W.B., Brosens, I. & Dixon, H.G. (1967). The pathological response of the vessels of the placental bed to hypertensive pregnancy. *Journal of Pathology and Bacteriology*, **93**, 581–92.

Robertson, W.B., Brosens, I. & Dixon, H.G. (1975). Uteroplacental vascular pathology. *European Journal of Obstetrics, Gynecology and Reproductive Biology*, **5**, 47–65.

Robertson, W.B & Khong, T.Y. (1987). Pathology of the uteroplacental bed. In *Hypertension in Pregnancy. Proceedings of the 16th Study Group of the Royal College of Obstetricians and Gynaecologists.* ed. F. Sharp & E.M. Symonds. pp. 101–113. Perinatalogy Press, Ithaca.

Robertson W.B., Khong T.Y., Brosens I., De Wolf F., Sheppard B.L. & Bonnar, J. (1986). The placental bed biopsy. A review from three European centers. *American Journal of Obstetrics and Gynecology*, **155**, 401–12.

Russell, P. (1980). Inflammatory lesions of the human placenta. III: The histopathology of villitis of unknown aetiology. *Placenta*, **1**, 227–44.

Sheppard, B.L. & Bonnar, J. (1981). An ultrastructural study of utero-placental spiral arteries in hypertensive and normotensive pregnancy and fetal growth retardation. *British Journal of Obstetrics and Gynaecology*, **88**, 695–705.

Thorbert, G., Alm, P., Björklund, A.B., Owman, C. & Sjöberg, N-O. (1979). Adrenergic innervation of the human uterus. *American Journal of Obstetrics and Gynecology*, **155**, 223–6.

Wallenburg, H.C.S., Stolte, L.A.M. & Janssens, J. (1973). The pathogenesis of placental infarction. I. A morphologic study in the human placenta. *American Journal of Obstetrics and Gynecology*, **116**, 835–40.

Zeek, P.M. & Assali, N.S. (1950). Vascular changes in the decidua associated with eclamptogenic toxemia of pregnancy. *American Journal of Clinical Pathology*, **20**, 1099–109.

Zuspan, F.P., O'Shaughnessy, R.W., Vinsel, J. & Zuspan, M. (1981). Adrenergic innervation of uterine vasculature in human term pregnancy. *American Journal of Obstetrics and Gynecology*, **139**, 678–80.

8

Human fetal blood gases, glucose, lactate and amino acids in IUGR

RODOLFO MONTEMAGNO and
PETER SOOTHILL

Introduction

Intrauterine growth retardation (IUGR) implies failure to achieve the genetic growth potential for fetal size, but is a definition that encompasses a heterogeneous group. It is an important cause of mortality and morbidity in the perinatal period (Haas, Balcazar & Caulfield, 1987; Villar et al., 1990) and is associated with diseases in adult life such as non-insulin-dependent diabetes, hypertension and stroke (Barker et al., 1989). Although as yet there is no effective intrauterine treatment, assessment and management is important and has improved in the last two to three decades as a result of the introduction of ultrasound imaging, Doppler technology and ultrasound guided needle aspiration of fetal blood (cordocentesis). The latter enables investigation to confirm or refute a suspected diagnosis such as chromosomal abnormality, but has also improved our understanding of the pathology of growth retardation. Before this technique, information concerning the human fetal intrauterine environment and growth came predominantly from studies of umbilical cord blood samples at delivery or during labour from the capillaries of the presenting part following cervical dilatation and rupture of membranes. However, both these approaches provide samples which may reflect acute changes associated with delivery and not a steady state.

In this chapter we will review the techniques of fetal blood sampling before labour and the data on blood gases, glucose, lactate and amino acids obtained by cordocentesis in IUGR. We will also briefly consider the implications of the results for clinical practice.

Fetal blood sampling

History

Access to the fetal circulation was originally achieved by exposing the fetus at the time of hysterotomy (Freda & Adamson, 1964) but such

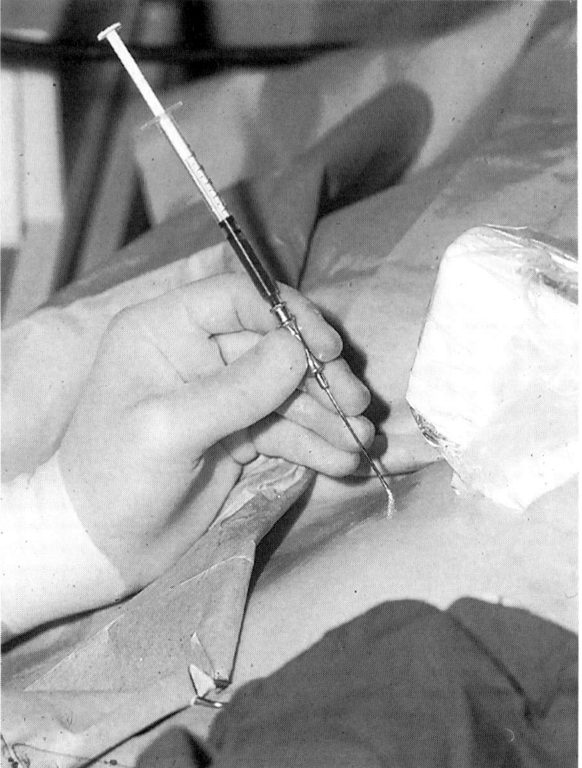

Fig. 8.1. Fetal blood sampling by ultrasound guided needle aspiration of umbilical cord blood (Cordocentesis).

surgery would alter fetal oxygenation at least as much as Caesarean section. In the 1970s, percutaneous fetoscopy was developed and used to visualize and sample from vessels on the chorionic plate or the umbilical cord (Rodeck & Campbell, 1978). However, this is a difficult technique associated with a fetal loss rate of 2–4% and the sedation and analgesia used has been shown to cause a mild fetal respiratory acidosis as a result of maternal hypoventilation (Soothill et al., 1986*a*). In the 1980s ultrasound-guided needling of umbilical cord vessel (cordocentesis) rapidly became the most widely used technique, and it is particularly suited to studies of fetal oxygenation (Nicolaides et al., 1986).

Techniques

Cordocentesis is an outpatient, ultrasound-guided procedure (Fig. 8.1) for which maternal fasting, sedation, antibiotics, tocolysis or fetal paralysis are not required and should be avoided. A 20–22 G needle is passed transplacentally or transamniotically, depending on the position of the placenta, but the advantage of the former is that it allows aspiration of 'intervillous' blood from placental lakes (Nicolaides et al., 1986) which may be useful for the study of placental transfer. Simply as a result of its larger size, the umbilical vein is sampled more often (80%) than an umbilical artery (20%) and the vein is probably safer with a lower incidence of fetal bradycardia (Weiner et al., 1991). Since it is not always possible to choose the vessel sampled prospectively it is essential when studying fetal oxygenation to identify it after obtaining blood, by a small injection of saline which causes a turbulence in the intravascular flow visible on the ultrasound screen. The volume of blood that can be safely removed from the fetal circulation depends on gestational age but is generally 1–4 ml. Sampling sites other than umbilical cord have been described (such as the intrahepatic vein (Nicolini et al., 1990*b*) or the heart (Hansmann, et al., 1991) but these have the potential problem of sampling a mixture of blood from different sources so, for studies of oxygenation, cordocentesis is preferred by the authors.

Risks

Direct maternal complications are negligible except for red cell iso-immunization, and anti-D prophylaxis should be offered to rhesus-negative women. However chorio-amnionitis or emergency Caesarean section in the fetal interest can result in secondary maternal problems. Fetal loss rates following cordocentesis have been approximately 1% in several large series (Soothill, 1994). This rate varies with gestational age, the experience of the operator and with fetal condition at the time of sampling, being significantly higher at earlier gestations and in sick, severely growth-retarded fetuses. Potential fetal complications are infection, premature rupture of membranes, haemorrhage, severe bradycardia, cord tamponade, thrombosis and abruptio placentae, but the exact cause of fetal loss following cordocentesis often cannot be determined, so it may be impossible to say if it would have happened anyway without the procedure.

Use in IUGR

Concern about fetal growth is one of the commonest problems in obstetric care. The causes of being small are numerous and fall into three broad categories: fetal disease such as chromosomal defects, malformation or infection (about 15% of cases referred to fetal medicine units), fetal starvation with or without hypoxia because of impaired placental function or maternal undernutrition or, by exclusion, a normal, constitutionally small fetus. The reason for offering cordocentesis to a pregnant woman with its risk of fetal loss is to identify the cause when this has not been possible non-invasively, because it may significantly change the obstetric management. For example, Caesarean section and iatrogenic premature delivery can be avoided if an IUGR fetus can be shown to have normal structure, chromosomes and placental function and so is presumed to be normal and constitutionally small. Invasive investigation has also enormously increased our understanding of the pathophysiology of impaired placental function by making samples available for study. When cordocentesis is undertaken in IUGR standard investigations should include karyotyping, a full blood picture and blood gases.

Normal ranges

It is impossible to interpret results from IUGR fetuses without having appropriate reference ranges, but these have been difficult to construct because of the very selected nature of pregnancies in which fetal blood sampling is indicated. There have been six publications presenting fetal blood gas reference ranges (Soothill et al., 1986*a*; Pardi et al., 1987; Cox et al., 1988; Nicolaides et al., 1989; Weiner & Williamson, 1989; Okamura et al., 1990) and all found similar values and changes with gestational age. However, Pardi et al. (1987), Cox et al. (1988) and Weiner and Williamson (1989) did not describe their cases in detail, simply giving the range in comparison with their pathological data. The values differed significantly from animal studies, human scalp blood in early labour and cord blood after delivery (Huch & Huch, 1984) but the results were compatible with measurements at hysterotomy in early gestation and at elective Caesarean section at term (Rudolph et al., 1971; Pardi et al., 1987).

A significant limitation of human data is that paired umbilical arterial and venous blood samples are rarely available. Although paired samples are the only accurate way to assess placental or fetal uptake/production of a substance in the blood, in the human we have to rely on differences in the mean concentrations of groups. A possible advantage of the human data is the ability to obtain maternal blood from placental lakes (intervillous blood) although this has only been studied by one group so far (Soothill et al., 1986*a*). The exact relationship between blood values at this site and the uterine veins is unknown and may vary depending on the

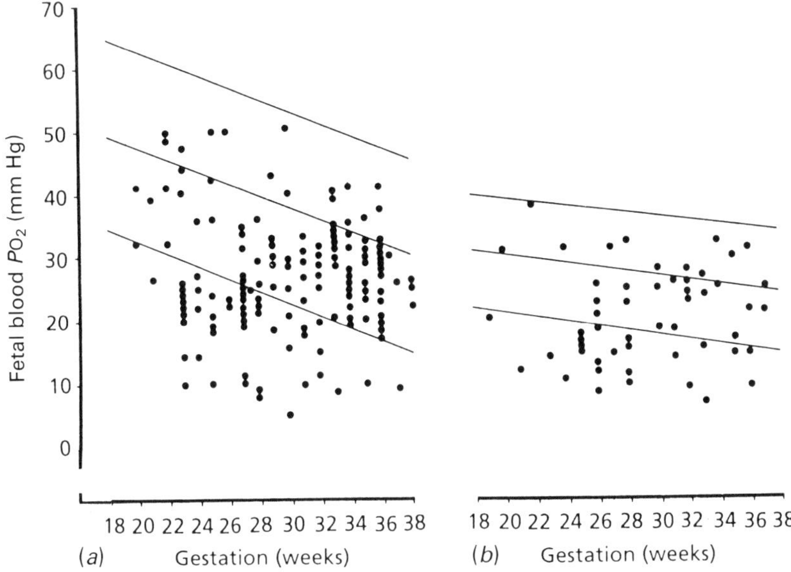

Fig. 8.2. Umbilical venous and arterial PO_2 values for IUGR fetuses plotted against reference ranges. (Nicolaides et al., 1989.)

part of the placenta sampled but the intervillous blood PO_2 was about 10 mm Hg higher than the umbilical venous blood values. In the future, this technique may prove to be extremely useful to assess placental transfer.

Since many factors in the fetus change significantly with gestational age, spurious correlations can be reported unless the raw data is adjusted for gestational age (Soothill & Nicolaides, 1987). The usual way is to express the data in multiples of standard deviation from the normal mean for gestational age (a z-score). Alternatively, analysis of variance can be used.

PO_2

Umbilical venous and arterial PO_2 fall with gestational age (Soothill et al., 1986*a*; Pardi et al., 1987; Cox et al., 1988; Nicolaides et al., 1989; Weiner et al., 1991) from about 50 and 37 mm Hg at 18 weeks to 35 and 30 mm Hg at 36 weeks gestation, respectively (Fig. 8.2). Although the oxygen tension in fetal blood is higher than expected from sheep studies, it is much lower than in maternal blood, either because of incomplete venous equilibration between the uterine and umbilical circulations or due to placental oxygen consumption. The fall in PO_2 with gestation is steeper in umbilical venous than arterial blood and, since the utero-placental blood flow per kilogram remains the same (Gerson et al., 1987), it probably reflects increased placental oxygen consumption with advancing gestational age (Soothill et al., 1986*a*; Nicolaides et al., 1989). Indeed the umbilical venous–arterial difference decreases with gestational age.

Two possible compensatory mechanisms for the decrease in fetal PO_2 have been described. The umbilical venous blood oxygen content may increase slightly throughout gestation as a result of a rise in fetal blood haemoglobin concentration (Soothill et al., 1986*a*). There is also a significant rise in the mean velocity of blood in both the aorta and the middle cerebral artery with advancing gestation in normal pregnancies (Bilardo, Nicolaides & Campbell, 1990). Both of these adaptations would be expected to maintain tissue oxygen delivery.

PCO_2

Fetal PCO_2 levels rise from 16 weeks in both umbilical arterial and venous blood (Soothill et al., 1986*a*; Pardi et al., 1987; Cox et al., 1988; Nicolaides et al., 1989; Weiner et al., 1989; Okamura et al., 1990) and are significantly higher than in the mother. The mean and 95% confidence intervals for umbilical venous and arterial blood are shown in Fig. 8.3. The rise in PCO_2 could be the result of increased production or decreased placental clearance of carbon dioxide. Comparison with the discussion of the fall in PO_2 suggests that the rise is due to increased placental consumption of oxygen and so increased production of carbon dioxide.

Lactate

Fetal umbilical venous and arterial lactate concentrations probably do not change significantly with gestational age in normal pregnancies (Soothill et al., 1986*a*; Pardi et al., 1988; Nicolaides et al., 1989; Okamura et al., 1990) and the values obtained at cordocentesis are similar to those obtained at elective Caesarean section at term (Pardi et al., 1987; Marconi et al., 1990). Animal studies have demonstrated that lactate is produced by the placenta under physiological conditions (Holzman, Phillips & Battaglia, 1979) and that the fetus is a net lactate consumer. The finding in human third trimester pregnancies of higher blood lactate concentration in the umbilical vein than in the umbilical artery (Soothill et al., 1986*a*) supports the suggestion that lactate is also produced by the

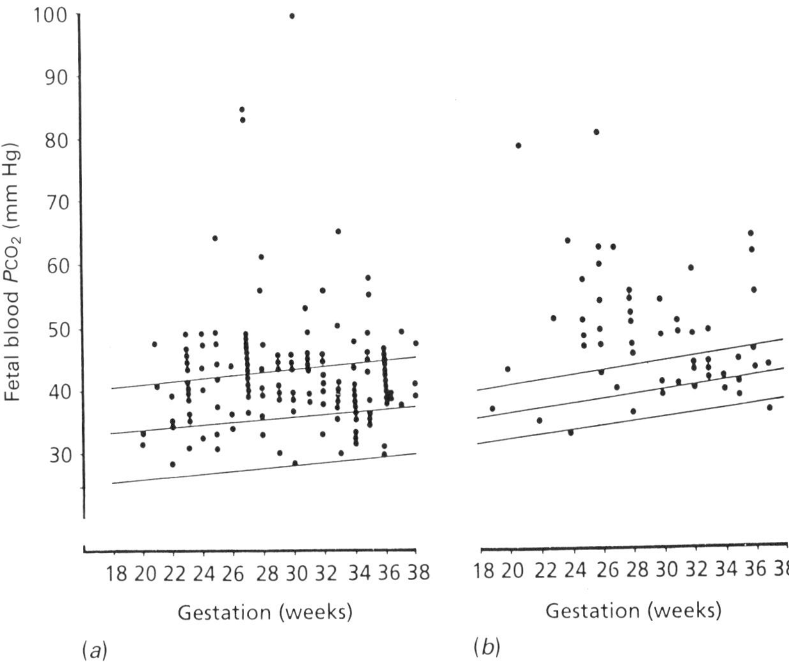

Fig. 8.3. Umbilical venous and arterial PCO_2 values for IUGR fetuses plotted against reference ranges. (Nicolaides et al., 1989.)

placenta and consumed as an energy substrate by the human fetus under physiological conditions. However, lactate is clearly an excretory product of fetal metabolism in tissue hypoxia and so placental clearance of lactate may help repay a fetal 'oxygen debt' (Soothill et al., 1987). Therefore, in human fetal life, lactate can be either a substrate or excretory product depending on tissue oxygenation.

pH, bicarbonate and base excess

Following the rise in PCO_2, it is not surprising that the umbilical venous and arterial pH decrease significantly with gestational age. Reference ranges for pH (mean and individual 95% confidence intervals) are shown in Fig. 8.4 (Soothill et al., 1986*a*; Pardi et al., 1987; Cox et al., 1988; Nicolaides et al., 1989; Weiner et al., 1989). Bicarbonate and base excess show a small but significant positive correlation with gestational age in the umbilical venous blood (Soothill et al., 1986*a*; Pardi et al., 1987; Cox et

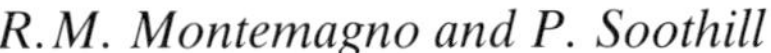

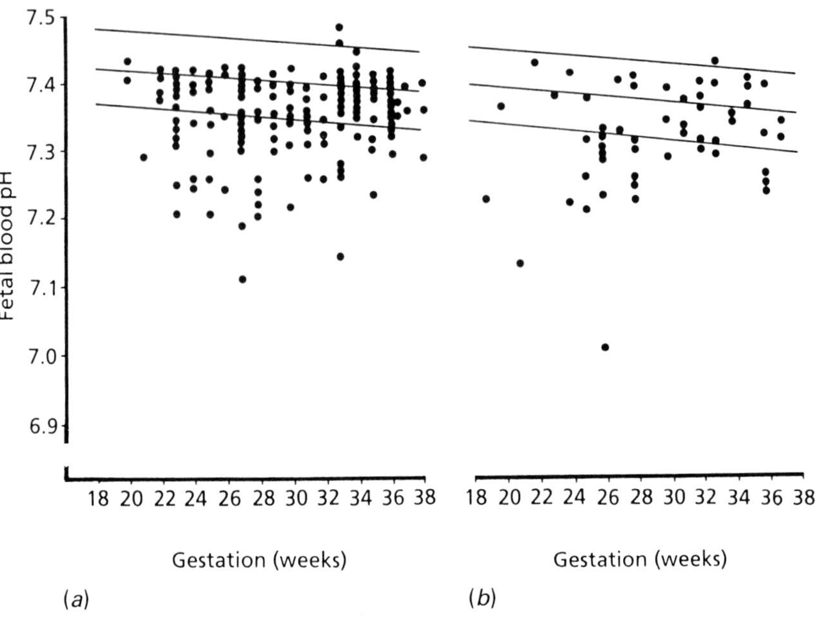

Fig. 8.4. Umbilical venous and arterial pH values for IUGR fetuses plotted against reference ranges. (Nicolaides et al., 1989.)

al., 1988). These indices are calculated to give an indication of whether an acid–base disturbance is of respiratory or metabolic origin and are derived from the pH and PCO_2 (e.g. 'actual' bicarbonate = constant × PCO_2/pH). The same information can be obtained by examination of the measured parameters from which these indices are derived (e.g. if the pH is low but the PCO_2 is normal, then the acidosis is not respiratory but metabolic).

Glucose

Glucose transport across the placenta is by carrier-mediated facilitated diffusion and, until saturation of the carrier molecule, the glucose uptake into the umbilical venous blood from the placenta is directly related to the maternal glucose concentration and to the placental glucose gradient (Spellacy et al., 1964; Hay et al., 1984). The mean umbilical venous blood glucose concentration is higher than umbilical arterial which indicates there is a fetal glucose uptake from the placenta. Similarly, the maternal glucose concentration is higher than that in the fetus, and levels in the two compartments are significantly correlated, which confirms that the major source of fetal glucose is the mother. However, maternal and fetal glucose levels do not change significantly with gestational age (Economides, Proudler & Nicolaides, 1989*a*).

The umbilical venous plasma insulin concentration and the fetal insulin to glucose ratio increases exponentially with gestation (Economides et al., 1989*a*), presumably reflecting the progressive maturation of fetal endocrine activity. Although insulin has been demonstrated in the fetal plasma as early as 10 weeks of gestation, it has been suggested that pancreatic insulin release is glucose insensitive before 28 weeks (Hill, 1978). Furthermore, it has been shown that, between 17 and 38 weeks of gestation, fetal glucose levels correlate better with the maternal glucose concentration than with fetal insulin levels, suggesting that the primary determinant of fetal blood glucose level is the maternal blood glucose concentration.

Amino acids

Amino acids have been measured in the umbilical circulation of chronically catheterized fetal lambs (Lemons et al., 1976) and a significant fetal uptake of most neutral and basic amino acids was found but there was a significant release of glutamic acid and serine from the fetus to the placenta. The fetal amino acid uptake far exceeds the rate needed for protein synthesis (Battaglia & Meschia, 1986) and, with the high production of urea (Gresham et al., 1972), this suggests that amino acids are utilized for oxidation during intrauterine life.

In the human, fetal levels of most amino acids are higher than maternal in normal pregnancies suggesting active transport across the placenta (McIntosh, Rodeck & Heath, 1984), but there is a strong correlation between fetal and maternal levels (Cetin et al., 1988, 1990; Economides et al., 1989*b*). The concentrations of most amino acids and total amino-nitrogen are higher in umbilical venous than arterial blood samples obtained at Caesarean section (Cetin et al., 1988) suggesting fetal uptake. Although the total maternal venous plasma concentration of amino acids does not change significantly with gestational age, the fetal–maternal ratio of amino acids decreases implying increased consumption by the fetal–placental unit (Economides et al., 1989*b*). The increased amino acid consumption is compatible with the increased oxygen use and carbon dioxide production suggesting increased metabolic activity with advancing gestation (Soothill et al., 1986*a;* Nicolaides et al., 1989). The alternative explanation of reduced placental uptake as a result of decreased placental perfusion with maternal blood or impaired placental active transport is unlikely because the blood flow to the uterus and its contents in ml/kg per minute do not change with gestational age (Gerson et al., 1987).

Data from IUGR fetuses

PO_2

Many IUGR fetuses with a normal karyotype and structure are remarkably hypoxaemic with PO_2 levels even <10 mm Hg (Fig. 8.2) (Soothill et al., 1987; Cox et al., 1988; Nicolaides et al., 1989; Weiner et al., 1991; Pardi et al., 1993). This finding could be due to reduced supply of oxygen as result of impaired exchange between the uteroplacental and fetal circulations or increased fetal consumption. The latter is not the cause because the umbilical venous PO_2 is reduced as much as the umbilical arterial blood PO_2 and the former explanation is suggested by Doppler studies that show high resistance in the uterine (Soothill et al., 1986*c*) and umbilical arteries (Nicolaides et al., 1988) in hypoxic IUGR. Indeed histopathological studies have shown a failure of the normal change of maternal placental bed arteries into low resistance vessels (Sheppard & Bonnar, 1976).

The low PO_2 is a chronic longstanding hypoxia and the human fetus is not passive but exhibits biochemical and cardiovascular responses. In hypoxic IUGR fetuses there is an increase in the erythroblast count (Soothill et al., 1987) associated with raised erythropoietin levels (Snijders et al., 1993), which is a haematological adaptation tending to improve oxygen carrying capacity. Furthermore, the human fetus, like that of the sheep (Peeters et al., 1979), responds to chronic hypoxia with a redistribution of blood flow to the fetal heart, brain and adrenal glands at the expenses of lungs, kidneys, spleen, gut and carcass. This has been shown in the human by Doppler studies with a high resistance patterns and low blood velocity in the descending aorta (Soothill et al., 1986*b*) but a low resistance pattern and high blood velocity in the vessels supplying the brain (e.g. middle cerebral artery) (Wladimoroff, Tonge & Stewart, 1986). This process, called 'brain sparing', helps maintain brain oxygenation at the risk of subsequent ischaemic complications in other organs such as necrotizing enterocolitis in the gut.

PCO_2

PCO_2 is significantly raised (sometimes to levels above 60 mmHg) (Fig. 8.3) in many cases of IUGR and strongly correlates with hypoxaemia so the same cases tend to be both hypoxic and hypercapnic (Soothill et al., 1987; Cox et al., 1988; Nicolaides et al., 1989; Weiner et al., 1991; Pardi et al., 1993). Although umbilical venous blood hypoxaemia may be present to a mild degree in the absence of hypercapnia or acidosis, as the umbilical arterial blood becomes hypoxaemic there is a linear increase in the degree of hypercapnia. Therefore, in mild uteroplacental insufficiency the carbon dioxide that accumulates in the umbilical arterial blood is cleared by a single passage through the placenta reflecting the greater speed of diffusion of this molecule compared to oxygen.

Lactate

Some IUGR fetuses are hyperlacticacidaemic and this can be found even with borderline hypoxaemia, so hyperlacticacidaemia is an early biochemical sign of oxygen deficit (Soothill et al., 1987; Pardi et al., 1987; Nicolaides et al., 1989). One possible mechanism of hyperlacticacidaemia is increased placental production of lactate to be used by the fetus as an alternative substrate to glucose. Alternatively, it could be that impaired gluconeogenesis results in decreased utilization of lactate by the fetus, and indeed some other gluconeogenic substrates (such as alanine and glycine) are increased in hypoxaemic IUGR fetuses. However, the most likely explanation is that hyperlacticacidaemia is caused by reduced oxygen supply, inhibition of the Krebs cycle and increased conversion of pyruvic acid to lactic acid as an anaerobic source of energy for the stressed fetus. Marconi et al. (1990) showed at the time of elective Caesarean section that IUGR fetuses with increased impedance in the umbilical circulation (umbilical Doppler PI > 4) had significantly higher levels of both umbilical venous and arterial lactate than in IUGR with PI < 4.

pH, base excess and bicarbonate

Some hypoxic IUGR fetuses are acidotic (Soothill et al., 1987; Cox et al., 1988; Nicolaides et al., 1989; Weiner et al., 1991; Pardi et al., 1993) and this can be to astonishingly low levels (Fig. 8.4); even pH values <7.1 have been detected. The degree of fetal acidosis correlates significantly with both hypercapnia and hyperlacticacidaemia indicating a mixed respiratory and metabolic acidosis (Soothill et al., 1987; Nicolaides et al., 1988). As expected, base excess and bicarbonate values reflect the changes in PCO_2 and pH but these calculations do not substantially improve the assessment of blood gases and acid–base balance (Soothill et al., 1986; Pardi et al., 1993).

Glucose

IUGR fetuses are hypoglycaemic (Soothill et al., 1987; Economides et al., 1989*a*; Nicolini et al., 1989) but the maternal glucose levels in IUGR fetuses are also significantly lower than in controls. The degree of fetal smallness does not correlate with either the maternal–fetal glucose gradient or the degree of hypoxia (Economides et al., 1989*a*; Nicolini et al., 1990*a*). The lower maternal glucose levels are thought to be the result of decreased placental production of diabetogenic hormones (Khouzami et al., 1981) but changes in maternal levels do not account for the severity of fetal hypoglycaemia. The cause of low fetal glucose levels may be decreased placental perfusion (Hay et al., 1984), inadequate placental transfer (Economides & Nicolaides, 1989), decreased gluconeogenesis or increased consumption by anaerobic metabolism to lactate. The degree of hypoxaemia correlates with the maternal–fetal glucose gradient in both umbilical venous and umbilical arterial blood (Economides & Nicolaides, 1989). Animal studies suggest that the major cause of fetal hypoglycaemia is not likely to be decreased endogenous production or increased consumption of glucose but decreased supply (Owens, Falconer & Robinson, 1987; Jacobs et al., 1988). The maternal–fetal glucose gradient is likely to be a measure of impaired placental perfusion, and the degree of hypoglycaemia is related to the severity of abnormality in Doppler measurements in both the uterine and umbilical circulations (Economides, Nicolaides & Campbell, 1990; Nicolini et al., 1990*a*).

Some IUGR fetuses are hypoinsulinaemic and this also correlates significantly with the degree of hypoglycaemia (Economides et al., 1989*b*; Nicolini et al., 1990*a*). The low insulin levels could have been the response to low glucose levels but the fetal glucose/insulin ratio is also lower than normal (Economides et al., 1989*b*). It is possible that hypoxia may inhibit insulin release (Nicolini et al., 1990*a*) as a consequence of pancreatic beta cell dysfunction or ischaemia from the redistribution process, and at autopsy the pancreas is small in growth-retarded infants (Van Assche et al., 1977). Furthermore IUGR fetuses do not have a normal insulin release in response to an intravenous bolus of glucose but a fall in pH is observed which does not correlate with fetal PO_2 (Nicolini et al., 1990*a*). Therefore, attempts at fetal glucose supplementation to treat IUGR are likely to be harmful because, although they may increase blood glucose temporarily, cellular uptake may be impaired because of low insulin levels and hypoxia will predispose the fetus to lactic acidosis by anaerobic glycolysis.

Amino acids

In pregnancies complicated by hypoxaemic IUGR there is a significant disturbance of both maternal and fetal plasma amino acids profiles (Economides et al., 1989*b*). As with glucose metabolism there are significant correlations between the change in amino acid concentrations and the degree of umbilical venous hypoxaemia. Maternal plasma concentrations of both essential and non-essential amino acid are significantly increased in the presence of umbilical venous hypoxaemia, compatible with the concept that in uteroplacental insufficiency there is a reduced extraction from the mother of amino acids by the fetoplacental unit.

In IUGR the fetal plasma concentration and fetal–maternal ratio of essential amino acids are decreased and this finding correlates with the degree of fetal hypoxaemia (Economides et al., 1989*a*). Increased fetal–placental consumption or reduced transport across the placenta are possible mechanisms but the reduced supply of oxygen and glucose suggests that placental transfer and umbilical uptake of amino acids is reduced. In agreement with these findings, Cetin et al. (1988) showed that in paired umbilical venous and arterial samples at Caesarean section there is a smaller than normal fetal uptake of essential amino acids and total amino-nitrogen in IUGR.

Changes in the non-essential amino acids are variable. Some, like serine, tyrosine, taurine and ornithine, are significantly decreased, and it is possible that the biosynthetic pathways for these amino acids may not be fully established in intrauterine life; their supply may be dependent on placental transport and they may be ‘essential’ in the fetus. Other non-essential amino acids such as glycine increase in IUGR fetuses and this may be the result of:

1. tissue breakdown;
2. decreased utilization for protein synthesis (perhaps because of reduced supply of essential amino acids);

3. decreased utilization as an energy substrate as reported for alanine in babies asphyxiated at birth (Schultz, Mestyan & Soltesz, 1977);
4. decreased utilization for gluconeogenesis (Haymond, Karl & Pagliari, 1974).

Recently Bernardini suggested a 'concentrating index' based on the numeric mean of the fetal–maternal ratio of six amino acids (threonine, valine, methionine, tyrosine, phenylalanine and lysine). This parameter is independent of gestational age, is significantly reduced in IUGR fetuses and may indicate the severity of placental functional impairment (Bernardini et al., 1991).

IUGR with normal blood values

As described above, some fetuses with IUGR have significant metabolic changes with hypoxaemia, hypercapnia, hyperlacticacidaemia and disturbance of carbohydrate and protein metabolism. However, in the majority of cases all the measurements being discussed above are entirely normal (see Fig. 8.2, Fig. 8.3, and Fig. 8.4). It is the hypoxaemic fetus that has *all* the other changes described. Since the long-term epidemiological consequences of being light at birth seem to be independent of cause (Barber et al., 1989) understanding the mechanism of reduced growth in cases with normal placental function is important. There is much interest in the possible role of insulin-like growth factors (IGFs) I and II and their binding proteins (IGFBPs) in the regulation of intrauterine and extrauterine development. IGF mRNA is present in virtually all human fetal tissues (Han et al., 1988) and significant correlations have been reported between IGF levels in cord blood and both birthweight and length (Gluckman et al., 1983; Gluckman & Brinsmead, 1976). However, much further work is required to understand the causes of IUGR in cases with apparently normal placental function and fetal metabolism.

Fetal oxygenation and neuro-developmental outcome in IUGR

It is widely accepted that severe acute perinatal asphyxia can cause mortality in newborn infants and subsequent neurological disability (e.g. cerebral palsy) in survivors, but the associations are weak. Indeed, it is difficult to identify reliable predictors of subsequent neuro-development during pregnancy or after birth and, for example, there is very little association between acidaemia in cord blood or Apgar score at the time of

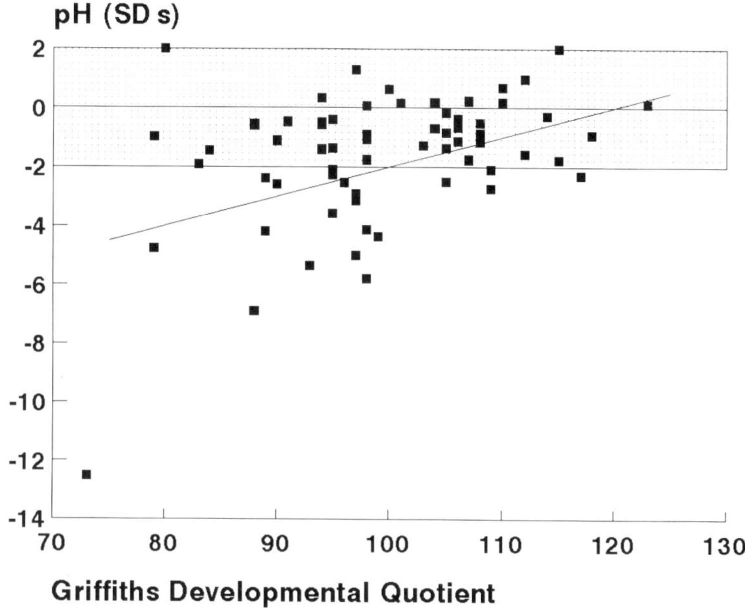

Fig. 8.5. Positive correlation between pH in utero at cordocentesis and subsequent neurodevelopment assessed by the Griffiths score at 1–5 years of age ($r = 0.41$, $n = 65$, $p = 0.0008$). All the neonates weighed less than −2 SD at birth and were born after 32 weeks gestation. Since pH changes with the gestational age in normal pregnancies, the results are expressed as multiples of SD. (Soothill et al, 1995.)

delivery and subsequent impaired neuro-development (Ruth & Ravjio, 1988). Indeed, it has been suggested that metabolic acidosis at birth may simply reflect good physiological adaptation to the stress of delivery (Sykes et al., 1982). The association between IUGR, chronic hypoxic injury and outcome is stronger. Children that were growth retarded as fetuses have lower intellectual performances in the first year of life (Watt, 1986), disturbances of sleep/wake organization, disturbances of social integration (Watt & Strongman, 1985), lower mental and physical developmental indices at 12 months (Vohr & Oh, 1983), lower developmental scores at 2 and 4 years and higher level of school failure (Francis-Williams & Davies, 1974) compared to controls. Therefore, chronic hypoxic injury, often well before labour or delivery, is likely to be more important for long-term consequences.

Recently, it has been shown that there is a significant association between pH at cordocentesis in IUGR fetuses after 32 weeks gestation and childhood neuro-development evaluated with the Griffiths neuro-development quotient (Fig. 8.5) (Soothill et al., 1995). Equally importantly, there was not a significant association between neuro-development and fetal PO_2, fetal size or gestational age. The relationship between chronic acidaemia and impaired neuro-development does not necessarily mean that acidaemia is the brain-damaging factor. Other abnormalities associated with chronic acidaemia include fetal hypothyroidism (Thorpe-Beeston et al., 1991) and thrombocytopenia (Van den Hoff & Nicolaides, 1991), either of which may be determinants of developmental delay. An hypothesis arising from these results is that, if IUGR fetuses are delivered when hypoxia is detected but before acidaemia develops, neurological damage might be avoided. Since current non-invasive tests detect acidaemia rather than hypoxia alone, present practice may be to deliver mature IUGR fetuses later than the ideal. However, before any change in management is instituted, this hypothesis needs to be tested by intervention trials using both neonatal condition and neuro-development as outcomes.

Summary

Human cordocentesis and assessment of oxygenation play a crucial role in the understanding of the possible causes of IUGR. Together with non-invasive tests such as Doppler studies and the biophysical profile, this technique can help guide the most appropriate clinical management. However, IUGR is not a diagnosis but a physical sign and ideally the term should be restricted to cases where a pathological process has been detected. A significant proportion of fetuses with severe early onset IUGR are chromosomally abnormal and, in these cases, detailed ultrasound scanning will often demonstrate the presence of fetal anatomical defects. Chromosomally normal IUGR fetuses without biochemical abnormalities seem to have normal neuro-development and are likely to be normal small individuals.

IUGR fetuses with evidence of impaired placental perfusion have reduced placental transfer of nutrients (e.g. oxygen, glucose and essential amino acids), reduced fetal metabolism leading to high levels of substrates (e.g. non-essential amino acids) and low levels of tissue products (e.g. thyroid hormone, insulin, platelets) (Table 8.1). In many ways IUGR resembles undernutrition in postnatal life because hypoinsulinaemia, hypoglycaemia and a high ratio of non-essential to essential amino acids are all reported in both IUGR and in subjects with chronic protein or calorie malnutrition (e.g. kwashiorkor) (Economides et al., 1989*b*).

Table 8.1. *Changes of blood gases, lactate, glucose and amino acid metabolism in human IUGR pregnancies compared to well-known controls*

	pO_2	pCO_2	Lactate	pH	Glucose	Insulin	Ess. AA
Maternal	=	=	⇑	⇓	⇓	=	⇑
Fetal	⇓	⇑	⇑	⇓	⇓	⇓	⇓

Ess. AA: essential amino acids; = unchanged; ⇑ increased; ⇓ decreased.

When metabolic and nutritional dysfunction is associated with significant fetal acidaemia subsequent neuro-development may be affected.

The ideal timing of delivery is an important aspect of the management of IUGR, and we must continue to develop techniques that identify poor placental function at an early stage and research into the sequence of associated secondary effects. Similarly, for pregnancies that are too premature for delivery, attempts to improve the intra-uterine environment must be evaluated. Logical delivery decisions will always require an understanding of the risk of morbidity or mortality to the fetus of remaining in utero compared to that of premature delivery. The data described in this chapter, by helping us understand the pathophysiology of IUGR, allow more accurate diagnosis of the cause and assessment of the risks in utero.

References

Barker, D., Osmond, C., Golding, J., Kuh, D. & Wadsworth, M. (1989). Growth in utero, blood pressure in childhood and adult life, and mortality from cardiovascular disease. *British Medical Journal*, **298**, 564–67.

Battaglia, F.C. & Meschia, G. (1986). *An Introduction to Fetal Physiology*, pp. 154–167. Academic Press, London.

Bernardini, I., Evans, M.I., Nicolaides, K.H., Economides, D.L. & Gahl, A.W. (1991). The fetal concentrating index as a gestational age-independent measure of placental dysfunction in intrauterine growth retardation. *American Journal of Obstetrics and Gynecology*, **164**, 1481–90.

Bilardo, C.M., Nicolaides, K.H. & Campbell, S. (1990). Doppler measurements of fetal and uteroplacental circulations: relationship with umbilical venous blood gases measured at cordocentesis. *American Journal of Obstetrics and Gynecology*, **162**, 115–20.

Cetin, I., Corbetta C., Sereni, L.P., Marconi, A.M., Bozzetti, P., Pardi, G. & Battaglia, C. (1990). Umbilical amino acids concentrations in normal and growth-retarded fetuses by cordocentesis. *American Journal of Obstetrics and Gynecology*, **162**, 253–61.

Cetin, I., Marconi, A.M., Bozzetti, P., Sereni, L.P., Corbetta C., Pardi, G. & Battaglia, C. (1988). Umbilical amino acid concentrations in appropriate and small for gestational age infants: a biochemical difference present in utero. *American Journal of Obstetrics and Gynecology*, **158**, 120–6.

Cox, W.L., Daffos, F., Forestier, F., Descombey, D., Aufrant, C., Auger, M.C. & Gaschard, J.C. (1988). Physiology and management of intrauterine growth retardation: a biologic approach with fetal blood sampling. *American Journal of Obstetrics and Gynecology*, **159**, 36–41.

Economides, D.L. & Nicolaides, K.H. (1989). Blood glucose and oxygen tension levels in small for gestational age fetuses. *American Journal of Obstetrics and Gynecology*, **161**, 1004–8.

Economides, D.L., Nicolaides, K.H. & Campbell, S. (1990). Relation between maternal-to-fetal blood glucose gradient and uterine and umbilical Doppler blood flow measurements. *British Journal of Obstetrics and Gynaecology*, **97**, 543–44.

Economides, D.L., Nicolaides, K.H., Gahl, W.A., Bernardini, I. & Evans, M.I. (1989*b*). Plasma amino acids in appropriate and small for gestational age fetuses. *American Journal of Obstetrics and Gynecology*, **162**, 382–6.

Economides, D.L., Proudler, A. & Nicolaides, K.H. (1989*a*). Plasma insulin in appropriate- and small-for-gestational age fetuses. *American Journal of Obstetrics and Gynecology*, **160**, 1091–4.

Francis-Williams, J. & Davies, P.A. (1974). Very low birthweight and later intelligence. *Developmental Medicine of Childhood Neurology*, **16**, 709–28.

Freda, V.J. & Adamson, K.J. (1964). Exchange transfusion in utero. *American Journal of Obstetrics and Gynecology*, **89**, 817–21.

Gerson, A.G., Wallace, D.A., Stiller, R.J., Paul, D.. Weiner, S. & Bolognese, R.J. (1987). Doppler evaluation of umbilical venous and arterial blood flow in the second and third trimesters of normal pregnancy. *Obstetrics and Gynecology*, **70**, 622–6.

Gluckman, P.D. & Brinsmead, M.W. (1976). Somatomedin in cord blood: relationship to gestational age and birth size. *Journal of Clinical Endocrinology and Metabolism*, **43**, 1378–81.

Gluckman, P.D., Johnson-Barret, J.J., Butler, J.H., Edgar, B.W. & Gunn, T.R. (1983). Studies of insulin-like growth factor I and II by specific radioligand assays in umbilical cord blood. *Clinical Endocrinology*, **19**, 405–13.

Gresham, E.L., James, E.J., Raye, J.R., Battaglia, F.C., Makowski, E.L. & Meschia, G. (1972). Production and excretion of urea by the fetal lamb. *Pediatrics*, **50**, 372–9.

Haas, J.D., Balcazar, H. & Caulfield, L. (1987). Variation in early neonatal mortality for different types of fetal growth retardation. *American Journal of Physical Anthropology*, **73**, 467–73.

Han, V.K.M., Lund, P.K., Lee, D.C. & D'Ercole, A.J. (1988). Expression of somatomedin/insulin-like growth factor messenger ribonucleic acids in the human fetus: identification, characterization, and tissue distribution. *Journal of Clinical Endocrinology and Metabolism*, **66**, 422–9.

Hansmann, M., Gembruch, U., Bald, R., Manz, M. & Redel, A. (1991). Fetal tachyarrhythmias: transplacental and direct treatment of the fetus – a report of 60 cases. *Ultrasound in Obstetrics and Gynecology*, **1**, 162–70.

Hay, H.W., Sparks, J.W., Randall B.W., Battaglia, F.C. & Mescia, G. (1984). Fetal glucose uptake and utilization as function of maternal glucose concentration. *American Journal of Physiology*, **240**, 662–8.

Haymond, M.W., Karl, I.E. & Pagliari, A.S. (1974). Increased gluconeogenic substrates in the small for gestational age infants. *New England Journal of Medicine*, **291**, 322–8.

Hill, D. (1978). Effect of insulin on fetal growth. *Seminars of Perinatology*, **2**, 319–28.

Holzman, I.R., Phillips, A.F. & Battaglia, F.C. (1979). Glucose metabolism, lactate and ammonia production by the human placenta in vivo. *Pediatric Research*, **13**, 117–20.

Huch, R. & Huch, H. (1984). Maternal and fetal acid-base balance and blood gas measurements. In *Fetal Physiology and Medicine*, ed. R. Beard & P. Nathanielsz. pp. 713–56. Marcel Dekker, New York.

Jacobs, R., Owens, J.A., Falconer, J., Webster, M.E.D. & Robinson, J.S. (1988). Changes to metabolite concentration in fetal sheep subjected to prolonged hypobaric hypoxia. *Journal of Developmental Physiology*, **10**, 113–21.

Khouzami, V.A., Ginsburg, D.S., Daikoku, N.H. & Johnson, J.W. (1981). The glucose tolerance test as a means of identifying intrauterine growth retardation. *American Journal of Obstetrics and Gynecology*, **139**, 423–6.

Lemons, J.A., Adcock, E.W.III, Jones, M.D., Naughton M.A., Meschia, G. & Battaglia, F.C. (1976). Umbilical uptake of amino acids in the unstressed fetal lamb. *Journal of Clinical Investigation*, **58**, 1428–34.

McIntosh, N., Rodeck, C.H. & Heath, R. (1984). Plasma amino acids of the mid-trimester human fetus. *Biology of the Neonate*, **45**, 218–24.

Marconi, A.M., Cetin, I., Ferrazzi, E., Ferrari, M.M., Pardi, G. & Battaglia, C. (1990). Lactate metabolism in normal and growth-retarded fetuses. *Pediatric Research*, **28**, 652–6.

Nicolaides, K.H., Bilardo, C.M., Soothill, P.W. & Campbell, S. (1988). Absence of end diastolic frequencies in umbilical artery: a sign of fetal hypoxia and acidosis. *British Medical Journal*, **297**, 1026–7.

Nicolaides, K.H., Economides, D.L. & Soothill, P.W. (1989). Blood gases, pH and lactate in appropriate and small for gestational age fetuses. *American Journal of Obstetrics and Gynecology*, **161**, 996–1001.

Nicolaides, K.H., Soothill, P.W., Rodeck, C.H. & Campbell, S. (1986). Ultrasound-guided sampling of umbilical cord and placental blood to assess fetal wellbeing. *Lancet*, **i**, 1065–7.

Nicolini, U., Hubinont C., Santolaya, N.M., Fisk, N.M. & Rodeck, C.H. (1990*a*). Effects of fetal intravenous glucose challenge in normal and growth retarded fetuses. *Hormone and Metabolic Research*, **22**, 426–30.

Nicolini, U., Nicolaidis, P., Fisk, N.M., Tannirandon, Y. & Rodeck, C.H. (1990*b*). Fetal blood sampling from the intrahepatic vein: analysis of safety and clinical experience with 214 procedures. *Obstetrics and Gynecology*, **76**, 47.

Okamura, K., Watanabe, I., Tanigawara, S. et al. (1990). Biochemical evaluation of fetus with hypoxia caused by severe pre-eclampsia using cordocentesis. *Journal of Perinatology Medicine*, **18**, 441–7.

Owens, J.A., Falconer, J. & Robinson, J.S. (1987). Effect of restriction of placental growth on fetal and utero-placental metabolism. *Journal of Developmental Physiology*, **9**, 225–38.

Pardi, G., Buscaglia, M., Ferrazzi, E., Bozzetti P., Marconi, A.M., Cetin, I., Battaglia F.C. & Makowski E. (1987). Cord sampling for the evaluation of oxygenation and acid–base balance in growth retarded human fetuses. *American Journal of Obstetrics and Gynecology*, **157**, 1221–8.

Pardi, G., Cetin, I., Marconi, A.M., Bozzetti P., Ferrazzi, E., Buscaglia, M., Battaglia F.C. (1993). Diagnostic value of blood sampling in fetuses with growth retardation. *The New England Journal of Medicine*, **11**, 692–6.

Peeters, L.L.H., Sheldon, R.E., Jones, M.D., Makowski, E.L.& Meschia, G. (1979). Blood flow to fetal organs as a function of arterial oxygen content. *American Journal of Obstetrics and Gynecology*, **135**, 639–46.

Rodeck, C.H. & Campbell, S. (1978). Sampling pure fetal blood by fetoscopy in the second trimester of pregnancy. *British Medical Journal*, **2,** 728.

Rudolph, A.M., Heyman, M.A., Teramo, K.A.W., Barrett, C.T. & Raiha, N.C.R. (1971). Studies on the circulation of the previable human fetus. *Pediatric Research*, **5**, 452–65.

Ruth, V.J. & Ravjio, K.O. (1988). Perinatal brain damage: predictive value of metabolic acidosis and the Apgar score. *British Medical Journal*, **297**, 24–7.

Schultz, K., Mestyan, J. & Soltesz, G. (1977). The effect of birth asphyxia on plasma-free amino acids in preterm newborn infants. *Acta Paediatrica Academica Scientiarum Hungaricae*, **18**, 123–30.

Sheppard, B.L. & Bonnar, J. (1976). The ultrastructure of the arterial supply of the human placenta in pregnancy complicated by fetal growth retardation. *British Journal of Obstetrics and Gynaecology*, **83**, 948.

Snidjers, R.J., Abbas, A., Melby, O., Ireland, M. & Nicolaides, K.H. (1993). Fetal plasma erythropoietin in severe growth retardation. *American Journal of Obstetrics and Gynecology*, **168**, 615–19.

Soothill, P.W. (1994). Fetal blood sampling before labor. In *High Risk Pregnancy, Management Options*. ed. D.K. James, P.J. Steer, C.P. Weiner & B. Gonik. pp. 745–55. W.B. Saunders Company, London.

Soothill, P.W., Ajayi, R.A., Campbell, S., Ross, E.M. & Nicolaides K.H. (1995). Fetal oxygenation, maternal smoking and childhood neurodevelopment. *European Journal of Obstetrics and Gynaecology*, in press.

Soothill, P.W. & Nicolaides, K.H. (1987). Fetal blood gas and acid–base measurements must be corrected for gestational age. *Obstetrics and Gynecology*, **70,** 429.

Soothill, P.W., Nicolaides, K.H., Bilardo, C.M. & Campbell, S. (1986*b*). Relationship of fetal hypoxia in growth retardation to mean blood velocity in the fetal aorta. *Lancet*, **ii**, 1118–20.

Soothill, P.W., Nicolaides, K.H., Bilardo, C.M. & Campbell, S. (1986*c*). Utero-placental blood velocity resistance index and umbilical venous PO_2, PCO_2, pH, lactate and erythroblast count in growth retarded fetuses. *Fetal Therapy*, **1**, 176–9.

Soothill, P.W., Nicolaides, K.H. & Campbell, S. (1987). Prenatal asphyxia, hyperlacticaemia, hypoglycaemia and erythroblastosis in growth-retarded fetuses. *British Medical Journal*, **i**, 1051–3.

Soothill, P.W., Nicolaides, K.H., Rodeck, C.H. & Campbell, S. (1986*a*). Effect of gestational age on fetal and intervillous blood gas and acid base values in human pregnancy. *Fetal Therapy*, **1**, 168–75.

Spellacy, W.N., Goetz, F.C., Greenberg, B.Z. & Ells, J. (1964). The human placental gradient for plasma insulin and blood glucose. *American Journal of Obstetrics and Gynecology*, **90**, 753–7.

Sykes, G.S., Molloy, P.M., Johnson P. et al. (1982). Do Apgar scores indicate asphyxia? *Lancet*, **i**, 494–6.

Thorpe-Beeston, J.G., Nicolaides, K.H., Snijders, R.J.M., Felton, C.V. & McGregor, A.M. (1991). Thyroid function in small for gestational age fetuses. *Obstetrics and Gynecology*, **77**, 701–6.
Van Assche, F.A., Deprins, F., Aerts, L. & Verjans, M. (1977). The endocrine pancreas in small-for-dates infants. *British Journal of Obstetrics and Gynaecology*, **84**, 751–3.
Van den Hoff, M.C. & Nicolaides, K.H. (1991). Platelet count in normal, small and anaemic fetuses. *American Journal of Obstetrics and Gynecology*, **162**, 735–9.
Villar, J., de Onis, M., Kestler, E., Bolanos, F., Cerezo, R. & Bernedes, H. (1990). The differential neonatal morbidity of the intrauterine growth retardation syndrome. *American Journal of Obstetrics and Gynecology*, **163**, 151–7.
Vohr, B.R. & Oh, W. (1983). Growth and development in preterm infants small for gestational age. *Journal of Pediatrics*, **103**, 941–5.
Watt, J. (1986). Interaction and development in the first year. Effects of intrauterine growth retardation. *Early Human Development*, **12**, 211–23.
Watt, J.E. & Strongman, K.T. (1985). The organization and stability of sleep states in full term, preterm and small for gestational age infants: a comparative study. *Developmental Psychobiology*, **18**, 151–62.
Weiner, C.P., Wenstrom, K.D., Sipes, S.L. & Williamson, R.A. (1991). Risk factors for cordocentesis and fetal vascular transfusion. *American Journal of Obstetrics and Gynecology*, **165**, 1020.
Weiner, C.P. & Williamson, R.A. (1989). Evaluation of severe growth retardation using cordocentesis: haematologic and metabolic alterations by aetiology. *Obstetrics and Gynecology*, **73**, 225–9.
Wladimiroff, J.W., Tonge, H.M. & Stewart, P.A. (1986). Doppler ultrasound assessment of cerebral blood flow in the human fetus. *British Journal of Obstetrics and Gynaecology*, **93**, 471–5.

9

Glucose and fetal growth derangement

JOHN M. BASSETT

Introduction

Fetal growth derangement is associated with abnormalities in the regulation of both maternal and fetal glucose homeostasis in many situations. The classic clinical example is the fetal macrosomia which frequently accompanies poor control of maternal diabetes, especially in the latter half of gestation (Metzger, 1991). It is equally evident, however, from the dramatic 30–70% reduction in the rate of increase of fetal girth and crown–rump length measurements which occurs in fetal lambs within 3 days of reducing maternal plasma glucose by severe undernutrition in late pregnancy (Mellor, 1984). Fetal hypoglycaemia is also observed in intrauterine growth retardation (IUGR) (Economides, Nicolaides & Campbell, 1991) and in many experimental models of fetal growth retardation (see Chapter 6 by Owens, Owens & Robinson). The delivery of glucose to the uterus therefore plays a very important role in determining the rate of fetal growth, but why should this be so?

The vital role of glucose as an essential substrate for oxidative metabolism in fetal tissues is well known (Battaglia & Meschia, 1978), but it is very unlikely that the rate of fetal tissue growth will depend in any simple way on the rate of glucose delivery to the conceptus. The programmed differential growth of organs and tissues within the conceptus from the earliest stages of embryogenesis makes it far more likely that mechanisms exist to regulate the delivery and availability of glucose and other substrates to meet the differing needs of these individual tissues. However, mechanisms must also exist to prioritize these requirements and to alter the pattern of glucose use when supply is either inadequate or in excess of requirement. Local control of tissue blood flow may contribute to the regulation of substrate distribution, but central regulation of cardiac output and its distribution among tissues seems likely to play the more important role in determining the actual delivery of glucose and other substrates to individual tissues throughout fetal development. Because of the vital importance of the central nervous system and the heart in coordinating bodily function during development, the needs of these organs take precedence over those of all other tissues. Sophisticated neural, neuroendocrine and endocrine mechanisms exist for protection of oxygen supply to the brain both before and after birth. It is therefore likely that the mechanisms which regulate the distribution of glucose use among tissues to maintain glucose homeostasis during post-natal life also participate in the control of glucose use within the developing conceptus and therefore participate in the regulatory changes which lead to growth derangement when glucose availability to the fetus is abnormal.

Integration of the functional roles of placental and fetal somatic tissues in glucoregulation

The role of the placenta and the mechanisms regulating glucose transfer to the developing conceptus are dealt with elsewhere in this volume (Chapter 1, Doughty & Sibley). However, if we are to understand how alterations in glucose availability to the conceptus might lead to growth derangement, it is necessary to recognize the importance of functional integration among all the tissues comprising the conceptus. Before birth the survival and growth of infants depends as much on the development and function of the extracorporeal structures derived from the trophectoderm of the blastocyst as it does on the functional organization and development of fetal somatic tissues. Too often because the placenta and fetal membranes are discarded at birth, their function during prenatal development is considered separately from that of the fetus, lumped together with that of the maternal uterine structures, or ignored altogether, despite the fact that the trophoblast is perfused by fetal blood and that the delivery of blood to the umbilical circulation accounts for close to 50% of fetal cardiac output near to term. The proportion of fetal cardiac output perfusing the placenta and membranes must be far greater earlier in gestation when the size of the fetus relative to that of the placenta and extraembryonic membranes is far less than later in gestation (Bell et al., 1986). The complex transport and secretory epithelia, with their supporting membranes and structures derived from the expanding trophoblast, provide the actual interface between the conceptus and the maternal intrauterine environment, and it is these tissues which are totally responsible for regulating the acquisition of glucose and other metabolic substrates essential to normal development of the whole conceptus, as well as for maintenance of the characteristic differences between mother and fetus in circulating concentrations of most blood constituents. It is necessary to remember, however, that the placental attachments comprise tissues from two separate individuals. Despite their complex and intimate association, tissues of the maternal placenta are perfused and nourished by blood from the uterine artery, while the trophoblast is perfused by blood from the umbilical circulation, but because of the problems of access to the vasculature on both sides of placental attachments and also because of difficulty in identifying separately their metabolic and transport functions, there is still very inadequate information about the regulation of metabolic activities which actually support and drive the processes of exchange in fetal placental tissue. Given the need for central coordination of development of the conceptus as a whole, it seems unlikely that the trophoblast is nourished by glucose or other nutrients in transit from the mother to the conceptus as so often supposed. Bassett, Burks and Pinches (1985) proposed, on the basis of radiochemical labelling patterns in fetal plasma lactate and fructose, that glucose utilized for oxidative metabolism by the fetal placenta at the site of fructose synthesis was provided by the umbilical arterial supply from the fetal glucose pool. The concept has been discussed elsewhere (Bassett, 1986, 1991) and support for it provided by Hodgson, Mellor and Field (1991). However, an increasing body of less direct evidence is also consistent with the concept, illustrated in Fig. 9.1, that the fetal placenta is nourished by glucose derived from the umbilical artery, and that its metabolic activity is therefore subject to regulation from within the conceptus.

Although the tracer methodology used does not permit unequivocal identification of the source of substrate used by maternal and fetal components of the 'uteroplacenta', Hay et al. (1990) observed that uteroplacental glucose utilization occurred primarily in tissues having access to glucose supplied by the umbilical circulation and concluded that the uteroplacental glucose metabolic rate and its dependence on fetal glucose concentration were major factors determining the magnitude and variability of glucose transfer between maternal and fetal plasma. Furthermore, observations of interorgan cycling of serine and glycine (Cetin et al., 1992) and of glutamate and glutamine (Marconi et al., 1989) between the fetal placenta and liver, as well as evidence that deamination

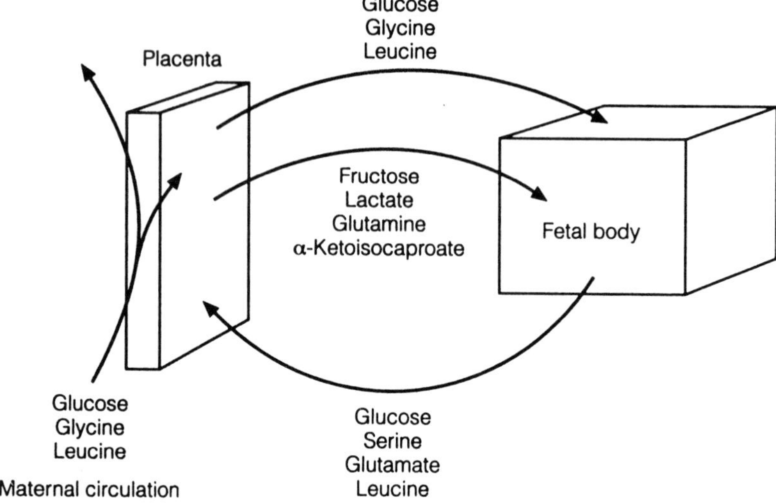

Fig. 9.1. A schematic illustration of the functional interdependence of fetal placental and somatic tissues to emphasize the metabolic integration of these components of the conceptus. Although the placenta is the site of metabolite and gas exchange with the maternal circulation, substrate for its nourishment and metabolic activity is provided and controlled from within the conceptus. (Based on observations by Bassett et al., 1985*a,b*; Cetin et al., 1992; Loy et al., 1990; Marconi et al., 1989.)

of leucine from the fetal blood pool occurs in the placenta while the α-ketoisocaproic acid released is returned to the fetus for decarboxylation (Loy et al., 1990), provides additional evidence that the tissues of the fetal placenta are extensively involved in interorgan substrate cycles with the liver or other tissues of the fetus (see Fig. 9.1). Perhaps the strongest evidence of all for the concept was provided by the observation by Owens, Falconer and Robinson (1987*a,b*) who showed that, although total fetal glucose consumption was reduced in growth-retarded fetuses from ewes which had had endometrial caruncles removed before conception, glucose consumption per kilogram of fetus was similar to that of control fetuses, yet uteroplacental consumption of glucose per kilogram of placenta was actually significantly reduced in the ewes carrying small fetuses. Lactate production per kilogram of placenta was also significantly higher in the ewes carrying small fetuses compared to that in controls, but neither fetal nor uteroplacental oxygen consumption per kilogram of tissue in the small fetuses differed from the values in normal controls. Uteroplacental production of lactate actually increased as the oxygen content of blood from the femoral artery of the fetus (i.e. umbilical arterial oxygen) decreased in control and carunclectomized sheep. Clearly, where substrate delivery to the maternal interface of the placenta is seriously reduced, it is placental metabolism and not fetal metabolism which is most seriously handicapped. This makes it seem most unlikely that the placenta uses significant amounts of substrates or even oxygen in transit from the mother. More likely, it depends on substrates and oxygen provided by the umbilical arterial supply. Indeed, we can only explain the remarkable constancy in the relationship between fetal and placental growth, and its regulation when nutrition of the conceptus is altered, if we accept that placental growth is controlled from within the conceptus itself. Whether nutrition of the conceptus is altered by variation in fetal number, maternal nutrition, pathological changes in maternal endocrine regulatory mechanisms, e.g. diabetes, or by limitation of uterine blood supply to the maternal placental attachment, the relative changes in placental and fetal tissue growth remain the same (see Fig. 9.2). Investigations over many species and in a variety of experimental models, where the growth of fetuses has been retarded or accelerated, show fetal size remains closely correlated with placental size, despite considerable diversity in placental structure and in the time of gestation at which experimental manipulations were applied. As reviewed earlier (Bassett, 1991) differences in placental size are also closely associated with substantial differences in uterine blood flow to the maternal placental interface and consequent differences in the delivery of glucose and other nutrients to the fetal circulation. Small placental size and reduced delivery of glucose may therefore be an important limitation to future growth of the whole conceptus. However, examination of the effects of fetal nutritional variation on the relative development of the placenta and fetal somatic tissues shows that experimental manipulations, just like natural variation consequent on differences in litter size (Michael, Ward & Moore, 1983; Bassett, 1986), which all limit nutrient delivery to the individual conceptus, result in proportionately larger reduction in placental size than in the size of the fetal brain or most other somatic tissues other than the liver. The great consistency in the differential responses of placenta and brain to experimental limitation of conceptus growth in the sheep by a variety of procedures imposed at different times during gestation is illustrated in Fig. 9.2. As observed elsewhere (Bassett, 1991), the relative effects on development of placenta and brain are remarkably similar whether the manipulations were imposed earlier or later in

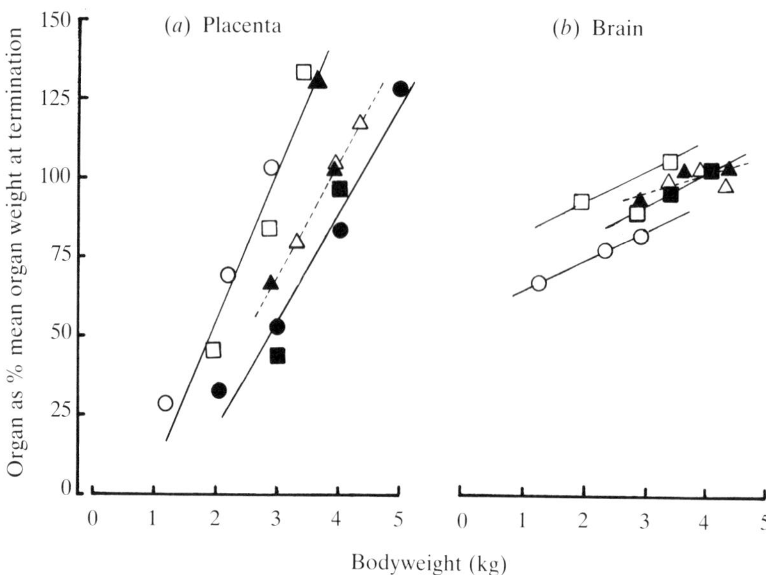

Fig. 9.2. Effects of experimental manipulation of nutrient delivery to the conceptus on the development of placenta and brain relative to body weight in normal and growth retarded fetal lambs. Variations in fetal nutrition were achieved by alterations in maternal nutrition during pregnancy (●, Mellor, 1985); by removal of uterine caruncles before conception (○, Harding et al., 1985; □, Owens et al., 1987*a,b*); by unilateral fetectomy at 50 days of gestation (△, Vatnick et al., 1991), by chronic heat stress from 64–141 days of gestation (■, Bell et al., 1989) or by repetitive uteroplacental embolization with, and without, fetal intravenous nutritional supplementation (▲, Charlton & Johengen, 1987). Placental and brain weights were expressed as a percentage of the mean weight for all fetuses in the study at termination and are plotted relative to fetal body weight at termination. Age at termination ranged between 120 days gestation and term (145 days).

gestation and despite clear evidence for placental compensatory hypertrophy which occurs following carunclectomy before pregnancy (Harding, Jones & Robinson, 1985; Owens et al., 1987*a,b*) or fetectomy after 50 days gestation (Vatnick et al., 1991) in sheep. Litter reduction in rabbits after 9 days gestation (Fletcher, Falconer & Bassett, 1982) also results in compensatory placental hypertrophy but does not alter the differential relationships (Bassett, 1986). The consistency of these relationships suggests the existence of an important underlying regulatory mechanism. Whatever this is, growth of the placenta, despite its location on the supply line between mother and fetus, does not depend on opportunistic utilization of glucose or other substrates being transported at the expense of fetal supply. The finding by Charlton and Johengen

(1987), that giving an intravenous supplement of glucose and a mixture of amino acids to fetuses whose uteroplacental circulation had been embolized (the filled triangle symbol well above the dotted line in Fig. 9.2) actually increased placental size significantly relative to fetal body weight, implies strongly that the availability of a nutrient, possibly glucose, within the umbilical arterial supply plays an important role in determining placental size even during late gestation when placental growth is generally considered to have ceased.

Regulation of glucose delivery to, and use within, the conceptus

Although glucose transfer across the placenta occurs by facilitated diffusion down a concentration gradient and the rate depends on both maternal and fetal concentration as well as the magnitude of the gradient (see Chapter 1, Doughty & Sibley), I hope to show that the conceptus is a very active participant in regulating both the rate at which this transfer occurs and in supporting the metabolic activity of the tissues involved. As reviewed elsewhere (Bassett, 1991), this active involvement of the conceptus actually begins with manipulation of the maternal environment by secretion of steroid and peptide hormones into the maternal circulation from the trophoblast. These alter the concentration of glucose in the maternal blood through antagonism of glucose use in tissues and increase the delivery of blood to the uterus and exchange surfaces of the placenta. However, while supporting the needs of the conceptus, these mechanisms remain essentially secondary or complementary to the principal endocrine and neural mechanisms responsible for maintenance of glucose homeostasis in the adult. It is the function, or dysfunction, of these which needs to be considered in relation to alterations in glucose availability to the conceptus.

Postnatal glucoregulatory systems

The role of insulin

During postnatal life increased secretion of insulin from the pancreatic β-cells is the principal endocrine mechanism regulating the blood glucose concentration close to its set point, and for ensuring optimum use and distribution of glucose among tissues when its availability increases following food ingestion. Insulin secretion may be regulated by increases in glucose concentration above a threshold value which varies among species, but its regulation also involves central neural, neuroendocrine and enteroendocrine anticipatory mechanisms. The relative importance of these mechanisms varies from species to species. Nevertheless, in all of them the stimulatory effect of increased glucose concentration on insulin secretion serves to provide a fail-safe mechanism to protect the body, and in particular the central nervous system, from the adverse effects of unregulated hyperglycaemia. The consequences of failure in this system in uncontrolled diabetes or in the face of insulin antagonism resulting from hormones secreted by the conceptus are clearly evident in the deranged fetal growth regulation seen in these situations (Metzger, 1991; Kalkhoff, 1991).

Glucose counter-regulation

When glucose concentration falls below the normal range there is an even more elaborate system concerned with restoration of normoglycaemia, coordinated by the central nervous system and involving a hierarchy of redundant glucose counter-regulatory mechanisms (Havel & Taborsky, 1989; Cryer, 1993). While parasympathetic activation and increased secretion of pancreatic polypeptide occur with CNS glucose deficits far smaller than those triggering increased release of adrenaline (Havel & Taborsky, 1989), the quantitative role of these parasympathetically mediated endocrine changes have been less clearly evaluated than the sympathetically mediated changes in glucagon and catecholamine release. It is now well established by the work of Cryer and associates (Cryer, 1993) that increased glucagon release is the primary mechanism by which hypoglycaemia is countered. However, other studies (De Feo et al., 1991) show that adrenergic mechanisms still play a key counter-regulatory role, even in the presence of appropriate glucagon responses. Although increased adrenaline release still permits a relatively normal recovery when the glucagon response is defective, the studies of De Feo et al. (1991) indicate that the lack of response of a single counter-regulatory hormone may not be compensated fully by greater responses of the other hormones. Important insulin-antagonist roles of cortisol or growth hormone only contribute significantly to restoration of normoglycaemia where hypoglycaemia is prolonged.

Prenatal glucoregulatory mechanisms

While the endocrine systems involved in maternal glucose homeostasis outlined above are present within the fetus throughout the latter half of gestation in most long-gestation species, their regulation, and the functional integrity of the sympathetic and parasympathetic neural control systems, remains uncertain. To understand how these systems may be involved in the derangement of pre-natal growth when glucose availability is altered it is important to recognize that the functional characteristics of the mechanisms by which glucose is transferred across the placenta dictate maintenance of a concentration gradient. Calculations based on investigations in sheep by Molina et al. (1991) indicate that, because fetal demand for glucose rises more rapidly than placental glucose transport capacity during the second half of gestation, an increased gradient is necessary to balance glucose supply and demand. The functioning of a glucose homeostatic mechanism directly comparable to that of the adult is therefore unlikely to be wholly appropriate for the fetus and it does raise questions about how changes in glucose concentration or availability are sensed by the pancreatic β-cells secreting insulin, or by the glucoregulatory cells of the fetal hypothalamus. Nevertheless, the importance of glucose to fetal metabolism is so great that it would be unlikely for its availability and utilization not to be monitored or regulated.

The increasing antagonism of maternal glucose utilization by placental steroids and hormonal peptides during the second half of gestation clearly contributes to the maintenance of the maternal supply to the placenta and may on occasion, as in gestational diabetes mellitus, result in excessive glucose supply. Nevertheless, fasting glucose concentrations in normal pregnant women are lower than those of non-pregnant women (Bleicher, O'Sullivan & Freinkel, 1964), while in sheep maternal glucose concentrations are frequently decreased chronically during late pregnancy, especially where two or more fetuses are present. Fetal regulatory mechanisms to promote the utilization of glucose are therefore essential to maintain the transplacental gradient and to promote fetal growth. Regulatory systems are also necessary to limit and redistribute fetal glucose utilization in the face of inadequate maternal glucose supply.

The role of insulin

Insulin is present in fetal plasma for a substantial part of gestation in most species and plays an important role in regulating prenatal growth as well as regulating glucose metabolism, so it is likely that interactions between glucose and insulin will be of great importance to any understanding of how glucose may alter fetal growth. Quantitative studies of glucose utilization by the fetal lamb during late gestation (Hay et al., 1988, 1989,

1990) show that increasing glucose and insulin concentrations have additive effects on fetal somatic tissue glucose utilization and oxidation and clearly establish that increases in insulin concentration play an important role in redistributing glucose use as the fetal glucose concentration increases. Observations by Milley, Papacostas and Tabata (1986) and by Philipps et al. (1990) show that increases in plasma insulin concentration result in decreased plasma concentrations of α-amino acid nitrogen and most individual amino acids as well as glucose, while Milley et al. (1986) also observed a positive relationship between insulin and umbilical α-amino acid nitrogen uptake. The observations of Philipps et al. (1990) suggest that regulation of amino acid uptake by insulin is complex. Nevertheless, insulin drastically decreased the rate of fetal urea excretion (Philipps et al., 1990), and Liechty et al. (1992) showed that insulin decreased the rate of fetal leucine oxidation when maternal substrate intake was limited. It is clearly evident that insulin is involved in redistributing amino acid utilization and in stimulating net protein accretion.

Numerous investigations have shown that changes in plasma insulin accompany changes in plasma glucose since the observations by Bassett and Madill (1974*a*) that changes in plasma insulin concentration of fetal lambs closely followed changes in fetal glucose throughout the 24 h following food ingestion and a subsequent 48 h fast, while brief or prolonged elevation of the fetal plasma glucose level by intravenous glucose infusion results in hyperinsulinaemia (Bassett & Thorburn, 1971; Bassett & Madill, 1974*b*). However, although most of the evidence confirms that hyperglycaemia and hyperinsulinaemia may increase glucose utilization in the fetal lamb, a number of investigations have shown that prolonged hyperglycaemia and/or hyperinsulinaemia can also result in arterial hypoxaemia in the fetus (Philipps et al., 1982; Milley et al., 1986), the hypoxaemia serving to limit hyperinsulinaemia where hyperglycaemia persists. The clinical significance of this remains uncertain. DiGiacomo and Hay (1990*b*) suggested that increases in plasma insulin of greater than 5 μU/ml were necessary to obtain demonstrable changes in fetal glucose utilization and also that there may be a threshold glucose concentration apparently above the normal concentration range necessary for stimulation of insulin release. However, experimental pancreatectomy of the fetus (Fowden, Silver & Comline, 1986*b*) or β-cell ablation by streptozotocin administration (Hay & Meznarich, 1988; Philipps et al., 1991) shows that fetal insulin is essential for maintenance of the normal fetal plasma glucose concentration, for preservation of the maternal to fetal glucose gradient and for normal rates of umbilical glucose uptake and clearly refutes the proposition of DiGiacomo and Hay (1990*b*).

A detailed discussion of the control by glucose of insulin release from the fetal pancreas is beyond the scope of this chapter, but it should be observed that both in vivo and in vitro studies in our laboratory (Bassett et al., 1973) confirmed that the glycaemic threshold for stimulation of insulin release from fetal lamb pancreas was far lower than that required to stimulate insulin secretion after birth, despite the attenuated magnitude of the prenatal response. However, it should be noted that major structural changes occur in the pancreatic islets of lambs during the perinatal period (Titlbach, Falt & Falkmer, 1985) and these may explain differences in functional responses of fetal and postnatal pancreas. In particular, the fetal insulin-secreting β-cells are structurally different from mature β-cells and disappear soon after birth. Hellerstrom and Swenne (1991) have also shown that there are major structural and functional differences between fetal and mature pancreatic β-cells in other species, with glucose being a strong stimulus to β-cell replication, despite evidence for attenuated efficacy as an insulin secretagogue, a finding which may explain the increased insulin/glucose ratios observed by Salvesen et al. (1993) in association with fetal macrosomia in pregnancies complicated by diabetes mellitus.

After pancreatectomy or streptozotocin administration, fetal plasma glucose concentration increases, yet umbilical glucose uptake is decreased by approximately 60%. By contrast, glucose uptake by the uteroplacental tissues which is not influenced by insulin was not significantly altered by pancreatectomy or β-cell ablation with streptozotocin (Fowden et al., 1986*b*; Hay & Meznarich, 1988). Fetal plasma α-amino acid nitrogen concentrations, like glucose also increased as insulin concentration decreased following pancreatectomy (Fowden, Mao & Comline, 1986*a*) while both pancreatectomy (Fowden et al., 1986*a*; Fowden, Hughes & Comline, 1989) or ablation of pancreatic β-cells with streptozotocin (Philipps et al., 1991) also significantly reduced the rate of fetal somatic growth, with body weight and protein accretion being more seriously reduced than skeletal growth. Fowden's investigations (Fowden et al., 1989) also show that growth can be restored in pancreatectomized lambs given replacement infusions of insulin, the extent of recovery being dependent on the rate of insulin infusions. These observations therefore provide compelling evidence for the active involvement of insulin in regulation of fetal glucose utilization at normal basal concentrations, while the observations of DiGiacomo and Hay (1990*b*) indicate that it also plays an important role in regulating the fetal disposal of glucose when maternal concentrations are elevated.

These observations thus provide strong support for the causal role of insulin in the regulation of prenatal growth inferred from the macrosomia of infants of diabetic mothers and the close relationships between plasma insulin concentration and fetal size at birth or earlier in gestation reported in a number of species. This role of insulin in regulation of fetal growth was comprehensively reviewed by Fowden (1989). The question of whether insulin regulates fetal growth directly, or through effects on tissue IGF-I production, remains an open one. Like insulin concentrations, fetal IGF-I concentrations are decreased by maternal fasting and IGF-I concentrations are positively related to plasma insulin (Gluckman et al., 1987). Recently, Oliver et al. (1993) have shown that fetal glucose, but not amino acid, infusion after 48 h maternal fasting increased fetal IGF-I and insulin concentrations and concluded that glucose may have a more important role than amino acids in the regulation of fetal plasma IGF-I. However, it is likely that this effect is mediated through insulin since IGF-I concentrations were low in pancreatectomized fetuses despite elevated glucose concentrations (Gluckman et al., 1987). Insulin therefore seems more likely than IGF-I to be the primary determinant of variations in growth rate, with tissue IGF-I production serving to act as a local amplifier of the endocrine signal.

Whatever the mechanism by which insulin may act to regulate protein synthesis and growth in individual tissues, these observations are very relevant to any interpretation of how variations in glucose supply and utilization may be associated with, or bring about, derangements in prenatal growth. If insulin is to be a positive regulator of the relationship between glucose availability to the conceptus and fetal somatic growth, its secretion and plasma concentration must be regulated by glucose or nutrient availability in some way, irrespective of whether the fetus has any glucose homeostatic mechanism maintaining glucose concentration independent of the maternal concentration and the rate of maternal glucose delivery to the placenta.

Interestingly, although data were limited Fowden et al. (1986*a*) reported that placental size was not decreased by pancreatectomy so, like the embolized fetuses supplemented with glucose and amino acids by Charlton and Johengen (1987) (and illustrated in Fig. 9.2), pancreatectomized fetal lambs with elevated umbilical arterial plasma glucose and α-amino acid nitrogen concentrations had enlarged placentas relative to body size. It may be significant that Gluckman et al. (1987) observed increased plasma IGF-II concentrations in pancreatectomized fetuses in association with the hyperglycaemia and speculated that IGF-II may play a role in the regulation of placental glucose metabolism.

Clearly, increased insulin secretion is a crucial determinant of accelerated fetal growth when the availability of glucose to the conceptus is increased. However, while the investigations of Hay et al. (1988, 1989) show that utilization of glucose by fetal tissues increases relative to glucose utilization in the placenta because the rate of placental glucose utilization is solely dependent on the fetal blood glucose concentration and because insulin has no effect on placental glucose utilization (DiGiacomo & Hay, 1990*a*), they say nothing about the redistribution of glucose use which must be occurring as a result of the non-uniform distribution of insulin receptors within the tissues, although it is presumed largely to reflect increased uptake by skeletal muscle. Information on this aspect of insulin action is very limited, but Milley (1987) reported that infusion of exogenous insulin into fetal lambs increased cardiac output and heart rate and selectively increased flow to the heart, stomach, carcass and placenta, while the fraction of cardiac output distributed to the carcass tissues increased by 7%, largely at the expense of delivery to the placenta. Since no attempt was made to prevent hypoglycaemia in the fetus it is not clear whether these changes were specific responses to insulin, although they were totally unlike reported responses to stimulation of sympathetic activity. In this context it is relevant that Jones and Ritchie (1978*a*) observed a positive relationship between plasma glucose and heart rate in fetal lambs, but although insulin values were not reported they might be expected to increase over this glucose concentration range. Recent observations on adult man also show that insulin increases cardiac output and heart rate and selectively decreases vascular resistance in the leg of lean subjects, effectively augmenting the proportion of cardiac output delivered to skeletal muscle (Baron & Brechtel, 1993). It is evident that selective effects of insulin on tissue vascular resistance play an important part in determining the redistribution of glucose use within the conceptus by a mechanism independent of effects on glucose transport across the cell membrane. However, the significance of these observations needs further delineation. Changes in glucose use among tissues of the carcass or in different regions of the carcass, with changing glucose availability, do not appear to have been studied, even though differential retardation of skeletal and muscular components of the carcass by undernutrition during fetal life is well recognized.

Insulin is therefore not just an important determinant of changes in tissue glucose utilization and protein accretion by the conceptus when uterine supply of glucose to the placental interface is not limiting, but significantly alters the distribution of glucose use within the conceptus. Also, because of the stimulatory effects of insulin on fetal growth, excessive supply of glucose to the conceptus over prolonged periods as in diabetes may lead to promotion of excessive tissue growth and the characteristic macrosomia. While insulin has no direct effect on placental glucose metabolism, it is likely that, in situations of large nutrient excess and stimulated metabolic activity, the concentration of glucose in blood returning to the placenta remains sufficiently high to support excessive placental growth too and thereby increases the opportunity for substrate delivery to the conceptus later in gestation. Clinically, however, situations where glucose supply to the conceptus is unlimited and in excess of requirements are likely to be far fewer than those where glucose supply is marginal or inadequate or where its utilization is compromised by hypoxaemia.

Glucose counter-regulation

While numerous investigations in experimental animals have shown that interference with the ability of the uterine vasculature to supply glucose and other nutrients to the placental interface results in reduced glucose consumption by the conceptus and slower fetal growth, far less is known about the fetal neural, neuroendocrine and endocrine responses which may contribute to restoration of metabolic balance in this situation.

It is widely recognized from studies on normal fetal lambs during maternal fasting or insulin-induced hypoglycaemia (Hay et al., 1984; DiGiacomo & Hay, 1989) and on small growth-retarded fetuses from carunclectomized ewes (Harding et al., 1985; Owens et al., 1987*b*) that, when glucose availability to the conceptus is severely reduced, oxidative metabolism is maintained by increased utilization of alternative substrates such as amino acids and lactate, as well as by an increase in fetal glucose production by glycogenolysis or gluconeogenesis. However, recent observations on growth-retarded human fetuses (Marconi et al., 1993) studied after overnight fasting of the mother at 30–36 weeks gestation provided no evidence for similar fetal gluconeogenesis at this stage of human pregnancy. Even in sheep, evidence for quantitatively significant gluconeogenesis remains weak. Dalinghaus, Rudolph and Rudolph (1991) reported that, after 4 days of maternal fasting, gluconeogenesis could account for only 8% of fetal glucose utilization.

In postnatal life, as already outlined, neural mechanisms sensing a reduction in glucose supply to the brain limit the utilization of glucose for less essential purposes by two methods. They inhibit the secretion of insulin and antagonize its actions. In this way, tissues where glucose uptake is determined primarily by insulin sensitive glucose transport mechanisms are forced to utilize alternative substrates for support of oxidative metabolism. They also promote increased glucose production from the liver by glycogenolysis and gluconeogenesis. Fetal hypoxia consequent on experimental reduction in uterine blood flow results in alterations in blood flow and in the proportion of fetal cardiac output delivered to the brain, heart and adrenal gland in order to maintain oxygen delivery to these organs at the expense of oxygen delivery to the carcass and the skin (Jensen, Roman & Rudolph, 1991). Like acute hypoxia induced by causing the mother to breathe a low oxygen gas mixture (Jones & Ritchie, 1983), it also results in a galaxy of endocrine and metabolic changes, many of which, like the cardiovascular changes, appear to depend on the large increases in adrenal output of adrenaline and noradrenaline which occur (Jones et al., 1988; Hooper et al., 1990). Although oxygen consumption by the fetus is maintained during prolonged hypoxaemia induced in this way (Bocking et al., 1992), one important consequence of the changes occurring is that there is a decrease in the rate of DNA synthesis in fetal muscle tissue, lung and thymus gland within the first 24 h (Hooper et al., 1991). However, while such experimental manoeuvres bring about dramatic neural, endocrine and metabolic changes consequent on a sudden reduction in blood PO_2, their relevance to the changes which occur during the development of growth retardation consequent on prolonged inadequacy in uterine delivery of blood to the maternal side of the placenta must be questionable.

The observations of Owens et al. (1987*a,b*), referred to earlier, suggest glucose availability to the fetus may become rate limiting sooner than oxygen, but whether the gradual reduction in glucose availability relative to requirements which must occur as the fetus develops, generates a neuroendocrine response comparable to that generated by acute hypoxaemia is less clear. Certainly, it is known that plasma catecholamine concentrations in experimentally growth-retarded fetal lambs which have become hypoxaemic may be maintained at very high levels for prolonged periods, possibly as a consequence of the concurrent hypoxaemia (Jones, 1980). Also, acute fetal hypoglycaemia consequent on maternal or fetal insulin infusion results in increased fetal plasma adrenaline and noradrenaline concentrations in rats (Phillippe & Kitzmiller, 1981) and sheep (Jones, 1980; Harwell et al., 1990; Cohen et al., 1991) and increased catecholamine output from the fetal adrenal in sheep (Cohen et al., 1991). In addition, increases in fetal plasma adrenaline following intracarotid infusion into the fetus of small amounts of 2-deoxyglucose, a non-metabolizable glucose analogue which blocks glucose utilization (Jones, 1991), show that hypothalamic glucose-sensing mechanisms are involved in modulating these responses. Substantial increases in the magnitude of the adrenaline response and the accompanying increase in plasma glucose which occurs during the period between 120 and 140 days gestation indicate that there is considerable maturation in the responsiveness of the system over this period. This may be related to adrenal maturation, but may possibly also involve changes in the set point regulation of the hypothalamic receptor mechanism. Jones and Ritchie (1978*a,b*) showed that infusion of adrenaline for 1 h into fetal lambs at 117–135 days gestation brought about a number of cardiovascular, metabolic and endocrine changes which mimicked those seen during hypoxia and which would aid the recovery of the blood glucose and so maintain glucose supply to the brain and myocardium in the face of acutely reduced supply. Adrenaline increased plasma glucose, lactate, α-amino acid nitrogen and free fatty acid concentrations in fetal lambs between 117–125 days gestation and, like administration of adrenaline to postnatal animals (Bassett, 1970), decreased plasma insulin concentrations. Indeed, it appeared that inhibition of insulin secretion by adrenaline could largely explain its effects on plasma glucose concentration. The ability of adrenaline to inhibit insulin release and to counteract its actions also plays an important part in its role as a counter-regulatory hormone in postnatal life (De Feo et al., 1991; Cryer, 1993). However, the most important distinction between pre- and postnatal responses is the extent to which adrenaline and noradrenaline alter the proportionate distribution of blood flow to the brain. In postnatal life, brain blood flow alters little so the plasma glucose concentration is the principal determinant of glucose delivery to the brain, but before birth alterations in brain blood flow may be of greater significance in maintaining glucose delivery during hypoglycaemia.

While most investigations into the action of adrenaline in the fetus have only used very short-term infusions lasting an hour or less, and have examined only the initial phase of response to the hormone dominated by β_2-receptors mediated actions, recent studies in our laboratory have shown that adrenaline infusions maintained for 8–12 days at similar rates to those used by Jones and Ritchie (1978*a,b*) result in a prolonged

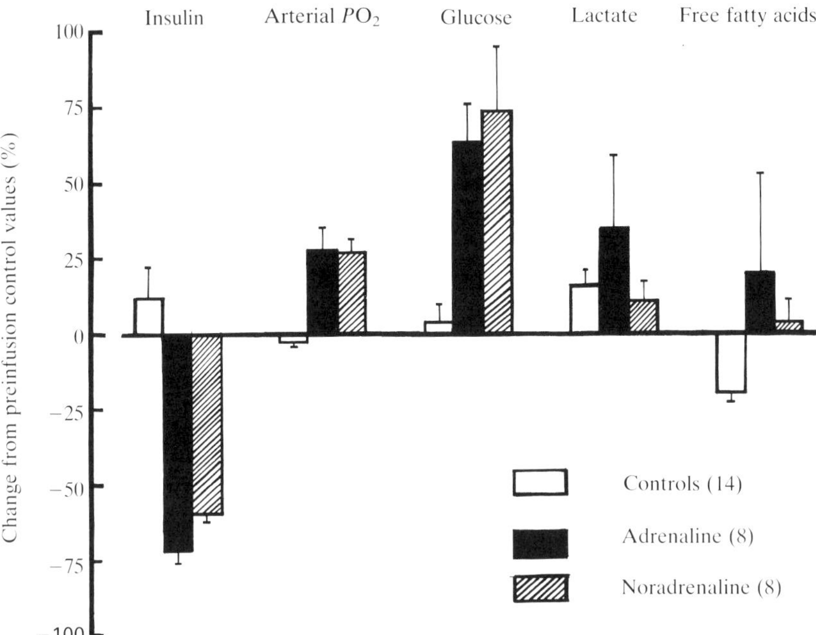

Fig. 9.3. Femoral arterial PO_2, insulin, glucose, lactate and free fatty acid concentrations in chronically cannulated twin fetal lambs during infusion of adrenaline (filled bars $n = 8$) or noradrenaline (hatched bars $n = 8$) compared with values in control twins infused with acidified saline diluent (open bars $n = 14$). Mean PO_2, hormone and metabolite concentration values in daily prefeeding samples 2–10 days after the start of infusion at 125–126 days gestation have been expressed as a percentage of the mean value in samples collected during 4 days before the start of infusion. Adrenaline was infused at 1 μg/min for 48 h then at 2 μg/min. Noradrenaline was infused at 2 μg/min for 48 h then at 4 μg/min.

inhibition of insulin release which was sustained for the entire duration of the infusion (Bassett, 1993), while initial increases in plasma lactate and free fatty acid concentrations were rapidly attenuated. In contrast to insulin, fetal plasma glucose was maintained at a significantly higher level than in uninfused control twins throughout the infusion, once the initial rapid increase had dissipated (Fig. 9.3).

Prolonged noradrenaline infusion over similar periods also inhibited insulin release and increased plasma glucose to a comparable degree (Fig. 9.3) even though short-term investigations (Jones & Ritchie, 1978*b*) had not demonstrated inhibitory effects of noradrenaline on insulin release.

Also, while Jones and Ritchie (1978*a*) did not observe any change in fetal PO_2 during their short infusions, long-term infusion of adrenaline

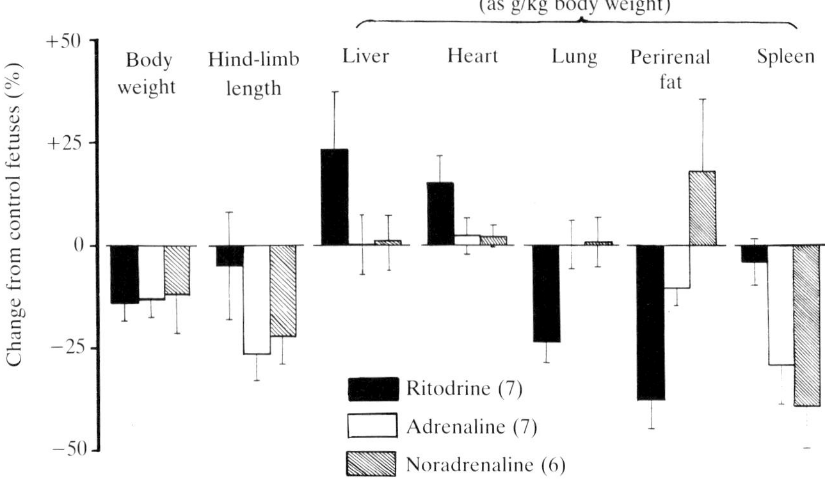

Fig. 9.4. Effects of prolonged intravenous infusion of the β_2-agonist ritodrine (solid bars $n = 8$), adrenaline (open bars $n = 8$) or noradrenaline (hatched bars, $n = 8$) into chronically cannulated twin fetal lambs on body weight, hind-limb length growth and on the size of organs expressed relative to body weight. Mean (±SE) values in infused lambs are shown as a percentage of values in control twins. Ritodrine was infused at 10 μg/min 12–14 days. Adrenaline and noradrenaline were infused at rates given in Fig. 9.3 for 9 ± 1 days and 12 ± 0.5 days respectively.

and noradrenaline both increased the oxygenation of fetal blood (Fig. 9.3). During the first 72 h of infusion PO_2 values in descending aortic blood increased by 25–30% by comparison with values in uninfused control twins and then remained higher until the end of the infusion.

Despite the hyperglycaemia and better oxygen status, growth of adrenaline and noradrenaline-infused fetuses was clearly retarded. Body weights of the infused fetuses were 12–15% less than those of control twins while a measurement of hind-limb length made at the time of fetal cannulation and again at termination suggested linear growth was decreased more. Supposing growth to have been similar in both twins during the control period before the start of infusion, calculations suggest growth may actually have been retarded by 40% or more during infusion (Fig. 9.4). While the magnitude of this decrease in growth was rather less than that observed in pancreatectomized or streptozotocin-treated fetuses (Fowden et al., 1986*b*; Phillipps et al., 1991) it seems likely that adrenergic inhibition of insulin release and the redistribution of cardiac output away from the insulin-sensitive carcass tissues may account for the effects on both growth and blood oxygenation, although other more direct inhibitory effects on tissue growth cannot be dismissed.

Despite these findings with substantially elevated adrenaline concentrations, it is not clear whether tonic sympathetic discharge or adrenal medullary secretion has any modulatory influence on insulin release in the fetus. Neither adrenal demedullation nor chemical sympathectomy significantly altered fetal insulin or glucose concentrations (Jones et al., 1987). In contrast, in vitro investigations have shown that insulin secretion from the ovine pancreas can be inhibited by adrenaline as early as 62 days gestation (Bassett, 1985), so immaturity of inhibitory α_2-adrenergic receptors is not likely to limit this important regulatory interaction between insulin and adrenaline. On the other hand, the timetable for development of islet innervation remains unknown. Interestingly, the in vitro investigations also suggested that glucagon secretion could be increased by adrenaline at this early stage but whether this was a direct effect, or a consequence of reduced intraislet insulin concentration, was not established. Hay and Meznarich (1988) observed that destruction of pancreatic β-cells by streptozotocin in fetal lambs also increased plasma glucagon concentrations, presumably because of the reduction in intraislet insulin concentrations. Harwell et al. (1990) did not observe any increase in fetal glucagon during hypoglycaemia induced by maternal insulin administration, despite increased catecholamine levels, but other investigators have shown that adrenaline administration can increase fetal glucagon secretion (Bassett, 1977; Sperling, Ganguli & Anand, 1980). This variation may be related to the high adrenaline concentration which Padbury et al. (1987) showed to be necessary for stimulation of glucagon secretion. Whether glucagon plays any physiological role in regulating plasma glucose concentration is also uncertain. Glucagon infusions increase fetal plasma glucose in a dose-dependent fashion (Philipps et al., 1983; Devaskar et al., 1984), but Devasker et al. (1984) concluded that the fetus, when compared to the newborn lamb, was relatively resistant to the glycogenolytic effects of glucagon. On the other hand, this response may be limited by developmental changes in hepatic glycogen reserves. In any case, while short-term acute responses to glucagon or adrenaline may be relevant responses to an acute reduction in glucose availability, to sudden asphyxia or short-term hypoxaemia, they are not necessarily directly relevant to combating the prolonged reduction in glucose availability consequent on chronic undernutrition, or the inadequate intrauterine delivery of substrates and oxygen associated with a small placenta. In these situations it seems far more likely that hypoinsulinaemia, consequent on the decreased glucose concentration and the increased secretion of the counter-regulatory hormone adrenaline, results in redistribution of cardiac output away from the insulin-sensitive tissues of the carcass and in increased utilization of alternative substrates such as amino acids to support oxidative metabolism both in fetal tissues and the placenta. However, the penalty for such adaptive alterations is a reduced rate of fetal growth. Our studies on the effects of prolonged catecholamine infusions in fetal lambs where metabolic responses were not limited by concurrent hypoxaemia (Fig. 9.3) are entirely consistent with this view. Indeed, they show clearly that one very important consequence of these actions is to increase the supply of both glucose and oxygen to the placenta via the umbilical circulation, as well as to maintain supply to the brain and heart. Increased redistribution of nutrients and oxygen to the fetal placenta in an attempt to maintain its transport and secretory functions is perhaps the most important adaptive response of all if the deficiency in uterine supply is to be overcome.

External environmental and pharmacological factors which influence plasma glucose and the rate of growth in the fetus

Variation in the supply of glucose to the conceptus is clearly the primary determinant of fetal plasma glucose concentration, but the complex endocrine mechanisms for regulating glucose distribution and utilization discussed above show this is only the initiator of a cascade of regulatory mechanisms which ultimately influence a wide range of functions in the fetus, including growth as well as the regulation of glucose utilization. However, while maternal nutrition is the principal determinant of this variation, the supply of glucose, oxygen and other substrates to the fetus may, as we have already seen, be determined by abnormalities in the maternal systems regulating glucose concentration or its delivery to the placental interface. Diabetes mellitus and gestational diabetes are the best known maternal abnormalities leading to fetal growth derangement through alterations in the availability of glucose for transfer to the fetus, while variation in fetal number or pathological alteration in the uterine vascular supply to the placenta are the principal factors limiting uterine placental flow. However, extreme variation in environmental temperature can also influence fetal nutrition and growth. Excessively high temperatures during early and mid-gestation have marked effects on placental growth with consequent severe limitation of glucose transfer to the fetus and restriction of fetal growth subsequently (Bell, Wilkening & Meschia, 1987; Bell et al., 1989). By contrast, cold exposure of late pregnant sheep, easily achieved by winter shearing 6–8 weeks before delivery, actually increases fetal growth significantly, the improved growth being attributable to increased fetal plasma glucose and insulin concentrations consequent on increased placental glucose transfer following an increase in maternal glucose concentration during adaptation to cold (Thompson et al., 1982). The benefits of the increased fetal growth and greater accumulation of energy reserves as glycogen and brown fat are discussed elsewhere in this volume (Chapter 5). Exercise during late pregnancy also brings about marked short-term alterations in maternal homeostasis which increase glucose transfer to the fetus and raise fetal glucose and insulin concentrations, an effect which may lead to increased lamb birthweights in sheep exercised regularly (Bell et al., 1983).

These mechanisms may be of great practical importance for commercial agriculture, but their direct clinical relevance is likely to be more limited. By contrast, passive manipulation of the fetal glucoregulatory control system by drugs administered to the mother for regulation of maternal conditions is likely to be of more direct clinical relevance. Under most circumstances the permeability characteristics of the placental barrier protect the developing conceptus against unregulated transfer of major hormones from the mother and thus permit virtual fetal autonomy in the control of metabolic homeostasis. Unfortunately, this is not always the case for synthetic analogues of catecholamine or steroid hormones. A broad discussion of this issue is beyond the scope of this chapter, but since the β_2-adrenergic-agonist drugs are widely used clinically as tocolytic agents for prevention of premature labour and they have profound effects on glucose metabolism and possibly on growth too, a consideration of their effects in the fetus is relevant to the present discussion.

Selective β_2-agonist drugs are administered during pregnancy primarily to reduce uterine contractility through selective stimulation of uterine β_2-adrenergic receptors, but they also influence maternal carbohydrate homeostasis, increasing blood glucose, lactate, insulin, free fatty acid concentrations and decreasing plasma bicarbonate and potassium concentrations during the first 12–24 h of administration, before returning to normal (Spellacy et al., 1978). Ritodrine has been the β_2-adrenergic agonist used most widely for tocolysis and is often given orally for a month or more after an initial period of intravenous administration.

Although cord samples obtained at delivery are indicative of extensive placental transfer of ritodrine, and fetal tachycardia is observed during the initial stages of treatment (Caritas et al., 1983), little is known about the metabolic effects of the β_2-agonist drugs on the human fetus in utero. Most information about what ritodrine or other β-agonist drugs may do to the fetus has therefore been derived from animal experiments. When ritodrine was administered to pregnant ewes with chronically cannulated fetuses, changes similar to those observed in pregnant women are observed in the ewe during the first 24–48 h of infusion (Bassett et al., 1985*a*). Largely similar changes also occurred in the fetus, with glucose, lactate and insulin increasing markedly while α-amino acid nitrogen and glucagon concentrations decreased. Most of these responses were greatly attenuated after the first 24 h of infusion, but fetal plasma lactate concentrations remained substantially elevated. However, Fujimoto et al. (1984) showed that the ovine placenta does not transfer significant amounts of ritodrine to the fetus in contrast to the ready transfer across the human placenta, so these changes in fetal metabolite and hormone concentration were consequent primarily on altered glucose transfer across the placenta and not on direct actions of ritodrine in the fetus. Subsequent investigations, in which ritodrine was infused directly into the fetus for up to 24 h (Warburton et al., 1987; Van der Weyde et al., 1992), or for periods of 2–10 days (Bassett, Hanson & Weeding, 1989; Bassett, Weeding & Hanson, 1990), have shown that fetal plasma glucose, insulin, lactate and free fatty acid concentrations remain markedly elevated for 48 h or longer and are accompanied by a severe hypoxaemia which only begins to abate when glucose and insulin concentrations return to the normal range. Van der Weyde et al. (1992) showed that this hypoxaemia was consequent on increased fetal tissue O_2 utilization sustained by an increase in the rate of O_2 extraction, since there was no effect of ritodrine on umbilical blood flow and the delivery of O_2 to the fetus declined. Despite the apparent normality of fetal metabolism once normoxaemia has been re-established, response to short infusions of adrenaline are indicative of selective attenuation of β-receptor-mediated responses to the endogenous catecholamines (Bassett et al., 1990). However, these investigations did not determine whether this results in compensatory changes in the level of sympathetic activity or adrenal medullary activity.

In our investigations the hypoxaemia has not been associated with any dramatic change in acid–base balance. In contrast the observations of Van der Weyde et al. (1992) had to be terminated after less than 24 h in several fetuses because of rapidly deteriorating acid–base status, but it is worthy of note that these investigations were carried out using antipyrine for measurement of umbilical blood flow to determine effects of ritodrine on fetal oxygen consumption. In fact, when we had attempted in our laboratory to determine umbilical blood flow using 4-amino antipyrine in fetuses infused with ritodrine, we also encountered a serious deterioration in fetal acid–base status within the first 6 h of ritodrine infusion, so abandoned the investigations (Bassett, Weeding & Hanson, unpublished observations). Thus the explanation for the difference between our published observations and those of Van der Weyde et al. (1992) appears to lie in the use of antipyrine for measurements of blood flow, since Andrianakis et al. (1989) and Hooper et al. (1992) have shown that 4-amino antipyrine and indomethacin, both of which inhibit prostaglandin synthesis, dramatically alter the responses of fetal lambs to hyperthermia and hypoxaemia and cause a significantly greater reduction in fetal pH. The results of Hooper et al. (1992) show that prostaglandin E_2 (PGE_2) produced by the placenta plays a very important role in moderating the deterioration in acid–base status during hypoxaemia, stimulating insulin secretion and attenuating the effects of catecholamines on fetal glucose and lactate concentrations.

More recently, Gull and Charlton (1993) have shown that antipyrine alters the metabolism of skeletal muscle in the hind limb, decreasing blood flow and utilization of glucose and oxygen, while increasing lactate production. Despite this, antipyrine has no effect on measured umbilical blood flows or uptakes of oxygen, glucose or lactate at the concentrations used for measurement of blood flow (Gull & Charlton, 1993). Nevertheless, the magnitude of the effects on skeletal muscle glucose use and effects of prostaglandin inhibitors on plasma insulin concentrations (Hooper et al., 1992) suggest that variation in the rate of prostaglandin production plays a very important role in regulating glucose use in some tissues of the conceptus. It is relevant in this context that PGE concentrations in the late pregnant ewe and fetus are closely related to the nutritional state of the ewe and there are strong negative correlations between plasma glucose and PGE_2 concentrations (Fowden et al., 1987). However, despite much speculation, effects of PGE_2 on fetal growth and maturation remain poorly defined. Our earlier investigations (Bassett et al., 1990) did not indicate that ritodrine altered fetal growth significantly, but subsequent studies in which ritodrine has been infused for 12–14 days have shown that ritodrine, like adrenaline and noradrenaline (Fig. 9.4), causes a significant decrease in fetal growth even though plasma metabolite and hormone concentrations had returned to the normal range after the third day of infusion (Bassett & Symonds, 1993). However, while the magnitude of the growth retardation was comparable to that caused by adrenaline and noradrenaline, there were some notable differences between ritodrine and the endogenous hormones in the way individual organs or tissues were influenced by prolonged drug infusion (Fig. 9.4). The most striking difference between ritodrine and the endogenous catecholamines is in their effect on perirenal brown fat. Consistent with the failure of attempts to 'switch on' brown fat in utero (see Chapter 5), neither adrenaline nor noradrenaline altered the amount of perirenal brown adipose tissue. By contrast, administration of ritodrine for 12–14 days stimulated the production of the uncoupling protein and caused virtually total depletion of the lipid content of the tissue (Bassett & Symonds, 1993). Lung weights were also reduced possibly as a consequence of specific receptor-mediated effects on the lung (Warburton et al., 1988), but the weights of the liver and heart were actually larger than those of the heavier untreated control twins. Warburton et al. (1987) observed marked depletion of hepatic glycogen stores after 24 h ritodrine infusion at a similar rate. Our observations, made after more prolonged infusion, imply that hepatic glycogen reserves, in contrast to brown fat lipid stores, are restored following attenuation of the initial β_2 receptor-mediated mobilization of glycogen during the first 24 h of infusion.

These observations indicate that β-agonist drugs administered passively to the fetus during maternal tocolysis may have profound effects on fetal development, despite the lack of clear clinical evidence for serious perinatal abnormalities in infants of mothers receiving tocolytic therapy. It should be borne in mind that fetal infusion of ritodrine does not mimic the effects of maternal drug administration and there are no significant changes in maternal metabolism comparable to those observed during maternal administration. Whether the concurrent administration of ritodrine to mother and fetus would worsen the fetal hyperglycaemia and hypoxaemia, or not, is a matter for conjecture. However, it is evident that possible effects on the welfare of the fetus should be given serious consideration before embarking on the administration of β-agonist tocolytic drugs. Quite clearly, the combined administration of β-agonist tocolytic drugs and prostaglandin inhibitors such as aspirin, indomethacin, etc. should be totally avoided.

Concluding comments

Viewed from a broad perspective there can be little doubt that glucose is the most important determinant of normality or derangement in the rate of prenatal growth. Because of its major importance as a substrate for oxidative metabolism, variations in glucose availability set in motion neural and endocrine responses either to increase or to limit its utilization, just as they do during postnatal life. It is these cascades of adaptive responses which initiate and amplify the changes in substrate use and distribution which lead to the alterations in glucose use and adjustments to development as its availability alters. However, it is still far from clear whether there is any optimum set point concentration for glucose within the conceptus and this does not appear to be an issue which has even been addressed specifically. If there is, it is obvious that it must differ among species to take account of the great differences among them in the normal range of plasma glucose concentrations. Certainly, the close relationship in fetal lambs between plasma glucose and insulin concentrations over the physiological glucose range of 0.5–1.5 μM, as well as the increases in adrenaline release which occur when glucose concentration decreases towards the lower end of this range, indicate that glucose thresholds for stimulation of insulin release by the pancreatic β-cell and for initiation of hypothalamic responses to hypoglycaemia differ greatly from those of adult sheep. Whether these are related to differences in glucose delivery is not known. It is a matter of conjecture whether similar changes in glucose concentrations or delivery thresholds also occur in human fetuses or those of other species, although the evidence suggests it must be so. This lack of information is surprising, given the acknowledged importance of fetal glucose concentration as a determinant of the endocrine secretions regulating its utilization and distribution among the tissues of the conceptus.

It is also surprising, given the extent of quantitative information about the transfer of glucose across the 'uteroplacenta' and its utilization within the fetus, that we still know little about the actual incorporation of glucose into the tissues as protein, glycogen or fat, or about the proportionate distribution of glucose use among the organs of the body other than the brain. Nothing seems to be known about the distribution of glucose use among tissues of the carcass itself nor about regional variations within these tissues, even though they are likely to be quantitatively the most important sites of insulin-regulated substrate use. Regional differences in the rate of development and maturation of the carcass tissues during fetal life have been well documented for most of the meat-producing animals. The effects of prenatal undernutrition and its consequences for postnatal growth on these patterns of development have also been determined. Barker et al. (1993) have recently drawn attention to the associations between prenatal developmental derangement and a variety of disease patterns in adult life (see Chapter 10), but it is evident that we still have little of the information necessary to determine how the causality of such relationships develops.

Much fetal research has been directed at understanding the nature of responses to hypoxaemia, yet the examination here suggests that hypoxaemia may be a correlate of fetal growth failure rather than the primary cause. In most situations, worsening hypoxaemia as fetal growth accelerates in late gestation (Soothill, Nicolaides & Campbell, 1987) appears to reflect a more generalized inadequacy of placental metabolic substrate supply dictated by small placental size or pathological changes in the maternal placental vasculature. As emphasized in an earlier review (Bassett, 1991), it is probable that far more attention needs to be given to understanding the means by which the conceptus initiates and enlarges the maternal vascularization of the placental attachments early in gestation, than to means for overcoming the later limitations imposed by inadequate placental development. Throughout gestation it is the ability of the maternal uterine vasculature to provide adequate glucose, oxygen and other nutrients to the exchange surface of the placenta which limits the availability of glucose and growth of the conceptus. Because of the differential growth of placental and fetal somatic tissues, early limitation in nutrient availability and placental development has long-term consequences for late fetal somatic development which are not readily overcome. Glucose may be essential as a substrate, but its role as a coordinator and regulator of normal prenatal development must not be underestimated.

Acknowledgements

I am very grateful to the many colleagues who have contributed to research carried out in my laboratory and to Christine Rathbone for assistance in preparation of the manuscript. Financial support for our research has been provided variously by the MRC, AFRC, The British Diabetic Association and the Wellcome Trust and their support is gratefully acknowledged.

References

Andrianakis, P., Walker, D.W., Ralph, M.M. & Thorburn, G.D. (1989). Effects of inhibiting prostaglandin synthesis in pregnant sheep with 4-aminoantipyrine under normothermic and hyperthermic conditions. *American Journal of Obstetrics and Gynecology*, **161,** 241–7.

Barker, D.J.P., Gluckman, P.D., Godfrey, K.M., Harding, J.E., Owens, J.A. & Robinson, J.S. (1993). Fetal nutrition and cardiovascular disease in adult life. *Lancet*, **341,** 941–4.

Baron, A.D. & Brechtel, G. (1993). Insulin differentially regulates systemic and skeletal muscle vascular resistance. *American Journal of Physiology*, **265,** E61–7.

Bassett, J.M. (1970). Metabolic effects of catecholamines in sheep. *Australian Journal of Biological Sciences*, **23,** 903–14.

Bassett, J.M. (1977). Glucagon, insulin and glucose homeostasis in the fetal lamb. *Annales de Recherches Veterinaires*, **8,** 362–73.

Bassett, J. M. (1985). Integration of pancreatic and gastrointestinal endocrine control of metabolic homeostasis during the perinatal period. In *Physiological Development of the Fetus and Newborn*, ed. C. T. Jones. pp. 123–33. Academic Press, London.

Bassett, J.M. (1986). Nutrition of the conceptus: aspects of its regulation. *Proceedings of the Nutrition Society*, **45**, 1–10.

Bassett, J.M. (1991). Current perspectives on placental development and its integration with fetal growth. *Proceedings of the Nutrition Society*, **50**, 311–19.

Bassett, J.M. (1993). Effects of prolonged adrenaline administration on metabolism in fetal lambs. *Journal of Physiology*, **459**, 326P.

Bassett, J.M., Burkes, A.H., Levine, D.H., Pinches, R.A. & Visser, G.H. (1985*a*). Maternal and fetal metabolic effects of prolonged ritodrine infusion. *Obstetrics and Gynecology*, **66**, 755–61.

Bassett, J.M., Burkes, A.H. & Pinches, R.A. (1985*b*). Glucose metabolism in the ovine conceptus. In *Physiological Development of the Fetus and Newborn*, ed. C. T. Jones. pp. 71–5. Academic Press, London.

Bassett, J.M., Hanson, C. & Weeding, C.M. (1989). Metabolic and cardiovascular changes during prolonged ritodrine infusion in fetal lambs. *Obstetrics and Gynecology*, **73**, 117–22.

Bassett, J.M. & Madill, D. (1974*a*). The influence of maternal nutrition on plasma hormone and metabolite concentrations of foetal lambs. *Journal of Endocrinology*, **61**, 465–77.

Bassett, J.M. & Madill, D. (1974*b*). Influence of prolonged glucose infusions on plasma insulin and growth hormone concentrations of foetal lambs. *Journal of Endocrinology*, **62**, 299–309.

Bassett, J.M., Madill, D., Nicol. D.H. & Thorburn, G.D. (1973). Further studies on the regulation of insulin release in foetal and postnatal lambs: the role of glucose as a physiological regulator of insulin release in utero. In *Foetal and Neonatal Physiology, Sir Joseph Barcroft Centenary Symposium*, ed. R. S. Comline, K.W. Cross, G.S. Dawes & P.W. Nathanielsz. pp. 351–9. Cambridge University Press, Cambridge.

Bassett, J.M. & Symonds, M.E. (1993). Effects of prolonged ritodrine or adrenaline administration on brown adipose tissue development in fetal lambs. *Journal of Physiology*, **459**, 325P.

Bassett, J.M. & Thorburn, G.D. (1971). The regulation of insulin secretion by the ovine foetus in utero. *Journal of Endocrinology*, **50**, 59–74.

Bassett, J.M., Weeding, C. & Hanson, C. (1990). Desensitization of β-receptor mediated responses to epinephrine in fetal lambs by prolonged ritodrine administration. *Pediatric Research*, **28**, 388–93.

Battaglia, F.C. & Meschia, G. (1978). Principal substrates of fetal metabolism. *Physiological Reviews*, **58**, 499–527.

Bell, A.W., Bassett, J.M., Chandler, K.D. & Boston, R.C. (1983). Fetal and maternal endocrine responses to exercise in the pregnant ewe. *Journal of Developmental Physiology*, **5**, 129–41.

Bell, A.W., Kennaugh, J.M., Battaglia, F.C., Makowski, E.L. & Meschia, G. (1986). Metabolic and circulatory studies of fetal lamb at midgestation. *American Journal of Physiology,* **250**, E538–44.

Bell, A.W., McBride, B.W., Slepetis, R., Early, R.J. & Currie, W.B. (1989). Chronic heat stress and prenatal development in sheep: 1. conceptus growth and maternal plasma hormones and metabolites. *Journal of Animal Science*, **67**, 3289–99.

Bell, A.W., Wilkening, R.B. & Meschia, G. (1987). Some aspects of placental function in chronically heat-stressed ewes. *Journal of Developmental Physiology*, **9**, 17–29.

Bleicher, S.J., O'Sullivan, J.B. & Freinkel, N. (1964). Carbohydrate metabolism in pregnancy. V. The interrelations of glucose, insulin and free fatty acids in late pregnancy and postpartum. *New England Journal of Medicine*, **271**, 866–72.

Bocking, A.D., White, S.E., Homan, J. & Richardson, B.S. (1992). Oxygen consumption is maintained in fetal sheep during prolonged hypoxaemia. *Journal of Developmental Physiology*, **17**, 169–74.

Caritas, S.N., Lin, L.S., Toig, G. & Wong, L.K. (1983). Pharmacodynamics of ritodrine in pregnant women during preterm labor. *American Journal of Obstetrics and Gynecology*, **147**, 752–9.

Cetin, I., Fennessey, P.V. Sparks, J.W., Meschia, G. & Battaglia, F.C. (1992). Fetal serine fluxes across fetal liver, hindlimb, and placenta in late gestation. *American Journal of Physiology*, **263**, E786–93.

Charlton, V. & Johengen, M. (1987). Fetal intravenous nutritional supplementation ameliorates the development of embolization-induced growth retardation in sheep. *Pediatric Research*, **22**, 55–61.

Cohen, W.R., Piasecki, G.J., Cohn, H.E., Susa, J.B. & Jackson, B.T. (1991). Sympathoadrenal responses during hypoglycaemia, hyperinsulinemia, and hypoxemia in the ovine fetus. *American Journal of Physiology*, **261**, E95–102.

Cryer, P.E. (1993). Glucose counterregulation: prevention and correction of hypoglycaemia in humans. *American Journal of Physiology*, **264**, E149–55.

Dalinghaus, M., Rudolph, C.D. & Rudolph, A.M. (1991). Effects of maternal fasting on hepatic gluconeogenesis and glucose metabolism in fetal lambs. *Journal of Developmental Physiology*, **16**, 267–75.

De Feo, P., Perriello, G., Torlone, E., Fanelli, C., Ventura, M.M., Santeusanio, F., Brunetti, P., Gerich, J.E. & Bolli, G.B. (1991). Contribution of adrenergic mechanisms to glucose counterregulation in humans. *American Journal of Physiology*, **261**, E725–36.

Devaskar, S.U., Ganguli, S., Styer, D., Devaskar, U.P. & Sperling, M.A. (1984). Glucagon and glucose dynamics in sheep: evidence for glucagon resistance in the fetus. *American Journal of Physiology,* **246,** E256–65.

DiGiacomo, J.E. & Hay, W.W., Jr. (1989) Regulation of placental glucose transfer and consumption by fetal glucose production. *Pediatric Research*, **25**, 429–34.

DiGiacomo, J.E. & Hay, W.W., Jr. (1990*a*). Placental-fetal glucose exchange and placental glucose consumption in pregnant sheep. *American Journal of Physiology*, **258**, E360–7.

DiGiacomo, J.E. & Hay, W.W., Jr. (1990*b*). Effect of hypoinsulinemia and hyperglycemia on fetal glucose utilization. *American Journal of Physiology*, **259**, E506–12.

Economides, D.L., Nicolaides K.H. & Campbell, S. (1991). Metabolic and endocrine findings in appropriate and small for gestational age fetuses. *Journal of Perinatal Medicine*, **19**, 97–105.

Fletcher, J.M., Falconer, J. & Bassett, J.M. (1982). The relationship of body and placental weight to plasma levels of insulin and other hormones during development in fetal rabbits. *Diabetologia*, **23**, 124–30.

Fowden, A.L. (1989). The role of insulin in prenatal growth. *Journal of Developmental Physiology*, **12**, 173–82.

Fowden, A.L., Harding, R., Ralph, M.M. & Thorburn, G.D. (1987). The nutritional regulation of plasma prostaglandin E concentrations in the fetus and pregnant ewe during late gestation. *Journal of Physiology*, **394**, 1–12.

Fowden, A.L., Hughes, P. & Comline, R.S. (1989). The effects of insulin on the growth rate of the sheep fetus during late gestation. *Quarterly Journal of Experimental Physiology*, **74**, 703–14.

Fowden, A.L., Mao, X.Z. & Comline, R.S. (1986*a*). Effects of pancreatectomy on the growth and metabolite concentrations of the sheep fetus. *Journal of Endocrinology*, **110**, 225–31.

Fowden, A.L., Silver, M. & Comline, R.S. (1986*b*). The effect of pancreatectomy on the uptake of metabolites by the sheep fetus. *Quarterly Journal of Experimental Physiology*, **71**, 67–78.

Fujimoto, S., Akahane, M., Uzuki, K., Inagawa, A., Sakai, K. & Sakai. A. (1984). Placental transfer of ritodrine hydrochloride in sheep. *International Journal of Gynaecology and Obstetrics*, **22**, 269–74.

Gluckman, P.D., Butler, J.H., Comline, R. & Fowden, A. (1987). The effects of pancreatectomy on the plasma concentrations of insulin-like growth factors I and II in the sheep fetus. *Journal of Developmental Physiology*, **9**, 79–88.

Gull, I. & Charlton, V. (1993). Effects of antipyrine on umbilical and regional metabolism in late gestation in the fetal lamb. *American Journal of Obstetrics and Gynecology*, **168**, 706–13.

Harding, J.E., Jones, C.T. & Robinson, J.S. (1985). Studies on experimental growth retardation in sheep. The effects of a small placenta in restricting transport to and growth of the fetus. *Journal of Developmental Physiology*, **7**, 427–42.

Harwell, C.M., Padbury, J.F., Anand, R.S., Martinez, A.M., Ipp, E., Thio, S.L. & Burnell, E.E. (1990). Fetal catecholamine responses to maternal hypoglycemia. *American Journal of Physiology*, **259**, R1126–30.

Havel, P.J. & Taborsky, J. Jr. (1989). The contribution of the autonomic nervous system to changes of glucagon and insulin secretion during hypoglycemic stress. *Endocrine Reviews*, **10**, 332–50.

Hay, W.W. Jr., DiGiacomo, J.E., Meznarich, H.K., Hirst, K. & Zerbe, G. (1989). Effects of glucose and insulin on fetal glucose oxidation and oxygen consumption. *American Journal of Physiology*, **256**, E704–13.

Hay, W.W. Jr. & Meznarich, H.K. (1988). Use of fetal streptozotocin injection to determine the role of normal levels of fetal insulin in regulating uteroplacental and umbilical glucose exchange. *Pediatric Research*, **24**, 312–17.

Hay, W.W. Jr., Meznarich, H.K., DiGiacomo, J.E., Hirst, K. & Zerbe, G. (1988). Effects of insulin and glucose concentrations on glucose utilization in fetal sheep. *Pediatric Research*, **23**, 381–7.

Hay, W.W. Jr., Molina, R.A., DiGiacomo, J.E. & Meschia, G. (1990). Model of placental glucose consumption and glucose transfer. *American Journal of Physiology,* **258**, R569–77.

Hay, W.W. Jr., Sparks, J.W., Wilkening, R.B., Battaglia, F.C. & Meschia, G. (1984). Fetal glucose uptake and utilization as functions of maternal glucose concentration. *American Journal of Physiology,* **246**, E237–42.

Hellerstrom, C. & Swenne, I. (1991). Functional maturation and proliferation of fetal pancreatic β-cells. *Diabetes,* **40(Suppl. 2)**, 89–93.

Hodgson, J.C., Mellor, D.J. & Field, A.C. (1991). Kinetics of lactate and glucose metabolism in the pregnant ewe and conceptus. *Experimental Physiology*, **76**, 389–98.

Hooper, S.B., Bocking, A.D., White, S., Challis, J.R.G. & Han, V.K.M. (1991). DNA synthesis is reduced in selected fetal tissues during prolonged hypoxemia. *American Journal of Physiology*, **261**, R508–14.

Hooper, S.B., Coulter, C.L., Deayton, J.M., Harding, R. & Thorburn. G.D. (1990). Fetal endocrine responses to prolonged hypoxemia in sheep. *American Journal of Physiology*, **259**, R703–8.

Hooper, S.B., Harding, R., Deayton, J. & Thorburn, G.D. (1992). Role of prostaglandins in the metabolic responses of the fetus to hypoxia. *American Journal Obstetric & Gynecology*, **166**, 1568–75.

Jensen, A., Roman, C. & Rudolph, A.M. (1991). Effects of reducing uterine blood flow on fetal blood flow distribution and oxygen delivery. *Journal of Developmental Physiology*, **15**, 309–23.

Jones, C.T. (1980). Circulating catecholamines in the fetus, their origin, actions and significance. In *Biogenic Amines in Development*, ed. H. Parvez & S. Parvez. pp. 63–86. Elsevier/North Holland Biomedical Press, Amsterdam.

Jones, C.T. (1991). Control of glucose metabolism in the perinatal period. *Journal of Developmental Physiology*, **15**, 812–89.

Jones, C.T. & Ritchie, J.W.K. (1978*a*). The cardiovascular effects of circulating catecholamines in fetal sheep. *Journal of Physiology*, **285**, 381–93.

Jones, C.T. & Ritchie, J.W.K. (1978*b*). The metabolic and endocrine effects of circulating catecholamines in fetal sheep. *Journal of Physiology*, **285**, 395–408.

Jones, C.T. & Ritchie, J.W.K. (1983). The effects of adrenergic blockade on fetal response to hypoxia. *Journal of Developmental Physiology*, **5**, 211–22.

Jones, C.T., Roebuck, M.M., Walker, D.W. & Johnston, B.M. (1988). The role of the adrenal medulla and peripheral sympathetic nerves in the physiological responses of the fetal sheep to hypoxia. *Journal of Developmental Physiology*, **10**, 17–36.

Jones, C.T., Roebuck, M.M., Walker, D.W., Lagercrantz, H. & Johnston, B.M. (1987). Cardiovascular, metabolic and endocrine effects of chemical sympathectomy and of adrenal demedullation in fetal sheep. *Journal of Developmental Physiology*, **9**, 347–67.

Kalkhoff, R.K. (1991). Impact of maternal fuels and nutritional state on fetal growth. *Diabetes*, **40(Suppl. 2)**, 61–5.

Liechty, E.A., Boyle, D.W., Moorehead, H., Liu, Y.M. & Denne, S.C. (1992). Effect of hyperinsulinemia on ovine fetal leucine kinetics during prolonged maternal fasting. *American Journal of Physiology*, **26**, E696–702.

Loy, G.L., Quick, A.N. Jr, Hay, W.W. Jr., Meschia, G., Battaglia, F.C. & Fennessey, P.V. (1990). Fetoplacental deamination and decarboxylation of leucine. *American Journal of Physiology*, **259**, E492–7.

Marconi, A.M., Battaglia, F.C., Meschia, G. & Sparks, J.W. (1989). A comparison of amino acid arteriovenous differences across the liver and placenta of the fetal lamb. *American Journal of Physiology*, **257**, E909–15.

Marconi, A.M., Cetin, I., Davoli, E., Baggiani, M. Fanelli, R., Fennessay, P.V., Battaglia, F.C. & Pardi, G. (1993). An evaluation of fetal glucogenesis in intrauterine growth retarded pregnancies. *Metabolism*, **42**, 860–4.

Mellor, D.J. (1984). Investigation of fetal growth in sheep. In *Animal Models in Fetal Medicine (IV),* vol 5, ed. P. W. Nathanielsz. pp. 149–73. Perinatology Press, New York.

Mellor, D.J. (1985). Nutritional and placental determinants of foetal growth rate in sheep and consequences for the newborn lamb. *British Veterinary Journal*, **139**, 307–24.

Metzger, B.E. (1991). Biphasic effects of maternal metabolism on fetal growth. Quintessential expression of fuel-mediated teratogenesis. *Diabetes*, **40(Suppl.2)**, 99–105.

Michael, K., Ward, B.S. & Moore, W.M.O. (1983). Relationship of fetal to placental size: the pig model. *European Journal of Obstetrics, Gynaecology and Reproductive Biology*, **16**, 53–62.

Milley, J.R. (1987). Effect of insulin on the distribution of cardiac output in the fetal lamb. *Pediatric Research*, **22**, 168–72.

Milley, J.R., Papacostas, J.S. & Tabata, B.K. (1986). Effect of insulin on uptake of metabolic substrates by the sheep fetus. *American Journal of Physiology*, **251**, E349–56.

Molina, R.D., Meschia, G., Battaglia, F.C. & Hay, W.W. Jr. (1991). Gestational maturation of placental glucose transfer capacity in sheep. *American Journal of Physiology*, **261**, R697–704.

Oliver, M.H., Harding, J.E., Breier, B.H., Evans, P.C. & Gluckman, P.D. (1993). Glucose but not a mixed amino acid infusion regulates plasma insulin-like growth factor-I concentrations in fetal sheep. *Pediatric Research*, **34**, 62–5.

Owens, J.A., Falconer, J. & Robinson, J.S. (1987*a*). Effect of restriction of placental growth on fetal and utero-placental metabolism. *Journal of Developmental Physiology*, **9**, 225–38.

Owens, J.A., Falconer, J. & Robinson, J.S. (1987*b*). Effect of restriction of placental growth on oxygen delivery to and consumption by the pregnant uterus and fetus. *Journal of Developmental Physiology*, **9**, 137–50.

Padbury, J.F., Ludlow, J.K., Ervin, M.G., Jacobs, H.C. & Humme, J.A. (1987). Thresholds for physiological effects of plasma catecholamines in fetal sheep. *American Journal of Physiology*, **252**, E530–7.

Philipps, A.F., Dubin, J.W., Matty, P.J. & Raye, J.R. (1982). Arterial hypoxemia and hyperinsulinemia in the chronically hyperglycemic fetal lamb. *Pediatric Research*, **16**, 653–8.

Philipps, A.F., Dubin, J.W., Matty, P.J. & Raye, J.R. (1983). Influence of exogenous glucagon on fetal glucose metabolism and ketone production. *Pediatric Research*, **56**, 51–6.

Philipps, A.F., Rosenkrantz, T.S., Clark, R.M., Knox, I., Chaffin, D.G. & Raye, J.R. (1991). Effects of fetal insulin deficiency on growth in fetal lambs. *Diabetes*, **40**, 20–7.

Philipps, A.F., Rosenkrantz, T.S., Lemons, J.A., Knox, I., Porte, P.J. & Raye, J.R. (1990). Insulin-induced alterations in amino acid metabolism in the fetal lamb. *Journal of Developmental Physiology*, **13**, 251–9.

Phillippe, M. & Kitzmiller, J.L. (1981). The fetal and maternal catecholamine response to insulin-induced hypoglycemia in the rat. *American Journal of Obstetrics and Gynecology*, **139**, 407–15.

Salvesen, D.R., Brudenell, J.M., Proudler, A.J., Crook, D. & Nicolaides, K.H. (1993). Fetal pancreatic β-cell function in pregnancies complicated by maternal diabetes mellitus: relationship to fetal acidemia and macrosomia. *American Journal of Obstetrics and Gynecology*, **168**, 1363–9.

Soothill, P.W., Nicolaides, K.H. & Campbell, S. (1987). Prenatal asphyxia, hyperlacticaemia, hypoglycaemia, and erythroblastosis in growth retarded fetuses. *British Medical Journal*, **294**, 1051–3.

Spellacy, W.N., Cruz, A.C., Buhi, W.C. & Birk, S.A. (1978). The acute effects of ritodrine infusion on maternal metabolism: measurements of levels of glucose, insulin, glucagon, triglycerides, cholesterol, placental lactogen, and chorionic gonadotropin. *American Journal of Obstetrics and Gynecology*, **131**, 637–42.

Sperling, M.A., Ganguli, R.A.C.S. & Anand, R. (1980). Adrenergic modulation of pancreatic hormone secretion in utero: studies in fetal sheep. *Pediatric Research*, **14**, 203–8.

Thompson, G.E., Bassett, J. M., Samson, D. & Slee, J. (1982). The effects of cold exposure of pregnant sheep on foetal plasma nutrients, hormones and birth weight. *British Journal of Nutrition*, **48**, 59–64.

Titlbach, M., Falt, K. & Falkmer, S. (1985). Postnatal maturation of the Islets of Langerhans in sheep. Light microscopic, immunohistochemical, morphometric, and ultrastructural investigations with particular reference to the transient appearance of argyrophil insulin immunoreactive cells. *Diabetes Research*, **2**, 5–15.

Van der Weyde, M.P., Wright, M.R., Taylor, S.M., Axelson, J.E. & Rurak, D.W. (1992). Metabolic effects of ritodrine in the fetal lamb. *Journal of Pharmacology and Experimental Therapeutics*, **262,** 48–59.

Vatnick, I., Schoknecht, P.A., Darrigrand, R. & Bell, A.W. (1991). Growth and metabolism of the placenta after unilateral fetectomy in twin pregnant ewes. *Journal of Developmental Physiology* , **15**, 351–6.

Warburton, D., Parton, L., Buckley, S., Cosico, L. & Saluna, T. (1987). Effects of beta-2 agonist on tracheal fluid flow, surfactant and pulmonary mechanics in the fetal lamb. *Journal of Pharmacology and Experimental Therapeutics*, **242**, 394–42.

Warburton, D., Parton, L., Buckley, S., Cosico, L. & Saluna, T. (1988). Effects of β-2 agonist on hepatic glycogen metabolism in the fetal lamb. *Pediatric Research*, **24**, 330–2.

10

Fetal programming of human disease

DAVID J.P. BARKER and H.Y. SULTAN

Introduction

Babies who are small at birth and during infancy are now known to be at increased risk of developing coronary heart disease, hypertension and diabetes during adult life. It is thought that these diseases are 'programmed' by an inadequate supply of nutrients or oxygen in utero or immediately after birth. The term 'programming' describes the process whereby a stimulus or insult at a critical period of development has lasting or lifelong significance (Lucas, 1991). The principle that the nutritional, hormonal, and metabolic environment afforded by the mother may permanently 'program' the structure and physiology of her offspring has long been established. Recent findings suggest that it is important in the development of human disease.

This chapter has three sections.

1. A summary of the phenomenon of programming.
2. A discussion of the ways in which maternal undernutrition may influence fetal growth and metabolism.
3. A review of the links between fetal undernutrition and adult disease in man.

Principles and mechanisms of programming

Animal studies have established three principles which appear to underlie the phenomenon of programming and point to several mechanisms which may mediate its effects. These are discussed in turn.

Permanent effects of early adverse influences

The primary concept of programming is that adverse influences acting early in life have permanent effects on the body's structure and physiology. One of the best examples of programming is the effect of early exposure to sex hormones on the development of sexual physiology and behaviour. A female rat injected with testosterone propionate on the fifth day after birth develops normally until puberty, but fails to ovulate or show normal patterns of female sexual behaviour thereafter (Barraclough & Gorski, 1961). Ovarian and pituitary function are normal, but the release of gonadotrophin by the hypothalamus has been irreversibly altered from the cyclical female pattern of release to the tonic male pattern. If the same injection of testosterone is given when the animal is 20 days old, it has no effect on reproductive function. Thus there is a critical time during development at which the animal's sexual physiology can be permanently changed. This is known as the 'sensitive' or 'critical' period. Numerous animal experiments have illustrated that hormones, undernutrition and other influences affecting development may permanently programme the structure and physiology of the body's tissues and systems when they act during sensitive periods (Winick & Noble, 1966; Osofsky, 1975; Roeder & Chow, 1971; Stephens, 1980; Swenne, Crace & Milner, 1987; Hahn, 1989; Mott, Lewis & McGill, 1991; Smart, 1991).

The body is more susceptible to programming when it is growing rapidly, and sensitive periods may correspond to phases of rapid cell replication (Widdowson & McCance, 1975). Tissues develop in a predetermined sequence from conception to maturity (Hammond & Appleton, 1932) and, according to this sequence, different organs and tissues undergo periods of rapid cell division at different times. The renal nephrons, for example, are laid down during the last trimester of pregnancy whereas the pancreatic β-cells continue to differentiate during infancy (Hellerström, Swenne & Andersson, 1988; Hinchliffe et al., 1992).

In some experimental animals, such as the pig and the rat, cell numbers increase most rapidly after birth, rather than before, and the animal can therefore recover to some extent from undernutrition in utero. Humans, however, accomplish a greater proportion of their growth before birth than do pigs. It has been calculated that the fertilized human ovum goes through some 42 rounds of cell division before birth (Milner, 1989), whilst after birth there need be only a further five cycles of division. In humans, the effects of intrauterine growth failure are therefore relatively severe (Widdowson, 1971).

The timing of the insult

The second principle established by experiments on animals is that exposure to an insult, such as undernutrition, during different stages of early life has different effects. This results from the existence of sensitive periods, and the fact that sensitive periods for different organs occur at different times.

Early in fetal life, growth is limited mainly by the supply of nutrients and oxygen. However, at some point before birth, or shortly after in some species, growth begins to 'track'. Animals who are small relative to others of the same age remain small, and large ones remain large. In humans, tracking is demonstrated by the way in which infants grow along centile curves (McCance & Widdowson, 1974). Once tracking is established, it is no longer possible to make animals grow faster by offering them unlimited food. Their rate of growth has become 'set', homeostatically controlled by feedback systems.

Numerous experiments on animals, including rats, mice, sheep and pigs, have shown that, when the protein or calorie intake of the mother during various stages of pregnancy and lactation is lowered, the offspring are smaller than they would otherwise have been (Chow & Lee, 1964; Dubos, Savage & Schaedler, 1966; Winick & Noble, 1967; Blackwell et al., 1969; Zeman & Stanbrough, 1969; Widdowson, 1971; Roeder, 1973). In general, the earlier in the life of an animal that undernutrition occurs, the more likely it is to have permanent effects on body weight and length. This was demonstrated by McCance and Widdowson in a series of experiments carried out 30 years ago. Rats which were undernourished from three to six weeks after birth, that is, immediately after weaning, lost weight. On resumption of full feeding at 6 weeks, they failed to return to the growth trajectory of the controls and remained permanently small. By contrast, rats who were not undernourished until 9 to 12 weeks after birth regained their growth trajectory when full feeding was resumed, and continued to grow normally thereafter (Widdowson & McCance, 1963; McCance & Widdowson, 1974).

Undernutrition early in intrauterine life tends to produce small but normally proportioned animals whereas undernutrition at later stages of development leads to selective organ damage and disproportionate growth (McCance & Widdowson, 1974). During undernutrition those tissues in which maturity is more advanced have a greater priority of growth and may continue to grow at the expense of other tissues (McCance & Widdowson, 1962). For example, when rats were undernourished immediately after weaning, the weight of the brain and skeletal muscle was unaffected but the weight of the liver, kidney and thymus was permanently reduced. When, however, undernutrition was delayed until 42 days after birth only the weight of the thymus was reduced (Winick & Noble, 1966).

In other rat experiments, growth impairment was brought about by ligation of the artery to one uterine horn and consequent uteroplacental ischaemia. In general, both undernutrition and ischaemia have similar effects on proportionate fetal growth if they are applied at the same time (Wigglesworth, 1964; Roux, Tordet-Caridroit & Chanez, 1970). It is the timing of the insult that determines which tissues and systems are damaged and hence the resultant disproportion in size and function. In addition, the pattern of disproportion is influenced by the relative sensitivity of different organs. Some aspects of maturation, such as the growth of the thymus, are markedly influenced by undernutrition whereas others, such as the growth of the eye, are less sensitive (Moment, 1933). The eye's development is less 'plastic' than that of most other tissues.

The influence of growth trajectory

The effect of undernutrition is influenced by the fetus's rate of growth. Rapidly growing fetuses are more vulnerable. In sheep, the response of the fetus to maternal undernutrition in late pregnancy depends on its growth rate (Harding et al., 1992). When rapidly growing fetuses are undernourished, their growth slows abruptly, whereas the more slowly growing fetuses continue to grow through the period of undernutrition. At birth the size of the lambs may be similar but their body compositions are found to differ; undernutrition has affected the proportions of the rapidly growing animals. Similarly, if rats are undernourished after weaning for a three-week period, those which were growing rapidly have different body compositions from those which were growing slowly – even if both groups of animals have the same final body weight. The bones of the fast-growing rats are longer, and the testes heavier, but the livers, spleens and small intestines are lighter (Widdowson & McCance, 1963). In humans, the growth trajectory in boys is more rapid than that of girls from early in embryonic life, and boys may therefore be more vulnerable to undernutrition.

The mechanisms which underlie programming

As yet, little is known about the cellular and molecular mechanisms which underlie programming.

Reduction in cell numbers of various organs following early undernutrition has frequently been observed in animal experiments. In rats, undernutrition before weaning permanently reduces the number of cells in many organs, including the brain, liver, kidneys and intestines (Winick & Noble, 1966, 1967; McLeod, Goldrick & Whyte, 1972). These animals do not regain their normal size when adequately nourished after weaning, which suggests that cell numbers may limit ultimate size. Growth-retarded human babies have reduced numbers of cells in their organs (Widdowson, Crabb & Milner, 1972). In some instances, reduction in cell numbers can be directly linked to limitations of function. In the rat, reduced numbers of pancreatic β-cells induced by a low protein diet during pregnancy may limit insulin secretion (Snoeck et al., 1990). Similarly, growth-retarded human neonates may have fewer β-cells and a lowered capacity for insulin secretion (Van Assche & Aerts, 1979).

The effects of early undernutrition may also be mediated through permanent changes in organ structure. In the rat, protein deficiency not only lowers β-cell numbers in the pancreas but also reduces the vascularization of the islets – which could further impair insulin secretion (Snoeck et al., 1990).

Nutrients may also effect permanent changes through altering hormonal axes, and this is of particular interest as a mechanism which may operate in the genesis of human disease (Barker et al., 1993*a*). Altered sensitivity to hormones may be brought about by 'setting' of hormone receptors in the cell membrane. Experiments suggest that the receptors are plastic during their maturation phase. At this time, exposure to a normal concentration of hormone seems to promote receptor development, while exposure to inappropriate levels of hormone, or to other hormones that are sufficiently similar to bind to the receptor, may permanently reduce the receptor response (Nagy & Csaba, 1980; Csaba & Török, 1991). The pattern of hormone release may also be programmed. Exposure to androgens determines the tonic pattern of gonadotrophin hormone release in males, as opposed to the cyclical pattern in females (Barraclough & Gorski, 1961).

Maternal undernutrition and fetal growth

Maternal constraint of fetal growth

It is well known that the mother constrains the growth of the fetus. This was first illustrated by the experiments of Walton and Hammond (1938), in which Shetland and Shire horses were crossed. The foals were smaller at birth when the Shetland pony was the mother than when the Shire horse was the mother. Since the genetic composition of the two crosses was similar, this suggested that the smaller Shetland mother had constrained the growth of her fetus. In humans, numerous studies have shown that the birthweights of mothers are related to those of their children and even their children's children (Klebanoff et al., 1984; Carr-Hill et al., 1987; Alberman et al., 1992; Emanuel et al., 1992). This has led to the conclusion that mothers constrain fetal growth and that the degree of constraint they exert is set when they themselves are in utero (Ounsted, Scott & Ounsted, 1986).

Maternal undernutrition may constrain fetal growth. The effects may be transmitted from one generation to the next, as was illustrated dramatically by the experience of the Dutch in western Holland during the famine of 1944–45. The famine began in October 1944 and ended suddenly seven months later, when Holland was liberated. The average food intake was approximately 1600 calories at the start of the famine, and fell to 1300 calories by the end. Babies who were exposed to famine during the latter half of gestation were born small, with an average birthweight 327 g lighter than that of babies born before the famine. Those who were undernourished earlier, during the first half of gestation, had normal birthweights themselves and grew to normal size but the mean birthweight of the women's own babies was reduced (Lumey, 1992).

Maternal constraint is thought to reflect the limited capacity of the mother to deliver nutrients to her fetus (Gluckman & Harding, 1992). The amount of nutrients reaching the fetus depends not only on the mother's diet during pregnancy, but also on the processes of digestion, absorption, transport in the blood and transfer across the placenta. The mother's nutrient stores prior to pregnancy are also important.

During the past 50 years numerous studies have examined whether the quality of the diet eaten by a pregnant woman influences the size of the baby at birth. Supplementation of protein, calories and minerals, and the effects of weight prior to pregnancy compared to weight gain during pregnancy have variously been considered. The results, however, have been inconsistent and contradictory (Burke, Harding & Stuart, 1948; Rosso, 1989; Doyle et al., 1990; Love & Kinch, 1965; Lechtig & Klein, 1981). In retrospect this is unsurprising since it is now known that the effects of diet interact with the mothers' prepregnant physiology and metabolism, to determine transport of nutrients to the fetus.

Maternal nutrition and the placenta

The fetus can become undernourished despite an adequate nutrient supply from the mother, if transport across the placenta is inadequate. This may result from poor implantation or breakdown of feedback control between fetus and placenta. If the nutrient supply to the placenta is reduced, not only is fetal growth suppressed but the placenta mediates secondary changes in maternal metabolism and cardiovascular function. In some circumstances, the placenta may adapt to reduced nutrient supply from the mother by enlarging. It has been shown that, in sheep, a restricted diet in mid-pregnancy stimulates placental enlargement, but only if nutrition was good at the time of conception. If the nutritional status immediately prior to pregnancy was poor, then the placenta is unable to enlarge (DeBarro et al., 1992).

A study in five countries has shown that increased placental size is associated with anaemia during pregnancy (Beischer et al., 1970). It is also known to be associated with mild hypoxaemia in women living at high altitude, and with maternal exercise in pregnancy (Mayhew, Jackson & Haas, 1990; Clapp & Rizk, 1992). In a study of 8684 pregnant women in Oxford, those whose haemoglobins fell to lower values during pregnancy had babies with larger placentas (Godfrey et al., 1991). Subsequent studies showed that placental size had become relatively high by 18 weeks of gestation in women with low haemoglobins (Howe & Wheeler, 1994). The association with haemoglobin is thought to reflect the effects of the oxygen content of maternal blood on placental development and function. Hypoxia may stimulate blood vessel formation in the growing placenta.

Fetal undernutrition and adult disease

As in animals, the growth of the human fetus is plastic. Its major adaptation to undernutrition is to slow its rate of growth. This enhances its ability to survive by reducing its substrate utilization and lowering its metabolic rate. Associated with this, there is a redistribution of blood flow which preserves the flow to tissues that are important for survival,

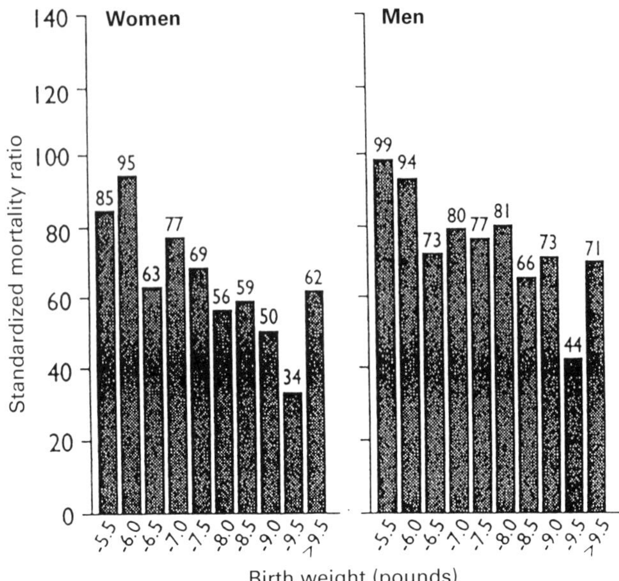

Fig. 10.1. Standardized mortality ratios for cardiovascular disease below age 65 according to birthweight.

including the brain (Widdowson, 1974). Although this ensures immediate survival, it may be at the price of long-term changes which cause disease and reduce survival in the postreproductive period. Undernutrition in late gestation, for example, may lead to reduced growth of the kidney which develops rapidly at that time. Reduced replication of kidney cells may permanently reduce cell numbers, since after birth there seems no capacity for renal cell division to 'catch-up' (Hinchliffe et al., 1992; Widdowson, 1974). Whether this reduced number of cells has long-term effects may depend on whether the system is stressed, for example, by high salt intake and therefore becomes unable to maintain the volume and composition of body fluids.

Birthweight and adult disease

Reduced early growth, as determined by birthweight or weight during infancy, has been linked to increased incidence of various diseases in adult life. In Hertfordshire, birth records were kept by health visitors detailing the birthweight of every baby born in the county from 1911 until the Second World War. Figure 10.1 shows the death rate from cardiovascular disease in the men and women born before 1930, in relation to

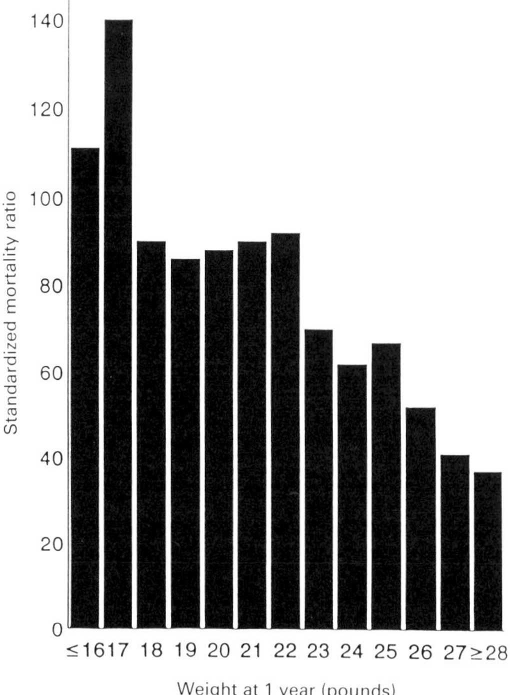

Fig. 10.2. Standardized mortality ratios for cardiovascular disease below age 65 according to weight at 1 year.

their birthweight (Barker et al., 1989; Osmond et al., 1993). In both sexes death rates fall as birthweight increases, though there is the suggestion of an upturn in the rates at the highest birthweights. Data from another study, in Sheffield, show that it is babies who are small for dates, rather than prematurely born, who are at increased risk (Barker et al., 1993*b*). Weight at one year, which is an indicator of growth in infancy, is also related to coronary heart disease in men, and predicts death rates more strongly than does birthweight. Death rates fall steeply between men who were small and those who were large at one year (Fig. 10.2).

These findings pose the question of what are the processes which link reduced early growth with adult disease. It is now known that people who were small have, as adults, raised blood pressure (Law et al., 1993), raised serum cholesterol (Barker et al., 1993*c*), raised plasma fibrinogen and factor 7 concentrations (Barker et al., 1992) and impaired glucose tolerance (Hales et al., 1991). Table 10.1 shows the mean systolic pressures of men and women aged 64–71 years. Systolic pressure falls

Table 10.1. *Mean systolic pressure (mm Hg) in men and women aged 64 to 71 years according to birthweight*

Birthweight (pounds)[a]	Men	Women
–5.5	171 (18)	169 (9)
–6.6	168 (53)	165 (33)
–7.5	168 (144)	160 (168)
–8.5	165 (111)	163 (48)
>8.5	163 (92)	155 (26)
Total	166 (418)	161 (184)
Standard deviation	24	26
p value for trend	0.02	0.01

[a] 1 pound = 454 g.
Figures in parentheses are numbers of subjects.

away progressively between those who were small at birth and those who were large (Law et al., 1993). The relation between birthweight and blood pressure has been demonstrated in a range of studies of children and adults (Barker et al., 1990; Law et al., 1991; Whincup, Cook & Papacosta, 1991), and there is a secure base for saying that impaired fetal growth is strongly linked to raised blood pressure at all ages except adolescence, when the tracking of blood pressure levels which began in early childhood is perturbed by the adolescent growth spurt.

Table 10.2 shows the prevalence of non-insulin-dependent diabetes and impaired glucose tolerance according to birthweight in a group of men. The prevalence falls sharply between men who were small at birth and men who were large (Hales et al., 1991). Similar trends have been observed in women, and the findings have been replicated in other studies in Britain (Phipps et al., 1993) and the USA (Valdez et al., 1994; McCance et al., 1994). It is thought that people who were small babies are insulin resistant and may also have reduced ability to produce insulin. The association between diabetes in adult life and low rates of fetal growth is perhaps unsurprising given that, during fetal life, insulin is central in the control of growth, linking maternal glucose supply to rates of cell replication (Fowden, 1989).

Body proportions and adult disease

Babies who are small at birth may either be proportionately small, that is 'perfect miniatures', or disproportionate. Consistent with the findings in

Table 10.2. *Prevalence of non-insulin-dependent diabetes and impaired glucose tolerance (2 h plasma glucose concentration >7.8 mmol/l) in men aged 59–70 years*

Birthweight pounds (kg)	Number of men	Impaired glucose tolerance or diabetes		Odds ratio adjusted for body mass index (95% CI)
		No.	%	
≤5.5 (2.50	20	8	40	6.6 (1.5 to 28)
–6.5 (2.95)	47	16	34	4.8 (1.3 to 17)
–7.5 (3.41)	104	32	31	4.6 (1.4 to 16)
–8.5 (3.86)	117	26	22	2.6 (0.8 to 8.9)
–9.5 (4.31)	54	7	13	1.4 (0.3 to 5.6)
>9.5 (4.31)	28	4	14	1.0
Total	370	93	25	χ^2 for trend = 15.4 ($p < 0.001$)

animals, the symmetrically small baby is thought to originate through undernutrition or some other adverse influence in early gestation. The disproportionate baby is thought to result from undernutrition in later gestation. Undernutrition in early gestation permanently affects body size, whereas undernutrition in late gestation has profound effects on body form. Different kinds of disproportion at birth have different long-term consequences, so that thin babies develop different disorders in adulthood from babies who are short (Barker, 1994).

Babies who are born thin, that is, with low ponderal index (birth weight/length^3) have an increased risk of developing insulin resistance in later life. The occurrence of insulin resistance in adults is characterized in a syndrome, called syndrome X, in which diabetes, hypertension and raised plasma triglyceride concentrations coincide in the same patient, together with insulin resistance and hyperinsulinaemia. The prevalence of this condition in men falls from 30% down to 6% between those who were small and those who were large at birth (Barker et al., 1993*d*), (Table 10.3). Further analysis shows that it is specifically the thin baby who develops syndrome X. Babies who are thin lack muscle as well as fat and muscle in adult life is the peripheral site of insulin action. Insulin tolerance tests carried out on men and women aged 50 have confirmed that those who were thin at birth are less sensitive to insulin (Phillips et al., 1994).

Table 10.3. *Prevalence of syndrome X (type 2 diabetes, hypertension and hyperlipidaemia) in men according to birthweight*

Birthweight pounds (kg)	Total number of men	% with syndrome X	Odds ratio adjusted for body mass index (95% confidence interval)
≤5.5 (2.50)	20	30	18 (2.6 to 118)
−6.5 (2.95)	54	19	8.4 (1.5 to 49)
−7.5 (3.41)	114	17	8.5 (1.5 to 46)
−8.5 (3.86)	123	12	4.9 (0.9 to 27)
−9.5 (4.31)	64	6	2.2 (0.3 to 14)
>9.5 (4.31)	32	6	1.0
Total	370	14	χ^2 for trend = 16.0 ($p < 0.001$)

Short babies are thought to have encountered undernutrition in late gestation and to have sustained brain growth at the expense of the trunk, including the abdominal viscera. Table 10.4 shows mean serum cholesterol concentrations in a group of men and women aged 50 to 53 according to abdominal circumference at birth. The concentrations of total low density lipoprotein (LDL) cholesterol fall between people who had small and large abdominal circumferences (Barker et al., 1993*c*). Abdominal circumference reflects liver size and an inference from these data is that babies who have impaired liver development reset their cholesterol metabolism, possibly by increased synthesis or reduced excretion, and this persists into adult life.

Reduced abdominal circumference at birth is also associated with raised plasma concentrations of fibrinogen, another strong predictor of coronary heart disease (Martyn et al., 1994). Babies who are short at birth tend to have low growth rates in infancy, and achieve only a low weight at one year. This may explain why poor infant growth is a strong predictor of death from coronary heart disease (Fig. 10.2).

Infant feeding

The method of infant feeding is also linked to adult disease. Amongst people in Hertfordshire, for whom details of infant feeding had been recorded, highest death rates from cardiovascular disease were observed

Table 10.4. *Mean serum lipid concentrations according to abdominal circumference at birth in men and women aged 50–53 years*

Abdominal circumference	Number of people		Total cholesterol (mmol/l)			Low density lipoprotein cholesterol (mmol/l)		
Men	Women	Men	Women	All	Men	Women	All	Men
−11.5	28	25	6.5	6.8	6.7	4.5	4.6	4.5
−12.0	22	21	6.8	6.9	6.9	4.8	4.4	4.6
−12.5	13	18	6.7	6.8	6.8	4.6	4.2	4.4
−13.0	21	24	6.0	6.5	6.2	3.8	4.2	4.0
>13.0	26	19	6.0	6.4	6.1	3.9	4.1	4.0
Total	110	107	6.4	6.7	6.5	4.3	4.3	4.3
p-value adjusted for gestational age by regression			0.009	0.16	0.003	0.003	1.12	0.0007

in two groups of people: those who had been breast fed beyond one year and those who had been exclusively bottle fed (Fall et al., 1992; Osmond et al., 1993). Serum lipids were measured in a group of men in Hertfordshire born 70 years ago (Fall et al., 1992). Table 10.5 shows that men who had been breast fed beyond one year, and those who had been exclusively bottle fed, had higher serum concentrations of total cholesterol in fasting and non-fasting samples, higher concentrations of low density lipoprotein (LDL) cholesterol, and higher low density lipoprotein to high density lipoprotein (HDL) cholesterol ratios (LDL:HDL) than men in the other two feeding groups. The feeding groups did not differ for other cardiovascular risk factors. These findings suggest that nutrition during infancy may have a permanent effect on lipid metabolism and the risk of coronary heart disease.

Placental weight

Placental weight is also correlated with adult disease, independently of birthweight. Babies with a placenta that is disproportionately large in relation to their birthweight are at increased risk of death from cardiovascular disease (Barker et al., 1993*b*), have increased rates of raised blood pressure (Barker et al., 1990; Law et al., 1991) impaired glucose tolerance (Phipps et al., 1993), and have raised plasma fibrinogen concentrations (Barker et al., 1992). Table 10.6 illustrates the strength of the association between placental weight and systolic blood pressure.

Conclusions

Babies who are small at birth and during infancy, or disproportionate, are now known to be at increased risk of developing coronary heart disease, hypertension and diabetes during adult life. The search for the causes of coronary heart disease has hitherto been guided by a 'destructive' model, in which the causes act in adult life and accelerate destructive processes – the formation of atheroma, rise in blood pressure, loss of glucose tolerance. A new 'developmental' model is now being explored. In adapting to undernutrition the baby restricts its growth in order to survive, but this occurs at the expense of its longevity. Premature death from coronary heart disease may be viewed as the price of successful adaptation in utero. A greater understanding of these adaptations is required: what they are, what induces them, how they leave a lasting mark upon the body, and how this gives rise to the diseases of later life.

Table 10.5. *Mean serum lipid concentrations in men aged 59 to 70 years according to infant feeding*

	Breast and bottle fed (1)	Breast fed, weaned before one year (2)	Breast fed, not weaned at one year (3)	Bottle fed only (4)	All	SD
Cholesterol mmol/l	6.6	6.6	6.9[a]	7.0[a]	6.7	1.2
Non-fasting cholesterol mmol/l	6.4	6.4	6.9[b]	7.1[b]	6.5	1.2
LDL cholesterol mmol/l	4.6	4.6	5.0[b]	5.1[a]	4.7	1.1
HDL cholesterol mmol/l	1.2	1.2	1.2	1.2	1.2	0.3
LDL/HDL ratio	3.8	3.8	4.2[b]	4.2	3.9	1.5
Triglyceride mmol/l	1.4	1.4	1.5	1.4	1.4	1.6
Apolipoprotein A1 g/l	1.31	1.30	1.29	1.35	1.30	1.2
Apolipoprotein B g/l	1.08	1.08	1.14	1.14	1.09	1.3
Number of men	116	253	91	25	485	

Comparison with groups (1) and (2) combined: [a] $p < 0.05$. [b] $p < 0.01$.

Table 10.6. *Mean systolic blood pressure (mmHg) of men and women aged 50, born after 38 completed weeks of gestation, according to placental weight and birthweight*

Birthweight (pounds)[a]	Placental weight (pounds)				
	≤1.0	−1.25	−1.5	>1.5	All
−6.6	149 (24)	152 (46)	151 (18)	167 (6)	152 (94)
−7.5	139 (16)	148 (63)	146 (35)	159 (23)	148 (137)
>7.5	131 (3)	143 (23)	148 (30)	153 (40)	149 (96)
All	144 (43)	148 (132)	148 (83)	156 (69)	149[b] (327)

[a] 1 pound = 454 g.
[b] Standard deviation = 20.4.
Figures in brackets are numbers of subjects.

References

Alberman, E.D., Emanuel, I., Filakti, H.& Evans, S.J.W. (1992). The contrasting effects of parental birthweight and gestational age on the birthweight of offspring. *Pediatric and Perinatal Epidemiology*, **6**, 134–44.

Barker, D.J.P. (1994). *Mothers, Babies, and Disease in Later Life*. BMJ Publishing Group, London.

Barker, D.J.P., Bull, A.R., Osmond, C. & Simmonds, S.J. (1990). Fetal and placental size and risk of hypertension in adult life. *British Medical Journal*, **301**, 259–62.

Barker, D.J.P., Gluckman, P.D., Godfrey, K.M., Harding, J.E., Owens, J.A. & Robinson, J.S. (1993*a*). Fetal nutrition and cardiovascular disease in adult life. *Lancet*, **341**, 938–41.

Barker, D.J.P., Hales, C.N., Fall, C.H.D., Osmond, C., Phipps, K. & Clark, P.M.S. (1993*c*). Type 2 (non-insulin dependent) diabetes mellitus, hypertension and hyperlipidaemia (Syndrome X): relation to reduced fetal growth. *Diabetologia*, **36**, 62–7.

Barker, D.J.P., Martyn, C.N., Osmond, C., Hales, C.N., Jespersen, S. & Fall, C.H.D. (1993*d*) Growth in utero and serum cholesterol concentrations in adult life. *British Medical Journal*, **307**, 1524–7.

Barker, D.J.P., Meade, T.W., Fall, C.H.D., Lee, A., Osmond, C., Phipps, K. et al. (1992). Relation of fetal and infant growth to plasma fibrinogen and factor VII concentrations in adult life. *British Medical Journal*, **304**, 148–52.

Barker, D.J.P., Osmond, C., Simmonds, S.J. & Wield, G.A. (1993*b*) The relation of small head circumference and thinness at birth to death from cardiovascular disease in adult life. *British Medical Journal*, **306**, 422–6.

Barker, D.J.P., Winter, P.D., Osmond, C., Margetts, B. & Simmonds, S.J. (1989). Weight in infancy and death from ischaemic heart disease. *Lancet*, **ii**, 577–80.

Barraclough, C.A. & Gorski, R.A. (1961). Evidence that the hypothalamus is responsible for androgen-induced sterility in the female rat. *Endocrinology*, **68**, 68–79.

Beischer, N.A., Sivasamboo, R., Vohra, S., Silpisornkosal, S. & Reid, S. (1970). Placental hypertrophy in severe pregnancy anaemia. *Journal of Obstetrics and Gynaecology of the British Commonwealth* **77**, 398–409.

Blackwell, B-N., Blackwell, R.Q., Yu, T.T.S., Weng, Y-S. & Chow, B.F. (1969). Further studies on growth and feed utilisation in progeny of underfed mother rats. *Journal of Nutrition*, **97**, 79–84.

Burke, B.S., Harding, V.V. & Stuart, H.C. (1948). Nutrition studies during pregnancy. IV. Relation of protein content of mother's diet during pregnancy to birth length, birth weight, and condition of infant at birth. *Journal of Pediatrics*, **32**, 506–15.

Carr-Hill, R., Campbell, D.M., Hall, D.M. & Meredith, A. (1987). Is birth weight determined genetically? *British Medical Journal*, **295**, 687–9.

Chow, B.F. & Lee, C-J. (1964). Effect of dietary restriction of pregnant rats on body weight gain of the offspring. *Journal of Nutrition*, **82**, 10–18.

Clapp, J.F.III & Rizk, K.H. (1992). Effect of recreational exercise on midtrimester placental growth. *American Journal of Obstetrics and Gynecology*, **167**, 1518–21.

Csaba, G. & Török, O. (1991). Influence of insulin and biogenic amines on the division of Chang liver cells after primary exposure (inprinting) and repeated treatments. *Cytobios*, **66**, 153–6.

DeBarro, T.M., Owens, J., Earl, C.R. & Robinson, J.S. (1992). Nutrition during early/mid pregnancy interacts with mating weight to affect placental weight in sheep. *Australian Society for Reproductive Biology, Adelaide* (Abstract).

Doyle, W., Crawford, M.A., Wynn, A.H.A. & Wynn, S.W. (1990). The association between maternal diet and birth dimensions. *Journal of Nutritional Medicine*, **1**, 9–17.

Dubos, R., Savage, D. & Schaedler, R. (1966). Biological Freudianism – Lasting effects of early environmental influences. *Paediatrics*, **38**, 789–800.

Emanuel, I., Filkarti, H., Alberman, E. & Evans, S.J.W. (1992). Intergenerational studies of human birthweight from the 1958 birth cohort. I. Evidence for a multigenerational effect. *British Journal of Obstetrics and Gynaecology*, **99**, 67–74.

Fall, C.H.D., Barker, D.J.P., Osmond, C., Winter, P.D., Clark, P.M.S. & Hales, C.N. (1992). Relation of infant feeding to adult serum cholesterol concentration and death from ischaemic heart disease. *British Medical Journal*, **304**, 801–5.

Fowden, A.L. (1989). The role of insulin in prenatal growth. *Journal of Developmental Physiology*, **12**, 173–82.

Gluckman, P. & Harding, J. (1992). The regulation of fetal growth. In *Human Growth: Basic and Clinical Aspects*. eds. M. Hernandez & J. Argente. pp. 253–59. Elsevier, Amsterdam.

Godfrey, K.M., Redman, C.W.G., Barker, D.J.P. & Osmond, C. (1991). The effect of maternal anaemia and iron deficiency on the ratio of fetal weight to placental weight. *British Journal of Obstetrics and Gynaecology*, **98**, 886–91.

Hahn, P. (1989). Late effects of early nutrition. In *Atherosclerosis: A Pediatric Perspective*, ed. M.T.R. Subbiah. pp. 155–164. CRC Press, Florida.

Hales, C.N., Barker, D.J.P., Clark, P.M.S., Cox, L.J., Fall, C., Osmond, C. & Winter, P.D. (1991). Fetal and infant growth and impaired glucose tolerance at age 64 years. *British Medical Journal*, **303**, 1019–22.

Hammond, J. & Appleton, A.B. (1932). *Growth and the Development of Mutton Qualities in the Sheep*. Oliver and Boyd, Edinburgh.

Harding, J.E., Liu, L., Evans, P.C., Oliver, M. & Gluckman, P.D. (1992). Intrauterine feeding of the growth retarded fetus: can we help? *Early Human Development*, **29**, 193–7.

Hellerström, C., Swenne, I. & Andersson, A. (1988). Islet cell replication and diabetes. In *The Pathology of the Endocrine Pancreas in Diabetes*, 37th edn, ed. P.J. Lefebvre & D.G. Pipeleers. pp. 141–170. Springer-Verlag, Heidelberg.

Hinchliffe, S.A., Lynch, M.R.J., Sargent, P.H., Howard, C.V. & Van Velzen, D. (1992). The effect of intrauterine growth retardation on the development of renal nephrons. *British Journal of Obstetrics and Gynaecology*, **99**, 296–301.

Howe, D. & Wheeler, T. (1994). Maternal iron stores and placental growth. *Journal of Physiology* (In press)

Klebanoff, M.A., Graubard, B., Kessel, S.S. & Berendes, H.W. (1984). Low birth weight across generations. *Journal of the American Medical Association*, **252**, 2423–7.

Law, C.M., Barker, D.J.P., Bull, A.R. & Osmond, C. (1991). Maternal and fetal influences on blood pressure. *Archives of Disease in Childhood*, **66**, 1291–5.

Law, C.M., de Swiet, M., Osmond, C., Fayers, P.M., Barker, D.J.P., Cruddas, A.M. & Fall, C.H.D. (1993). Initiation of hypertension in utero and its amplification throughout life. *British Medical Journal*, **306**, 24–7.

Lechtig, A. & Klein, R.E. (1981). Pre-natal nutrition and birth weight: is there a causal association? In *Maternal Nutrition in Pregnancy – Eating for two?*, ed. J. Dobbing. pp. 131–83. Academic Press, London.

Love, E.J. & Kinch, R.A.H. (1965). Factors influencing the birth weight in normal pregnancy. *American Journal of Obstetrics and Gynecology*, **91**, 342–9.

Lucas, A. (1991). Programming by early nutrition in man. In *The Childhood Environment and Adult Disease*, ed. G.R. Bock & J. Whelan. pp. 38–55. John Wiley & Sons, Chichester.

Lumey, L.H. (1992). Decreased birth weights in infants after maternal in utero exposure to the Dutch famine of 1944–45. *Pediatric and Perinatal Epidemiology*, **6**, 240–53.

McCance, D.R., Pettit, D.J., Hanson, R.L., Jacobsson, L.T.M., Knowles, W.C. & Bennet, P.H. (1994). Birthweight and non-insulin dependent diabetes. 'Thrifty genotype', 'thrifty phenotype' or 'surviving small baby genotype'. *British Medical Journal*, **308**, 942–5.

McCance, R.A. & Widdowson, E.M. (1962). Nutrition and growth. *Proceedings of the Royal Society of London (Biological)*, **156**, 326–7.

McCance, R.A. & Widdowson, E.M. (1974). The determinants of growth and form. *Proceedings of the Royal Society of London (Biological)*, **185**, 1–17.

McLeod, K.I., Goldrick, R.B. & Whyte, H.M. (1972). The effect of maternal malnutrition on the progeny in the rat. *Australian Journal of Experimental Biology and Medical Science*, **50**, 435–46.

Martyn, C.N., Meade, T.W., Stirling, Y. & Barker, D.J.P. (1994). Plasma concentrations of fibrinogen and factor VII in adult life and their relation in intra–uterine growth. *British Journal of Haematology*, in press.

Mayhew, T.M., Jackson, M.R. & Haas, J.D. (1990). Oxygen diffusion conductances of human placentae from term pregnancies at low and high altitudes. *Placenta*, **11**, 493–503.

Milner, R.D.G. (1989). Mechanisms of overgrowth. In *Fetal Growth. Proceedings of the 20th Study Group of the Royal College of Obstetricians and Gynaecologists*, ed. F. Sharp, R.B. Fraser & R.D.G. Milner. pp. 139–148. Royal College of Obstetricians and Gynaecologists, London.

Moment, G.B. (1933). The effects of rate of growth on the post-natal development of the white rat. *Journal of Experimental Zoology*, **65**, 359–93.

Mott, G.E., Lewis, D.S. & McGill, H.C. (1991). Programming of cholesterol metabolism by breast or formula feeding. In *The Childhood Environment and Adult Disease*, ed. G.R. Bock & J. Whelan. pp. 56–76. Wiley, Chichester.

Nagy, S.U. & Csaba, G. (1980). Dose dependence of the thytrophin (TSH) receptor damaging effect of gonadotrophin in the newborn rats. *Acta Physiologica Academiae Scientiarum Hungaricae*, **56**, 417–20.

Osmond, C., Barker, D.J.P., Winter, P.D., Fall, C.H.D. & Simmonds, S.J. (1993). Early growth and death from cardiovascular disease in women. *British Medical Journal*, **306**, 472–6.

Osofsky, H.J. (1975). Relationships between nutrition during pregnancy and subsequent infant and child development. *Obstetrical and Gynaecological Survey*, **30**, 227–41.

Ounsted, M., Scott, A. & Ounsted, C. (1986). Transmission through the female line of a mechanism constraining human fetal growth. *Annals of Human Biology*, **13**, 143–51.

Phillips, D.I.W., Barker, D.J.P., Hales, C.N., Hirst, S. & Osmond, C. (1994). Thinness at birth and insulin resistance in adult life. *Diabetologia*, **37**, 150–4.

Phipps, K., Barker, D.J.P., Hales, C.N., Fall, C.H.D., Osmond, C. & Clark, P.M.S. (1993). Fetal growth and impaired glucose tolerance in men and women. *Diabetologia*, **36**, 225–8.

Roeder, L.M. (1973). Effect of the level of nutrition on rates of cell proliferation and of RNA and protein synthesis in the rat. *Nutrition Reports International*, **7**, 271–87.

Roeder, L.M. & Chow, B.F. (1971). Influence of the dietary history of test animals on responses in pharmacological and nutritional studies. *American Journal of Clinical Nutrition*, **24**, 947–51.

Rosso, P. (1989). *Nutrition and Metabolism in Pregnancy – Mother and Fetus.* Oxford University Press, Oxford.

Roux, J.M., Tordet-Caridroit, C. & Chanez, C. (1970). Studies on experimental hypotrophy in the rat. I. Chemical composition of the total body and some organs in the rat foetus. *Biology of the Neonate*, **15**, 342–7.

Smart, J.L. (1991). Critical periods in brain development. In *The Childhood Environment and Adult Disease*, ed. G.R. Bock & J. Whelan. pp. 109–28. Wiley, Chichester.

Snoeck, A., Remacle, C., Reusens, B. & Hoet, J.J. (1990). Effect of a low protein diet during pregnancy on the fetal rat endocrine pancreas. *Biology of the Neonate*, **57**, 107–18.

Stephens, D.N. (1980). Growth and the development of dietary obesity in adulthood of rats which have been undernourished during development. *British Journal of Nutrition*, **44**, 215–27.

Swenne, I., Crace, C.J. & Milner, R.D.G. (1987). Persistant impairment of insulin secretory response to glucose in adult rats after limited periods of protein-calorie malnutrition early in life. *Diabetes*, **36**, 454–8.

Valdez, R., Athens, M.A., Thompson, G.H., Bradshaw, B.S. & Stern, M.P. (1994). Birth weight and adult health in a biethnic US population. *Diabetologia*, **37**, 624–31.

Van Assche, F.A. & Aerts, L. (1979). The fetal endocrine pancreas. *Contributions to Gynaecology and Obstetrics*, **5**, 44–57.

Walton, A. & Hammond, J. (1938). The maternal effects on growth and conformation in Shire horse–Shetland pony crosses. *Journal of the Proceedings of the Royal Society of London, Series B*, **125**, 311–35.

Whincup, P.H., Cook, D. & Papacosta, O. (1991). Do maternal and intrauterine factors influence blood pressure in childhood? *Archives of Disease in Childhood*, **67**, 1423–9.

Widdowson, E.M. (1971). Intra-uterine growth retardation in the pig. *Biology of the Neonate*, **19**, 329–40.

Widdowson, E.M. (1974). Immediate and long-term consequences of being large or small at birth: a comparative approach. In *Size at Birth (Ciba Symposium 27)*, ed. K. Elliott & J. Knight. pp. 65–82. Elsevier, Amsterdam.

Widdowson, E.M., Crabb, D.E. & Milner, R.D.G. (1972). Cellular development of some human organs before birth. *Archives of Disease in Childhood*, **47**, 652–5.

Widdowson, E.M. & McCance, R.A. (1963). The effect of finite periods of undernutrition at different ages on the composition and subsequent development of the rat. *Proceedings of the Royal Society of London (Series B)*, **158**, 329–42.

Widdowson, E.M. & McCance, R.A. (1975). A review: new thoughts on growth. *Pediatric Research*, **9**, 154–6.

Wigglesworth, J.S. (1964). Experimental growth retardation in the foetal rat. *Journal of Pathology and Bacteriology*, **88**, 1–13.

Winick, M. & Noble, A. (1966). Cellular response in rats during malnutrition at various ages. *Journal of Nutrition*, **89**, 300–6.

Winick, M. & Noble, A. (1967). Cellular response with increased feeding in neonatal rats. *Journal of Nutrition*, **91**, 179–82.

Zeman, F.J. & Stanbrough, E.C. (1969). Effect of maternal protein deficiency on cellular development in the fetal rat. *Journal of Nutrition*, **99**, 274–82.

Part Three

Clinical applications

11

Clinical assessment of placental function

JAMES F. PEARSON

Introduction

Growth – conceptual concerns

In any discussion regarding the assessment of fetal size and fetal growth, it is absolutely essential to differentiate between 'small for gestational age' (SGA) and 'intrauterine growth retardation' (IUGR). This distinction between size and growth is critical. A single estimate of fetal size in the third trimester is of little clinical usefulness as a measure of the adequacy of growth. For instance, if such an estimate of weight indicates that the fetus is below, say, the tenth centile for gestational age, the suggestion that this may indicate IUGR is quite unjustified because 10% of all babies born will lie below the tenth centile of a normal Gaussian distribution. Furthermore, other babies with weights well above the tenth centile may be suffering IUGR as a result of failing to achieve their full growth potential. It therefore follows that IUGR cannot be diagnosed from birthweight and gestational age alone (Thomson & Billewicz, 1976). This term should be restricted to those fetuses in whom there is clear evidence that the rate of intrauterine growth has faltered. It follows that many growth-retarded fetuses would have a weight above the tenth centile of the population range. A considerable but unknown proportion of these infants will have no adverse sequelae.

Growth cannot be estimated from less than two measurements of size. The clinician ideally would wish to know whether the fetal growth rate has deviated from its normal progression, therefore serial measurements are desirable. It is well within the capability of present-day imaging technology to distinguish the small infant growing at a normal rate from a larger infant whose rate of growth is severely diminished. Because the magnitude of the growth deficit is unknown for any given infant, it is likely that only the most disadvantaged infants will be identified, but this is probably enough for practical purposes. For instance, Kramer et al. (1990) showed increased mortality rates associated with IUGR only among babies whose birthweight was less than the 1.7th centile.

From a clinical point of view, the presence of specific maternal complications such as pre-eclampsia, rather than low birthweight alone, might be of fundamental importance in the genesis of neuro-developmental disabilities (Taylor & Howie, 1989), and no randomized trial has ever demonstrated clinical benefit simply from identifying small fetuses by screening in pregnancy (Altman & Hytten, 1989).

Furthermore, even after identification of IUGR there is a continuing need for tests of fetal well-being to avoid unnecessary intervention on the grounds of IUGR alone, as the outlook is favourable in the vast majority of cases.

Clinical methods

Symphysis–fundal height

Abdominal palpation as a means of estimating fetal weight remains a traditional part of the antenatal examination, despite the fact that it has been shown that 20–25% of clinical predictions after 36 weeks gestation were more than 450 g in error (Loeffler, 1967; Beazley & Kurjak, 1973). It is only in the last 20 years that symphysis–fundus height (SFH) charts have become a regular feature of antenatal care. This might seem surprising when one considers that, as long ago as 1886, Galabin's *Manual of Midwifery* published tables of SFH measurements made both by calipers and by tape measure.

Technique of measurement

Most workers have stressed the need for standardized technique to aid consistency in measurement. The technique of Calvert et al. (1982) is as follows:

The measurement is taken along the longitudinal axis of the uterus with the mother supine, legs straight and bladder empty. The position of the uterine fundus is determined on the skin and that point is gently marked with ballpoint. One end of the tape measure is pressed against the upper border of the symphysis pubis, and the distance to the mark measured to the nearest half centimetre keeping the tape smoothly in contact with the natural curve of the abdomen.

Using this technique the observer and interobserver coefficients of variation were 4.5% and 6.4% respectively, which confirms that SFH measurements are not precise and that, in clinical practice, neither endpoint is always easy to identify.

On the other hand, when these measurements were made, such as to avoid the effects of memory, anticipated result, or terminal digit preference, experience did not aid consistency. The implication is that the technique may be used by medical and paramedical staff without loss of accuracy – a considerable benefit where ultrasound is not readily available.

Results of the application of SFH

Several studies have shown quite good sensitivity and specificity for predicting low birthweight for gestation, but others have not. The prediction of SGA in 12 studies using SFH have shown differences of sensitivity (17–86%), specificity (64–95%) and positive predictive value (2–79%) (Jacobsen, 1992).

The only prospective randomized trial which has been reported showed a 28% prediction of SGA in the SFH group and 48% in the group using abdominal palpation only (Lindhard et al., 1990), not a good performance by any standards!

In clinical practice, results have been mixed. Backe and Nakling (1993) detected only 14% of infants below the tenth centile at birth. On the other hand, Pearce and Campbell (1987) found the diagnosis of low birthweight based on fundal height was nearly as good as that based on ultrasound measurement of abdominal circumference, but serial fundal height data were not presented and, thus far, the relationship between falling or static values of SFH and fetal growth failure has not been satisfactorily evaluated. Even if the results from this study (i.e. sensitivity and specificity of 76% and 79%, respectively) were universally achieved, it has been calculated that about 100 cases of SGA would be missed every year and 720 fetuses would be falsely labelled as SGA in a unit of 4000 deliveries per year.

Other applications of SFH

Using SFH as a surrogate measure of fetal weight, very little work has been done at the other end of the weight spectrum but Hughes et al.

(1987) showed a direct relationship between increased symphysis–fundus height and dystocia, second stage delay, Caesarean section rate and the incidence of fetal distress. The value of these observations is likely to be best exploited in developing countries, especially those where poor childhood nutrition, resulting in poor maternal pelvic growth, coincides with good fetal growth due to recent socioeconomic improvement. In these circumstances, SFH charts would be of use to identify those women at high risk of obstructed labour in time for appropriate arrangements to be made. Indeed, since the introduction of SFH charts in Botswana the perinatal mortality rate has halved in an area where it had been static for the previous 20 years. This is to say nothing of the avoidance of maternal genital fistulae, an all-too-common result of obstructed labour in third-world countries (Kennedy & Stephens, 1984).

SFH is a surrogate measurement of fetal weight. It is also influenced by obesity and the amount of amniotic fluid. The best results are obtainable using a standardized technique; even so the method is far from precise, but represents a great improvement on random abdominal palpation. The detection of SGA infants varies considerably from series to series owing to many possible confounding factors. SFH measurements have not been assessed at present as a means of screening for failure of fetal growth as opposed to the detection of small babies.

Ultrasound and fetal growth

Over the last 20 years, considerable efforts have been made to establish nomograms for almost every possible measurement of the fetus. Unfortunately many of the standards produced have been derived from cross-sectional data and, surprisingly, there has been very little work aimed at producing true growth charts based upon longitudinal measurements.

One of the earliest studies (Campbell & Dewhurst, 1971) identified 73% of SGA babies by repeated measurement of the biparietal diameter. Neilson, Whitfield and Aitchison (1980) later showed that a two-stage measurement of abdominal circumference between 34 and 36 weeks of pregnancy had a sensitivity of 81% and specificity of 89% in predicting SGA babies – the superiority of this measurement reflected the fact that the abdominal viscera, notably the liver, are most affected by IUGR and that there is also a 'brain sparing effect' which tends to maintain fetal head growth.

Ultrasound estimation of fetal weight is popular at present, but it is important to realize that such estimations are composite expressions of ultrasound data which, of themselves, have an inherently large variability. The general view is that ultrasound estimates of fetal weight are within 10% of the 'birthweight' in 70% of cases and even further adrift in 30% of cases. This would mean that a baby estimated as weighing 4000 g could actually weigh anything between 3600 g and 4400 g, the error being even greater in 30% of cases. This degree of accuracy is not much different from that originally reported for abdominal palpation. More importantly, failure to appreciate the magnitude of the potential error of such estimations can lead the clinician into errors of judgement. For instance, an overestimate of fetal weight may result in a woman with a previous Caesarean section performed for 'failure to progress' having a second, possibly unnecessary, elective Caesarean section if the estimated fetal weight was significantly greater than that of her first baby.

Symmetrical and asymmetrical growth retardation

For some years now, it has been considered that placental failure in late pregnancy leads to 'asymmetrical' growth retardation where the growth of the head is spared relative to that of the abdominal viscera. 'Symmetrical' growth retardation, on the other hand, is generally said to occur where the insult to the fetus is of early onset. Typical examples of the latter include fetal chromosomal abnormalities and those infants who have been infected in early pregnancy and in whom the global complement of cells is reduced, thus leading to diminished fetal size.

These observations led to the calculation of head:abdomen ratios, which it was hoped would discriminate between 'symmetrical' and 'asymmetrical' growth retardation (Campbell & Thoms, 1977).

This rather attractive concept has recently been recognized as being largely artefactual. A review of fetal growth in fetuses with abnormal chromosome complement (aneuploidy) indicated that 'symmetrical' growth retardation probably does not exist as an aetiologically distinct entity and that the occurrence of early onset uteroplacental insufficiency in a fetus with normal chromosome complement (euploidy) may subsequently result in a 'symmetrically' growth-retarded fetus (Droste, 1992).

The identification of fetal growth potential

Ideally, the clinician would wish to know the growth potential for each individual fetus in early pregnancy, so as to provide a firm basis for the sensible interpretation of ultrasound data and to help differentiate between those SGA babies who are IUGR and those who are not and, just as importantly, to discover growth failure in larger infants. Utilizing data with respect to gestational age, fetal sex, maternal weight, height, ethnic group, parity and birthweight, (and gestational age and sex of previous babies for parous women), a computer program has been devised by Gardosi et al. (1992) which can generate and print out customized antenatal growth charts for any given mother. As yet, the degree of growth failure which needs to be detected using such methods in order to lead to beneficial obstetrical intervention has not been determined. Almost certainly the identification of such an infant would indicate the performance of further biophysical testing.

Biophysical tests of fetal well-being

There are four attributes of the fetoplacental unit which are relatively easily amenable to evaluation and which to a greater or lesser extent reflect the degree of hypoxic compromise suffered by the fetus. These include:

1. fetal behaviour (fetal body movements, fetal breathing movements and fetal tone);
2. fetal heart rate monitoring (CTG);
3. amniotic fluid volume;
4. umbilical arterial blood velocity.

Maternal fetal movement counting, CTG tests and Doppler velocimetry are often used as discrete tests and thus will be discussed separately. Fetal breathing, tone and amniotic fluid volume are more commonly evaluated as part of the biophysical profile and will be discussed under that heading.

Fetal movement counting

The basis for using fetal movement count as a test of fetal well-being is the observation that reduction or cessation of fetal movements may precede fetal death by a day or more (Sadovsky & Yaffe, 1973). Normal fetal activity, on the other hand, has been associated with good clinical outcome and provides reassurance that delivery can be deferred to gain further fetal maturity (Pearson & Weaver, 1976). However, not all antepartum fetal deaths are potentially preventable by fetal movement counting, as some are not preceded by a reduction in fetal movement; in other cases, there may be insufficient time between the reduction of fetal movements and fetal death to allow for effective intervention – for instance, about 15% of late antepartum fetal deaths are due to placental abruption.

Fetal movements are first felt by the mother at about the 18th week of pregnancy and they increase to a maximum between 29 and 38 weeks, after which time they tend to decrease, possibly because of the relative diminution in the volume of liquor amnii at and beyond term.

Normal fetal activity is episodic. Phases of active body movement lasting on average 40 minutes are interspersed with quiet phases, characterized by absent body movements lasting on average 23 minutes which may represent sleep states. Patrick et al. (1982) found that only 1% of quiet phases lasted longer than 45 minutes and it has been suggested that quiet phases lasting longer than 60 minutes are abnormal (Timor-Tritsch et al., 1978). Further non-random variation may be introduced by a host of extrinsic factors such as maternal smoking and medication, meals, maternal posture, maternal physical activity, gestational age, time of day, sound and light stimulation and uterine palpation.

There is considerable variation in activity between individual fetuses. Some fetuses are consistently vigorous and others sluggish. As a group, fetuses with malformations are more likely to have reduced movements than normally formed infants. Rayburn and Barr (1982) found that 28% of 58 cases with major fetal malformations had reduced movements.

Methods of counting

Many methods of maternal fetal movement counting have been described, many clinicians simply informally requesting the mother to note fetal movement reduction.

As far as formal counting is concerned there are two approaches. One is for the mother to count for a fixed length of time each day – 'fixed time counting'. Examples of these techniques vary from 12 hours of counting to short periods of time of 1 hour or less, sometimes repeated 2, 3 or 4 times each day according to the system used. The other is the concept of 'fixed number counting'. The Cardiff 'count-to-ten' system (Pearson, 1977) is the best known example of this method. It is theoretically attractive because mothers with active fetuses count for a short length of time whereas mothers with quiet fetuses will count longer. This protocol has been demonstrated to be efficacious in the study by Liston et al (1982), and early studies indicated that the introduction of systematic daily fetal movement counting (DFMC) into primary care pregnancies is well accepted and reassuring to most patients (Eggertsen & Benedetti, 1987), but this study astutely predicted that the universal use of DFMC would increase the use of antepartum fetal heart rate testing because of the high false positive rate.

Neldam (1983) studied 2250 pregnant women in a hospital-based obstetric service, half of whom formally counted fetal movements, and found that of infants weighing more than 1500 g, there were 8 intrauterine deaths in the control group and no deaths in the 'counting' group. Based on the local stillbirth rate, 6 deaths would have been expected in each group. This latter study has, however, been criticized, mainly on the grounds of its size. For example, to cause a 50% reduction in a stillbirth rate of 3 per 1000 at a P value of 0.05, a study population of at least 3700 is required (using the z-test approximation to the binomial for difference between proportions). By far the largest trial yet performed is that of Grant et al. (1989) who enrolled 68 000 women in a trial of self-reported fetal movement counting. This showed no reduction in antepartum fetal deaths among counting women. However, in none of the 17 cases reporting low fetal movements where the fetuses were ill but alive when admitted was emergency delivery attempted, which indicates that it was not so much that fetal movement diminution was a poor predictor of bad outcome but that the other tests (mainly CTGs) used in conjunction with it did not confirm imminent fetal demise and were either poor tests or the test was improperly used or misinterpreted.

This result illustrates a major difficulty with large randomized trials of tests of fetal well-being. It is important to appreciate that such tests are not performed in isolation, and the test under investigation is usually interpreted by means of other tests, the reliability of which may not have been properly evaluated. Furthermore the degree of interdependence of the different tests is unlikely to be known.

Fetal heart rate monitoring in pregnancy

The original work on the interpretation of fetal heart rate (FHR) was performed during the course of labour. Changes and characteristic patterns in response to asphyxia and fetal acidosis were recognized, which led to the monitoring of the FHR during pregnancy as a means of assessing fetal well-being. Because the good quality recordings available using a scalp electrode could not be employed during pregnancy, Doppler ultrasound equipment is used to process the FHR transabdominally.

Attempts have been made to record the fetal ECG transabdominally but reliable equipment is still not available because of technical problems.

Fetal heart rate testing has developed somewhat differently on each side of the Atlantic. The oxytocin challenge test (OCT) became very popular in North America. This test depended on the interpretation of the fetal heart rate in the presence of oxytocin-induced uterine contractions, the rules for interpretation being the same as those for intrapartum monitoring. The OCT was time-consuming to perform, not readily reproducible and resulted in a high number of false positive tests, as well as being intrinsically unsafe, depending as it did on the deliberate induction of uterine contractions, which might provoke hypoxia in a fetus that may already be seriously compromised. Because of this, the OCT is now less frequently used. The OCT has now been largely replaced by the non-stress test (NST) (Evertson & Paul, 1978).

Interpretation of the NST is relatively simple as it depends solely on the presence or absence of fetal heart rate accelerations occurring in response to fetal movements. The usual duration of the NST is 20 minutes and to be classified as 'reactive', or normal, a minimum of two accelerations of at least 15 bpm above baseline lasting at least 15 seconds need to be seen. If accelerations are not seen, the test is said to be 'unreactive' and indicates further investigation (sometimes an OCT). Confounding factors leading to false positive NSTs would include a fetus in quiet sleep and maternal sedation. In order to surmount these difficulties, an 'unreactive' stress test is often repeated following manual stimulation of the fetus in order to alter its sleep state.

Antepartum cardiotocography (CTG) as practised in Europe not only recognizes the FHR pattern and its response to fetal movements but also the FHR response to uterine contractions. The usual duration of recording is for 30 minutes and it is important that uterine contractions are recorded as the earlier signs of fetal compromise reside in the fetal heart response to contractions, and unless contractions are recorded this early sign may well be missed.

The minutiae of CTG interpretation is beyond the scope of this chapter, but several scoring systems have been designed to simplify interpretation of CTGs. Those in common use are shown in Tables 11.1 and 11.2.

One of the major problems of scoring systems is that each variable tested attracts a whole number score, whereas some features of the trace are more important than others. The use of scoring systems have, however, helped to determine the sequence of the CTG response to

Table 11.1. *10-point scoring system for antenatal CTGs adapted from Meyer Menk (Huch et al., 1977). The higher the score, the lower the risk of fetal hypoxia*

Fetal heart rate variable	0	1	2
Basal fetal heart rate (beats/minute)	<100 >180	100–120 160–180	120–160
Amplitude of variability (beats/minute)	<5	5–10 >25	10–25
Frequency of variability (cycles/minute)	<2	2–4	4
Accelerations	–	Not present with contractions	Present with contractions
Decelerations	Late or severe variable	Light or moderate variable	Early or none

Table 11.2. *The 'six-point' scoring system for antenatal cardiographs (Pearson & Weaver, 1978); maximum score 6. The higher the score, the lower the risk of fetal hypoxia*

	0	1	2
Baseline FHR (beats/minute)	less than 100 or more than 180	100–200 or 160–180	
Movements and FHR change	none –	Present No change	Present Acceleration
Contractions ± FHR change	Deceleration	No change	Acceleration

hypoxia. For example, by using an analysis of the frequency by which the various components of the Cardiff 'six-point' scoring system (Pearson & Weaver, 1978) combined to achieve any given score, it was shown that the likely order of fetal deterioration was as follows:

1. Fetal heart rate decelerations in response to contractions appeared first.
2. The fetal heart rate then failed to accelerate with fetal movements.
3. Fetal movements ceased.
4. This was followed by terminal alterations in baseline fetal heart rate, initially in the direction of a fetal tachycardia.

Table 11.3. *Interpretation of antepartum FHR records*

Description of trace	Interpretation
Normal variability Accelerations present, no decelerations	Normal
Reduced variability without decelerations Normal variability with decelerations	Suspicious
Reduced variability or sinusoidal pattern No accelerations No fetal movements	Abnormal

Adapted from Kubli et al., 1977.

More recently, Ribbert, Nicolaides and Visser (1993) have confirmed that fetal heart rate abnormalities precede cessation of fetal movements.

A simple CTG classification was proposed by Kubli et al. (1977) which incorporated the above features. This is set out in Table 11.3 and represents a sound common-sense approach to the interpretation of CTGs.

Recognizing the considerable difficulty with subjective interpretation of CTGs the System 8000 (Oxford Sonicaid Limited, Chichester, UK) was produced. The signals are processed by an online computer system that averages the pulse intervals over consecutive 3.75 s epochs, constructs a baseline and identifies and quantifies accelerations and decelerations. Heart rate variation is calculated as the minute-by-minute range in the pulse intervals. A low mean range of less than 20 ms over one hour is associated with a high likelihood of fetal hypoxaemia (Smith et al., 1988). The major advantage of this system is that the analysis is uniform and has a consistency not attainable by visual methods.

Clinical use of CTGs

It is important to recognize that the fetal heart rate pattern can only be considered to reflect the state of fetal well-being at the time it is performed. The CTG may alter dramatically within a relatively short space of time. There can be few clinicians who have not experienced such a rapid deterioration of fetal cardiovascular control or even fetal death relatively shortly after a satisfactory CTG. Such 'one-off' experiences have tended to result in the performance of CTGs at ever more frequent intervals. This is even more understandable when considering that failure to diagnose fetal distress currently accounts for 40% of clinical negligence claims in obstetrics dealt with by one London firm of solicitors, with average claims for damages per case of over £400 000 (Agnew & Wilder 1994).

On the other hand, it is known that the method is not an appropriate test for screening for fetal compromise in otherwise normal pregnancies, and routine testing in high risk pregnancy has not been shown to be of value (Kidd, Patel & Smith, 1983).

It would therefore appear to be sensible to regard the CTG as one of a number of diagnostic tools which are of value in cases of acute and chronic placental dysfunction such as occur in oligohydramnios, suspected placental abruption, and fetal growth retardation. There are other relative indications for CTG testing such as 'postdates' pregnancy and during the latter weeks of pregnancy in diabetic women. In these situations CTGs are frequently used but their value in reducing fetal mortality has not been established.

It has also to be recognized that not all cases of fetal compromise are due to placental dysfunction and there is a small number of fetuses who fall victim to non-predictable haphazardly occurring events such as cord accidents.

Wheble et al. (1989) surveyed UK consultant obstetricians and found that 92% considered the CTG, alone or in combination with other tests, to be the most reliable method of detecting fetal distress in pregnancy.

Doppler ultrasound

The Doppler effect first reported in 1842 describes the phenomenon whereby soundwaves emitted from a moving source increase in frequency when moving towards a stationary observer and decrease in frequency when moving away. This phenomenon also applies to ultrasound where this phenomenon has been exploited so as to measure the velocity of blood flow. The ability to record the velocity waveforms from the umbilical vessels of the human fetus was first reported by Fitzgerald and Drumm (1977).

Normal placentation is characterized by a low vascular resistance as a result of trophoblast invasion of the uterine spiral arteries, thereby replacing the elastic lamina and smooth muscle by trophoblast, the resistance to blood flow in umbilical arteries reflecting vascular resistance in the placenta. Continuous ultrasound is usually used and the peak systolic flow is related to the end-diastolic flow (EDF). Reduction of

EDF reflects an increase in vascular resistance within the placenta due to obliteration of the small muscular arteries in the tertiary stem villi (Giles, Trudinger & Baird, 1985).

A number of indices of blood flow have been described:

1. The systolic (S)/diastolic (D) ratio.
2. The resistance index (RI) which is calculated according to the formula S-D/S.
3. The pulsatility index (PI) calculated by the formula S-D/mean.

The major drawback of Doppler ultrasound indices when examining the fetal circulation is that there are substantial intra- and interobserver errors when measuring PI in umbilical artery, descending aorta and internal carotid arteries. Because of these errors, values of indices tend to be unreliable and, for clinical purposes, it is better simply to use an endpoint such as absent EDF because observers commonly agree with respect to this finding (Scherjon et al., 1993).

As fetuses demonstrating absent EDF are at high risk of developing abnormal fetal heart rate patterns, this finding should alert the clinician and hopefully improve fetal outcome by leading to more aggressive management. Experience has shown that absent EDF occurs most frequently in cases of pre-eclampsia and in fetuses who are the victims of IUGR (Pattison, Normal & Odendaal, 1994). It follows from this that small-for-gestational-age infants who exhibit normal Doppler indices may benefit from a more conservative form of management as these infants are likely to be small but healthy and can generally expect a normal outcome.

Commenting on the findings of the National Institute of Health Consensus Conference (1986) on Doppler Ultrasound, Lowe (1991) concluded 'that no evidence had emerged during the last 5 years to support routine use of maternal or blood flow velocity determinations as a diagnostic test in the general obstetric population'.

To date, there have been four randomized control trials testing the value of Doppler velocimetry in the management of high-risk pregnancies (Trudinger et al., 1987; Tyrrell et al., 1990; Newnham et al., 1991; and Pattison et al., 1994). All interpreted their findings as showing that knowledge of the Doppler velocimetry result might improve the management but any improvement was slight and often not clinically significant. The study by Pattison et al. (1994) showed that, in a subset of women with absent EDF in the umbilical artery where the result was known to the clinicians, there was one death out of ten. In the ten patients in the control group where the ultrasound result was not known to the clinicians, five intrauterine deaths and one perinatal death occurred. All 20 cases had pregnancies which were either complicated by pre-eclampsia or had infants who were small for gestational age.

Soothill et al. (1993) studied those non-invasive tests which have been shown to identify fetuses at risk of fetal acidosis in 191 fetuses, 30 of whom were <2.5th centile (SGA). These included measurements of fetal abdominal circumference, fetal heart rate variability, biophysical profile score and umbilical artery pulsatility index. The fetal abdominal circumference was the best indicator of which fetuses were SGA. Morbidity at birth in SGA infants was best predicted by abnormal umbilical blood flow studies. In contrast, fetal heart rate variability and the biophysical profile did not predict perinatal morbitity. Among the 161 fetuses who were appropriately grown for gestational age, 27 of these infants had morbidity at birth, but this morbidity was not predictable by heart rate variability, biophysical profile or umbilical Doppler studies.

Nevertheless, pulsatility index and resistance index as measures of blood flow remain useful in clinical research and these have been used to interrogate most major vessels in the fetus. Most recently, it has been recognized that changes in cerebral blood flow may predate changes in fetal heart rate pattern in the hypoxic fetus. It has been shown that both the CTG and middle cerebral artery blood flow are equally good in predicting acidaemia at delivery and identifying the fetus at risk for interventricular haemorrhage in the first week of life. As the onset of fetal hypoxaemia is associated with preferentially increased fetal cerebral blood flow (the brain-sparing effect), the middle cerebral artery blood flow was increased in all the infants with hypoxaemia at birth, and in about half of these hypoxaemic infants this was evident for up to 4 days before any fetal heart abnormality was seen. The specificity of this test was, however, only 50% in this series (Chandran et al., 1993).

Although Doppler recording of umbilical artery blood flow is a good detector of fetal compromise, the results of its introduction into clinical practice have been disappointing (Davies, Gallivan & Spencer, 1992). A recent study of 2289 'at risk' pregnancies referred for Doppler studies showed that obstetricians did not use the test to modify their risk assessment and thus the need for fetal monitoring (Johnstone et al., 1993). It follows that, unless criteria are agreed for its role in management, Doppler ultrasound may simply consume additional resources without benefit.

The present state of the art appears to be that:

1. Absent EDF (rather than changes in RI or PI) is the best indicator of fetal hypoxia and precedes changes in the fetal heart rate pattern and biophysical profile.
2. Absent EDF is most likely to occur in those fetuses who are the victims of IUGR and/or severe maternal hypertension.
3. The presence of normal Doppler indices should help the clinician to differentiate between the 'small normal' fetus and the 'small sick' fetus.
4. As biophysical methods do not appear to be able to predict morbidity in normally grown infants, it would appear sensible in these days of increasingly limited resources to reserve biophysical testing for the more vulnerable infants in the population.
5. There is no place for serial Doppler measurements in a normal population.

Fetal biophysical profile scoring systems (BPS)

CTG scoring systems taking into account, as they do, both heart rate and fetal activity, can be considered to have been the precursors of more complex biophysical testing using ultrasound. The BPS devised by Manning, Platt and Sipos (1980) is one of the earliest and remains the most popular system used today.

The features observed include the presence or absence of fetal breathing movements, fetal body movements, estimation of fetal tone, the NST and a qualitative estimate of amniotic fluid volume. Apart from the NST all these features are monitored simultaneously by ultrasound and are scored 2 or 0 according to fixed criteria (Table 11.4).

Manning et al. (1987*a*) reported on over 44 000 tests in just over 19 000 patients. A normal score (BPS = 8–10) was observed in 97.5% of tests, an equivocal score (BPS = 6) in 1.7% and an abnormal score (BPS < 4) in 0.8% of instances. The false negative rate for this test, defined as a stillbirth occurring within a week of the last normal test result, remains low at approximately 1 per 1000. Modifications have been made to this scoring system and Manning et al. (1987*b*) have shown that the omission of the NST does not affect test accuracy but does improve its efficiency. Furthermore, the criteria for reduced amniotic fluid has been changed from less than 1 cm to less than 2 cm.

Table 11.4. *Biophysical profile score: technique and interpretation**

Biophysical variable	Normal (score = 2)	Abnormal (score = 0)
Fetal breathing movements	At least 1 episode of FBM of at least 30 s duration in 30 min observation	Absent FBM or no episode ⩾30 s in 30 min
Gross body movement	At least 3 discrete body/limb movements in 30 min (episodes of active continuous movement)	Two or fewer episodes of body/limb movement in 30 min
Fetal tone	At least 1 episode of active extension with return to flexion of fetal limb(s) or trunk. Opening and closing of hand considered normal tone	Either slow extension with return to partial flexion or movement of limb in full extension or absent fetal movement
Reactive FHR	At least 2 episodes of FHR acceleration of ⩾15 beats/min and of at least 15 s duration associated with fetal movement in 30 min	Less than 2 episodes of acceleration of FHR or acceleration of <15 beats/min in 30 min
Qualitative AFV†	At least 1 pocket of AF that measures at least 1 cm in 2 perpendicular planes	Either no AF pockets or a pocket <1 cm in 2 perpendicular planes

*FBM, fetal breathing movement; FHR, fetal heart rate: AFV, amniotic fluid volume; AF, amniotic fluid.
†Modification of the criteria for reduced amniotic fluid from <1 cm to <2 cm is now acceptable.

It is important in the interpretation of the BPS to be aware that fetal behaviour alters during gestation among both normal fetuses and SGA fetuses. For instance, the percentage of the time that the normal fetus shows active behaviour decreases from 100% at 14–19 weeks to about 60% at term and SGA fetuses tend to spend 5% more time showing active behaviour than normal fetuses (Pillai, 1992).

As with all scoring systems, some items of the BPS are more important than others. A comparison was made between quantified fetal activity and biophysical profile score in the prediction of fetal acidaemia in infants with IUGR (Ribbert et al., 1993). Nineteen growth-retarded fetuses were studied within 24 hours of Caesarean section for decelerative fetal heart rate patterns. Total fetal activity (that is generalized fetal movements plus fetal breathing movements) was a better predictor of fetal acidaemia than the other biophysical variables measured. The data also indicated that reduction in fetal body movements was likely to precede reduction in fetal breathing movements, and it was postulated that the decrease in body movements may mark continuing fetal adaptation to impaired oxygen delivery, fetal breathing movements only ceasing with the onset of acidaemia. This finding is in contrast to those of James, Parker and Smoleniec (1992) who found that, using the BPS, fetal breathing movements were the first variable to disappear but acknowledged that this may have been due in part to the episodic nature of breathing movements. It is important to distinguish between acidaemic and non-acidaemic fetuses, especially in those cases with equivocal fetal heart rate patterns where further in utero fetal maturation is desirable. The data of Ribbert et al. (1993) indicated that quantification of generalized fetal movements using ultrasound would probably be more precise than the all-or-none criteria adopted in the traditional BPS. Whilst this may well be true, only experience will determine whether or not it is justifiable to await unequivocal evidence of fetal acidosis before removing the fetus from its unfavourable environment.

References

Agnew, R. & Wilder, G. (1994). Back to the future II, Beachcroft Stanleys, *Health Law Bulletin*, **27**, 1–3.

Altman, G.D. & Hytten, F.E. (1989). Assessment of fetal size and fetal growth. In *Effective Care in Pregnancy and Childbirth*, ed. I. Chalmers, M. Enkin & M.J.N.C. Keirse. pp. 411–418. Oxford University Press, Oxford.

Backe, B. & Nakling, J. (1993). Effectiveness of antenatal care; a population based study. *British Journal of Obstetrics and Gynaecology*, **100**, 727–32.

Beazley, J.M. & Kurjak, A. (1973). Prediction of foetal maturity and birthweight by abdominal palpation. *Nursing Times*, **14 June**, 763–5.

Calvert, J.P., Crean, E.E., Newcombe, R.G. & Pearson, J.F. (1982). Antenatal screening by measurement of symphysis–fundus height. *British Medical Journal*, **285**, 846–9.

Campbell, S. & Dewhurst, C.J. (1971). Diagnosis of the small-for-dates fetus by serial ultrasonic cephalometry. *Lancet*, **ii**, 1002–6.

Campbell, S. & Thoms, A. (1977). Ultrasound measurement of the fetal head to abdomen circumference ratio in the assessment of growth retardation. *British Journal of Obstetrics and Gynaecology*, **84**, 165–74.

Chandran, R., Serra-Serra, V., Sellers, S.M. & Redman, C.W.G. (1993). Fetal cerebral Doppler with recognition of fetal compromise. *British Journal of Obstetrics and Gynaecology*, **100**, 139–44.

Davies, J.A., Gallivan, S. & Spencer, J.A.D. (1992). Randomised controlled trial of Doppler ultrasound screening of placental perfusion during pregnancy. *Lancet*, **340**, 1299–303.

Droste, S. (1992). Fetal growth in aneuploid conditions. *Clinical Obstetrics and Gynaecology*, **35**, 119–25.

Eggertsen, S.C. & Benedetti, T.J. (1987). Maternal response to daily fetal movement counting in primary care settings. *American Journal of Perinatology*, **4**, 327–30.

Evertson, R.L. & Paul, R.H. (1978). Antepartum fetal heart rate testing; The non-stress test. *American Journal of Obstetrics and Gynecology,* **132**, 895–900.

Fitzgerald, D.E. & Drumm, J.E. (1977). Non-invasive measurement of human fetal circulation using ultrasound: a new method. *British Medical Journal*, **2**, 1450–1.

Galabin, A.L. (1886). The duration and hygiene of pregnancy. In *A Manual of Midwifery*. pp. 131. J. & A. Churchill,London.

Gardosi, J., Chang, A., Kalyan, B., Sahota, D. & Symonds, E.M. (1992). Customised antenatal growth charts. *Lancet*, **339**, 283–7.

Giles, W.B., Trudinger, B.T. & Baird, P. J. (1985). Fetal umbilical flow velocity waveforms and placental resistance: pathological correlation. *British Journal of Obstetrics and Gynaecology,* **92**, 31.

Grant, A., Elbourne, D., Valentin, L. & Alexander, S. (1989). Routine formal fetal movement counting and risk of antepartum late death in normally formed singletons. *Lancet*, **ii**, 345–9.

Huch, A., Huch, R., Schneider, H. & Rooth, G. (1977). Continuous transcutaneous monitoring of fetal oxygen tension during labour. *British Journal of Obstetrics and Gynaecology*, **84**, 1–39.

Hughes, A.B., Jenkins, A., Newcombe, R.G. & Pearson, J.F. (1987). Symphysis–fundus height, maternal height, labor pattern and mode of delivery. *American Journal of Obstetrics and Gynecology*, **156**, 644–8.

Jacobsen, G. (1992). Prediction of fetal growth deviations by use of symphysis-fundus height measurements. *International Journal of Technology Assessment in Health Care,* **8**, 1152–9.

James, D., Parker, M. & Smoleniec, J. (1992). Comprehensive fetal assessment using three ultrasound chacteristics. *American Journal of Obstetrics and Gynecology,* **166**, 1486–95.

Johnstone, F.D., Prescott, R., Hoskins, P., Green I.A., McGlew, T. & Compton, M. (1993). The effect of introduction of umbilical Doppler recordings to obstetric practice. *British Journal of Obstetrics and Gynaecology,* **100**, 733–41.

Kennedy, I. & Stephens, B. (1984). Antenatal records: do they help us? A new record for watching fetal growth. *Tropical Doctor*, **14**, 130–2.

Kidd, L.C., Patel, N.B. & Smith, R. (1983). Non-stress antenatal cardiotocography – a prospective randomised clinical trial. *British Journal of Obstetrics and Gynaecology*, **92**, 1156–9.

Kramer, M.S., Olivier, M., McLean, F.H., Dougherty, G.E., Willis, D.M. & Usher, R.H. (1990). Determinants of fetal growth and body proportionality. *Paediatrics*, **86**, 18–26.

Kubli, F., Boos, R., Ruttgers, H., Hagens, C.V. & Vanselow, H. (1977). Antepartum fetal heart rate monitoring. In *The Current Status of Fetal Heart Rate Monitoring and Ultrasound in Obstetrics,* ed. R.W. Beard & S. Campbell, pp. 28–45. Royal College of Obstetricians & Gynaecologists, London.

Lindhard, A., Nielsen, P.V., Mouritsen, L.A., Zachariassen, A., Sorensen, H.U. & Roseno, H. (1990). The implications of introducing the symphyseal–fundal height measurement. A prospective randomized controlled trial. *British Journal of Obstetrics and Gynaecology,* **97**, 675–80.

Liston, R.M., Cohen, A.W., Mennuti, M.T. & Gabbe, S.G. (1982). Antepartum fetal evaluation by maternal perception of fetal movement. *Obstetrics and Gynaecology*, **60**, 424–6.
Loeffler, F.E. (1967). Clinical foetal weight prediction. *Journal of Obstetrics & Gynaecology of the British Commonwealth*, **74**, 675–7.
Lowe, J.A. (1991). The current status of maternal and fetal blood flow velocimetry (National Institute of Health Consensus Conference 1986). *American Journal of Obstetrics and Gynecology*, **164**, 1049–63.
Manning, F.A., Morrison, I., Lange, I.R. et al. (1987*a*). Fetal biophysical profile scoring: selective use of the non-stress test. *American Journal of Obstetrics and Gynecology*, **156**, 709.
Manning, F.A., Morrison, I., Harman, C.R., et al. (1987*b*). Fetal assessment by fetal BPS: experience in 19,221 referred high-risk pregnancies. II. The false negative rate by frequency and etiology. *American Journal of Obstetrics and Gynecology*, **157**, 880.
Manning, F.A., Platt, L.D. & Sipos, L. (1980). Antepartum fetal evaluation: development of a new biophysical profile. *American Journal of Obstetrics and Gynecology*, **136**, 787–95.
Neilson, J.P., Whitfield, C.R. & Aitchison, T.C. (1980). Screening for the small-for-dates fetus: a two-stage ultrasonic examination schedule. *British Medical Journal*, **280**, 1203–6.
Neldam, S. (1983). Fetal movements as an indicator of fetal well-being. *Danish Medical Bulletin*, **30**, 274–80.
Newnham, J.P., O'Dea, M.R.-A., Reid, K.P. & Diepeveen, D.A. (1991). Doppler flow velocity waveform analysis in high risk pregnancies: a randomized controlled trial. *British Journal of Obstetrics and Gynaecology*, **98**, 956–63.
Patrick, J., Campbell, K., Carmichael, L., Natale, R. & Richardson, B. (1982). Patterns of gross fetal body movements over 24 hours observation intervals during the last 10 weeks of pregnancy. *American Journal of Obstetrics and Gynecology*, **142**, 363–71.
Pattison, R.C., Normal, K. & Odendaal, H.J. (1994). The role of Doppler velocimetry in the management of high risk pregnancies. *British Journal of Obstetrics and Gynaecology*, **101**, 114–20.
Pearce, J.M. & Campbell, S. (1987). A comparison of symphysis fundal height and ultrasound as screening tests for light-for-gestational-age infants. *British Journal of Obstetrics and Gynaecology*, **94**, 100–4.
Pearson, J.F. (1977). Fetal movements – a new approach to antepartum care. *Nursing Mirror*, **144**, 49–51.
Pearson, J.F. & Weaver, J.B. (1976). Fetal activity and fetal wellbeing: an evaluation. *British Medical Journal*, **1**, 1305–7.
Pearson, J.F. & Weaver, J.B. (1978). A six-point scoring system for antenatal cardiotocographs. *British Journal of Obstetrics and Gynaecology*, **85**, 321–7.
Pillai, M. (1992). The development of behaviour in the human fetus. MD Thesis, University of Bristol, England.
Rayburn, W.F. & Barr, M. (1982). Activity patterns in malformed fetuses. *American Journal of Obstetrics and Gynecology*, **142**, 1045–7.
Ribbert, L.S.M., Nicolaides, K.H. & Visser, G.H.A. (1993). Prediction of fetal acidaemia in intrauterine growth retardation: comparison of quantified fetal activity with biophysical profile score. *British Journal of Obstetrics and Gynaecology*, **100**, 653–6.

Sadovsky, E. & Yaffe, H. (1973). Daily fetal movement recording and fetal prognosis. *Obstetrics and Gynaecology*, **41**, 845–50.

Scherjon, S.A., Kok, J.H., Oosting, H. & Zoindervan, H.A. (1993). Intra-observer and inter-observer reliability of the pulsatility index calculated from pulsed Doppler flow velocity waveforms in three fetal vessels. *British Journal of Obstetrics and Gynaecology*, **180**, 134–8.

Smith, J.H., Anand, K.J.S., Cotes, P.M., Dawes, G.S., Harkness, R.A., Howlett, T.A., Rees, L.H. & Redman, C.W.G. (1988). Antenatal fetal heart rate variation in relation to the respiratory and metabolic status of the compromised human fetus. *British Journal of Obstetrics and Gynaecology*, **95**, 980–9.

Soothill, P.W., Ajayi, R.A., Campbell, S. & Nicolaides, K.H. (1993). Prediction of morbidity in small and normally grown fetuses by fetal heart rate variability, biophysical profile score and umbilical artery Doppler studies. *British Journal of Obstetrics and Gynaecology,* **100**, 742–5.

Taylor, D.J. & Howie, P.W. (1989). Fetal growth achievement and neurodevelopmental disability. *British Journal of Obstetrics and Gynaecology*, **96,** 789–94.

Thomson, A.M. & Billewicz, W.Z. (1976). The concept of the 'light for dates' infant. In *The Biology of Human Fetal Growth*. ed. D.F. Roberts & A.M. Thomson. pp. 69–79. Taylor & Francis, London.

Timor-Tritsch, I.E., Dierker, L.J., Hertz, R.H., Deagan, N.C. & Rosen, M.G. (1978). Studies of antepartum behavioural state in the human fetus at term. *American Journal of Obstetrics and Gynecology,* **132**, 524–8.

Trudinger, B.J., Giles, W.B., Cook, C.M., Connely, A. & Thompson, R.S. (1987). Umbilical artery flow velocity waveforms in high-risk pregnancy; randomized controlled trial. *Lancet* **i**, 188–90.

Tyrrell, S.N., Lilford, R.J., MacDonald, H.N., Nelson, E.J., Porter, J. & Gupta, J.K. (1990). Randomized comparison of routine vs highly selective use of Doppler ultrasound and biophysical scoring to investigate high risk pregnancies. *British Journal of Obstetrics and Gynaecology,* **97**, 909–16.

Wheble, A.M., Gillmer, M.D.G., Spencer, J.A.D. & Sykes, G.S. (1989). Changes in fetal monitoring practice in the UK: 1977–1984. *British Journal of Obstetrics & Gynaecology*, **96**, 1140–7.

12

Measurement of human fetal growth

STEPHEN C. ROBSON and
TOU CHOONG CHANG

Introduction

Perinatal mortality and morbidity are linked not only to gestational age but also to fetal growth. The antenatal recognition of intrauterine growth retardation (IUGR) is therefore one of the primary aims of obstetric care. However, for years clinicians have confused size with growth. Size is an endpoint, typically weight at birth, whereas growth is the process by which this endpoint is reached. Size is determined by a combination of local factors in tissues and organs, together with systemic nutritional and endocrine factors. Genetic influences, which are the primary determinant of fetal size, probably act primarily at the local level. Systemic factors are, in a sense, secondary, because although they might direct the growth process they do not determine size other than at pathological extremes (Chard, 1989).

Ultrasound is the most accurate method of determining fetal gestational age and size. Thus clinical suspicion of abnormal fetal size should prompt ultrasound assessment. Reference standards for a variety of fetal biometric measurements exist. These are derived from cross-sectional studies in a 'representative' population of fetuses. Using appropriate standards, biometric measurements can be classified as appropriate-, small-, or large-for-gestational age. Assessment of fetal growth requires an assessment of the change in fetal size over time and therefore requires at least two measurements of fetal size. Reference standards for fetal growth can only be derived from serial biometric measurements.

This chapter discusses the ultrasound methods used to determine fetal size and the value of serial measurements in assessing fetal growth. The ability of various measurements to predict size at birth and the sequelae of growth retardation will be reviewed. As knowledge of gestational age is a prerequisite for determining whether fetal size is appropriate, the role of ultrasound in determination of gestational age will also be discussed.

Ultrasound measurements

Derivation of reference standards

To interpret a fetal measurement, it is necessary to compare it with a reference range. These standards are derived from a large number of normal fetuses and are generally presented as a mean with 5th and 95th centiles. Isolated measurements may be used to determine gestational age or fetal size, while serial measurements are required to quantify fetal growth. The reference standard used is clearly of great importance and, although hundreds of reference ranges and charts have been published, most of these have serious weaknesses in design or statistical analysis (Altman & Chitty, 1994). It is therefore appropriate to begin by considering the derivation of reference ranges for ultrasound fetal measurements.

Cross-sectional data

The methods used to construct reference ranges from cross-sectional fetal measurements have recently been reviewed (Altman & Chitty, 1994) and are summarized below. It is important to emphasize the difference between charts for estimating gestational age and those for estimating size. In the case of a dating curve, the ultrasound measurement is taken to be correct and is used to predict the gestational age assuming that the pregnancy is normal. For estimates of fetal size, gestational age is assumed to be known, and the measurement is used to establish whether fetal size is within some normal range.

Design. This should be cross-sectional with only one measurement from each patient and with an equal number of randomly selected women at each gestational week (stratified sampling). This necessitates a prospective collection of data with examinations performed specifically for the purpose of the study. Inclusion of data collected from examinations performed for some clinical indication, e.g. suspicion of a small fetus, should not be included. The method of performing measurements should be consistent.

Subject selection. The subjects chosen must represent a sample that is not significantly different from the general obstetric population with respect to race, age, height, weight and parity. Multiple pregnancies and those complicated by fetal malformation should be excluded as should pregnancies in women with disease or medication which is likely to affect the growth of the fetus (e.g. diabetes, renal disease, hypertension requiring treatment). It is controversial whether smokers and certain ethnic groups should be excluded.

In most cases gestational age is calculated from the date of the last menstrual period (LMP). To reduce errors only women with a recorded normal LMP and a regular cycle length who are not on the contraceptive pill are included. Even with a selected group such as this, more than 10% of women will have a difference of over 1 week between gestational age determined by early ultrasound and LMP (Geirsson, 1991). One method of avoiding this problem is to include only those subjects in whom gestational age determined from a routine first or second trimester ultrasound scan and LMP agree within 7 days. An alternative is to use data from women with a known date of ovulation or fertilization (Daya, 1993).

Analysis. A polynomial regression model is fitted to the data. This has the general form:

$$X = A + B(GA) + C(GA)^2 + \dots. \qquad (1)$$

where X is the ultrasound measurement, GA is the gestational age and $A, B \dots$ are constants which need to be calculated for each measurement. A quadratic or cubic curve usually gives an adequate fit. A plot of the residuals against gestational age will determine if the variability of the measurement changes with gestation. The next step is to model the variability as a function of gestational age to produce a regression equation for the standard deviation (SD). The 5th and 95th centiles can then be obtained as mean $\pm$ 1.645 SD (Altman & Chitty, 1994). This parametric method is based on the assumption that the data have a normal distribution and it is important to confirm this otherwise a transformation will be required. The process for deriving dating curves is similar except that they are based on regression of gestational age on the fetal measurement. A polynomial of the form $GA = A + B\,(X) + C\,(X)^2 \dots$ is therefore needed. This means that, for dating curves, the fetal measurement is on the horizontal axis and gestational age, which is unknown, is on the vertical axis. For curves of fetal size the gestational age, now known, is on the horizontal axis and the measurement is on the vertical axis.

Longitudinal data

Assessment of growth requires serial ultrasound measurements and thus reference standards need to be derived from longitudinally collected data so that growth patterns of individual fetuses can be examined (Gallivan et al., 1993). Longitudinal data are available primarily for abdominal circumference (AC) and estimated fetal weight (EFW), the two parameters most widely used to assess growth.

Design. This should be longitudinal with each fetus being measured at regular intervals (two- or four-weekly). The method of performing measurements must again be consistent.

Subject selection. As with cross-sectional data, the population studied must be representative of the general obstetric population. The same exclusions pertain to serial measurements. The comments regarding gestational age assignment discussed above also apply to longitudinally collected data.

Analysis. It is inappropriate to analyse longitudinal data by regression analysis in the manner described above for cross-sectional data because of the interdependence of repeated measurements on the same fetus. This will lead to an inappropriately low estimate of residual variance (Gallivan et al., 1993). It is necessary to determine the most appropriate mathematical model to describe the growth of individual fetuses. As the variance of measurements almost invariably increases with gestational age, log transformation of the data is usually required. Comparison of the standard deviation of the residual error is superior to the R^2 value in determining the goodness of fit (Gallivan et al., 1993). Several workers have found that fetal growth, at least as assessed by serial changes in $\log_{10}$(AC) and $\log_{10}$(EFW), is not linear but best described by a quadratic or cubic model (Larsen et al., 1990; Gallivan et al., 1993). The polynomial constants A, B and C are then used to produce a series of individual growth curves and these are used to interpolate values of $\log_{10}$(AC) and $\log_{10}$(EFW) for each fetus at a range of exact gestational ages (Gallivan et al., 1993). The mean and SD of the resulting $\log_{10}$(AC) and $\log_{10}$(EFW) values are then used to derive centile ranges.

Measurements for estimation of gestational age during the first and second trimester

Crown–rump length

Crown–rump length (CRL) can be measured from 6 to around 14 weeks and is the most accurate measurement for gestational dating in the first trimester. The longest axis of the fetus is measured as a straight line drawn between the two fetal poles. The 95% prediction interval (+2 SD) using CRL are consistently between ±4.7 days and ±6 days (Daya, 1993). Accuracy declines after around 11 weeks gestation.

Biparietal diameter

Biparietal diameter (BPD) is measured in a transverse plane of the fetal head. The section chosen should include the following landmarks: midline echo, thalami, cavum septum pellucidum and basal cisterns. Although several methods of measuring BPD have been described, the most commonly used is from the outer edge of the proximal parietal bone to the inner edge of the distal parietal bone. Measurements of BPD at between 14 and 24 weeks appear to be of comparable accuracy in predicting gestational age to CRL measurements (95% prediction interval ±5–7 days) (Chitty et al., 1994*a*). Head circumference (HC) is measured in the same plane as BPD around the outer edge of the skull. This can be done by either tracing around the perimeter of the skull or by derivation from the occipito-frontal and biparietal diameters. The 95% prediction interval for HC measurements between 14 and 24 weeks is between ±8–10 days (Chitty et al., 1994*a*).

Femur length

Femur length (FL) is measured between the two ends of the femoral diaphysis. To ensure that the whole of the femur is measured and that it is not foreshortened, the transducer is rotated until the longest possible image of the femur is obtained and the transducer is along the long axis of the femur. The predictive accuracy of FL measurements is slightly inferior to BPD measurements (95% prediction interval ±8–13 days) (Chitty et al., 1994*b*). We would recommend the BPD and FL dating curves of Chitty et al. (1994*a,b*) for assessment of gestational age.

Routine gestational age assignment

The most important consideration in clinically evaluating the size and growth of a fetus is the establishment of gestational age. In women with regular menstrual cycles the reliance on the first day of the LMP to determine the duration of pregnancy is widely accepted. However, in reality only approximately one-quarter of women have sufficiently accurate and regular cycles to allow the deduction that mid-cycle ovulation was reasonably likely. Even within this group some 12% of women will have a difference of over one week between early ultrasound and LMP (Geirsson, 1991). Ultrasound is subject to a certain degree of the same variation as LMP, but the variation is diminished by using reference standards from carefully chosen women, where there is a smaller and more normally distributed variation about the mean. Geirsson (1991) presents a persuasive argument for the routine adjustment of dates to ultrasound mean values suggesting that, while this may confer slight inaccuracy (of no real consequence compared to the real gestational age) in the individual, the practice will benefit the population at large. Most units within the UK have a policy of using ultrasound for dating if there is a 7- or 10-day difference between LMP and ultrasound estimation of gestational age providing the latter is performed before 24 weeks. However this will not correct the skew of LMP data (Geirsson, 1991) and failure to make allowance for differences of 7–10 days may also lead to misinterpretation of isolated measurements of fetal size during late pregnancy.

Measurements for estimation of fetal size during the second and third trimester

Abdominal circumference

Abdominal circumference (AC) is the most widely used measure of fetal size during the late second and third trimester of pregnancy. After finding the long axis of the fetus, the transducer is rotated through 90° to obtain a transverse image at the level where the umbilical vein enters the portal system of the liver. If the fetal cross-section is ovoid, or the aorta not circular, then the section is not perpendicular to the long axis and should not be used. The circumference should be measured around the outer edge of the image. This can be done directly using a tracker ball or indirectly using two sets of calipers. Alternatively, the AC can be calculated from the maximal abdominal diameters. Abdominal circumferences derived from diameter measurements are different from those measured directly and therefore it is crucial that the method is standardized and the appropriate reference ranges are used.

Estimated fetal weight

Size at birth is traditionally assessed by birthweight. It is therefore understandable why estimation of fetal weight has become widely used as a measure of fetal size. Several formulae based on different ultrasonic parameters can be used to estimate fetal weight. Initial formulae used BPD and AC measurements. Probably the most widely used two-parameter formula is that of Shepard et al. (1982):

$$\text{Log}_{10}\text{ weight} = -1.7492 + 0.166(\text{BPD}) + 0.046\,(\text{AC}) - 2.646(\text{AC} \times \text{BPD})/1000 \quad (2)$$

Subsequent formulae incorporated HC and FL. Hadlock et al. (1985) developed several multiparameter formulae although the one incorporating BPD, HC, AC and FL is the most popular:

$$\text{Log}_{10}\text{ weight} = 1.3596 - 0.00386\,(\text{AC} \times \text{FL}) + 0.0064\,(\text{HC}) + 0.00061(\text{BPD} \times \text{AC}) + 0.0424\,(\text{AC}) + 0.174\,(\text{FL}) \quad (3)$$

In a small prospective study the mean error of this four-parameter formula [−0.7 (SD 7.3)%] was significantly lower than that for the two-parameter Shepard formula [1.3 (SD 10.1) %] (Hadlock et al., 1985). The marginal superiority of the Hadlock four-parameter formula has been confirmed in larger prospective studies in unselected women. In most of these studies the SDs of the mean error have been larger than those reported by Hadlock et al. (1985) averaging 10–12% (Simon et al., 1987). Most formulae predict actual weight within 10% in approximately 60% of cases.

Both systematic and random prediction errors are greater when these general formulae are applied to small and large fetuses. In the small-for-gestational age (SGA) fetus weight is typically overestimated by around 5% although several studies have shown no systematic error with the Shepard formula (Simon et al., 1987). Conversely weight is consistently underestimated in large-for-gestational age (LGA) fetuses. In an attempt to incorporate the changes in fetal morphometry related to what the authors called 'aberrant growth', Sabbagha et al. (1989) developed weight formulae targeted to small-, appropriate-, and large-for-gestational age fetuses (defined by AC). Weight is determined from the appropriate table using the sum of the fetal parameters (GA [wk] + HC [cm] + 2 AC [cm] + FL [cm]). Across the birthweight range, use of the three targeted formulae resulted in a small reduction in birthweight

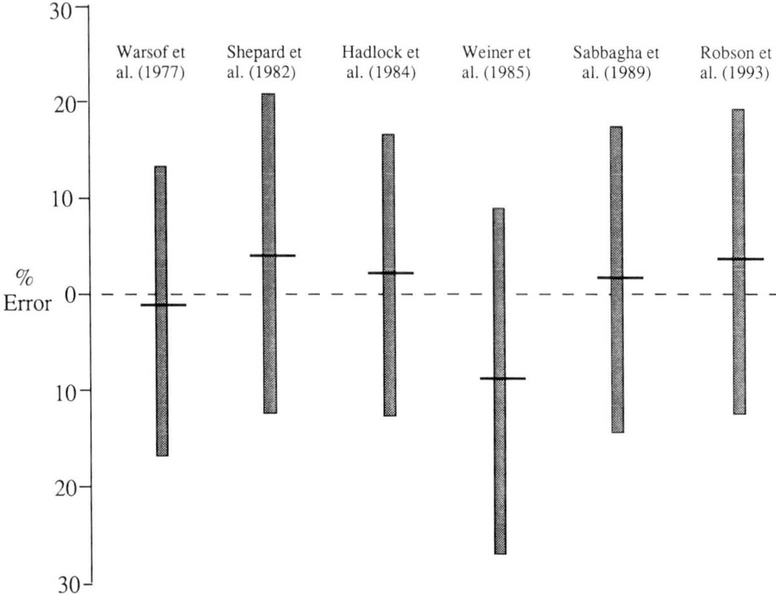

Fig. 12.1. Mean percentage errors with 95% prediction intervals for birthweight prediction errors using a variety of targeted and non-targeted EFW formulae in a group of 187 SGA fetuses. (Adapted from Robson et al., 1993.)

prediction error compared with the four-parameter Hadlock formula (mean error (2 SD); 0.0 (19.8)% versus −6.7 (21.6)%). However, the differences in prediction error were not significant in SGA and LGA fetuses. In a subsequent study of SGA fetuses, we were also unable to show any reduction in prediction error associated with the use of targeted formulae over general non-targeted formulae (Robson et al., 1993) (Fig. 12.1). It is worth noting that all the formulae had a small but statistically significant systematic error.

The choice of formula used to calculate weight will depend on the parameters available. The four-parameter formula of Hadlock et al. (1985) and the simpler targeted formula of Sabbagha et al. (1989) are probably the most appropriate for clinical use.

Several groups have reported normal ranges of AC and EFW derived from longitudinal data (for review, see Gallivan et al., 1993). Significant differences exist in the lower limits: at 40 weeks the lower limit for AC (2SD below the mean) ranges from 316 to 377 mm and for EFW from 1887 to 3031 g. Some of these differences relate to the method of statistical analysis. Two groups have analysed their data using least

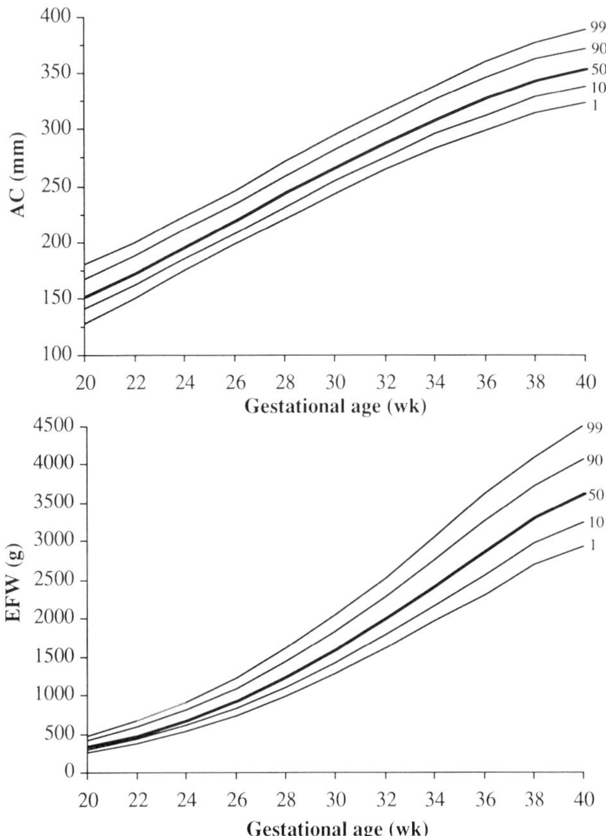

Fig. 12.2. Reference ranges (1st, 10th, 50th, 90th, 99th centiles) for abdominal circumference (*top*) and estimated fetal weight (*bottom*). (Adapted from Gallivan et al., 1993.)

squares fitting to obtain growth curves for individual fetuses (Deter et al., 1982; Gallivan et al., 1993). There are small differences between these reference ranges after 36 weeks gestation reflecting the different regression models used in the two studies. We would recommend the use of either of these standards. The AC and EFW data of Gallivan et al. (1993) are shown in Fig. 12.2.

It is important to note that fetal weight estimated by ultrasound is consistently greater than birthweight. At 34 weeks of pregnancy the tenth centile for EFW is 2170 g (Gallivan et al., 1993). The comparable value for birthweight in the Aberdeen population is 1880 g (Thomson, Billewicz & Hytten, 1968). At 40 weeks the values are 3240 g and 2840 g, respectively. Most studies in which EFW and birthweight data have been compared in the same population have found that weight differences tend to be more marked at gestational ages below 37 weeks. This reflects the fact that in around 50% of preterm labours, underlying conditions exist which cause uteroplacental insufficiency (Adelstein & Fedrick, 1978). Measurements of fetal weight should be compared with appropriate in utero reference ranges.

Reproducibility of measurements

Chang et al. (1993*a*) determined the reproducibility of AC and EFW measurements in third-trimester fetuses. The intraobserver standard deviations for AC and EFW measurements were small (4 mm and 63 g, respectively). While there were no systematic differences between observers, the 95% limits of agreement were wide: −17, 13 mm for AC and −160, 124 g for EFW. These results were obtained by two experienced observers using the average of three measurements in a selected group of small fetuses. Measurement variability is likely to be considerably larger when isolated measurements are performed on unselected fetuses in a busy ultrasound department. This will apply particularly to large-for-gestational age fetuses in which ultrasonic measurements may be more difficult to obtain.

Quantifying fetal growth from serial ultrasonic measurements

The appropriateness of fetal size can be determined by comparing isolated measurements of AC or EFW with appropriate reference standards. However, the change in fetal size between two time points is a direct measure of fetal growth. Growth rate may be abnormal even when individual values of fetal size are within the normal range. While simply eyeballing a plot of individual fetal measurements may give an impression of growth retardation or acceleration, a more objective definition is required. This requires the establishment of growth rate standards from longitudinally collected data. Since the upper and lower limits of growth are of most interest to the clinician, the method of deriving these is particularly important.

The simplest approach is to determine the increase in a fetal measurement over a defined period of time. Divon et al. (1986) suggested that an abnormal rate of AC growth was <10 mm/14 days. However, because fetal growth is not linear during the third trimester, changes in absolute measurements of AC or EFW are dependent on gestational age. Fescina et al. (1982) reported reference ranges for rate of growth of AC in the second and third trimesters based on serial data in 30 fetuses. The authors used data collected within 7 days of a defined gestation. This will lead to inappropriate estimations of standard deviation. Deter and Harrist (1992) studied 20 fetuses, and derived reference ranges for AC growth using the Rossavik growth model (see below) and the Hotellings T^2-statistic, a multivariate form of the t-test. Mean growth rate was 12 mm/week from 14 to 30 weeks and 11 mm/week thereafter. The limits of normal growth were particularly small: the lower limit (−2SD) ranging from 10 mm/week at 26 weeks gestation to 6 mm/week at 38 weeks.

Figure 12.3 shows the data from 43 fetuses in whom AC and EFW was measured within 2 days of exact gestational ages at fortnightly intervals between 26 and 40 weeks gestation (Chang, 1993). The data therefore reflect the real variation in growth velocity over a two-week period. Mean (SD) growth velocity of AC decreased from 11.3 (6.2) mm/wk at 30 weeks gestation to 7.1 (3.9) mm/wk at 38 weeks. The respective values for EFW were 219 (86) g and 194 (99) g. The marked difference in the lower limit of AC growth in this study and that of Deter and Harrist (1992) reflects the method of statistical analysis used to derive the SD.

An alternative method of quantifying serial ultrasound measurements is to use a change in standard deviation score (SDS) (Chang et al., 1993*b*). For each fetus, the SDS for AC at any gestational age is calculated using the formula: AC·SDS = (Measured AC − Mean AC at same gestation/SD of AC at same gestation). Mean and SD values are obtained from an appropriate reference range. Growth abnormalities may then be defined as a change in SDS greater than a predetermined threshold, e.g. 1.5 SDs. Thus a fetus with an AC that falls from the mean at 34 weeks gestation (SDS = 0) to −1.6 SDs at 37 weeks would be growth retarded while one whose AC increases from +1 SD to +2.6 SDs would have growth acceleration.

Larsen et al. (1990) measured EFW serially in 35 normal fetuses. Population growth curves were derived by weighted polynomial regression. Individual growth curves from 27 weeks gestation to delivery were then fitted to EFW as a percentage deviation from the population curve. They found that each fetus had a constant percentage deviation which they termed the growth channel. The individual growth channels were normally distributed with a SD of 10.2%. The 10th and 90th centiles were calculated to be +13.0%, corresponding to a weekly weight gain of 169 g/week and 221 g/week, respectively.

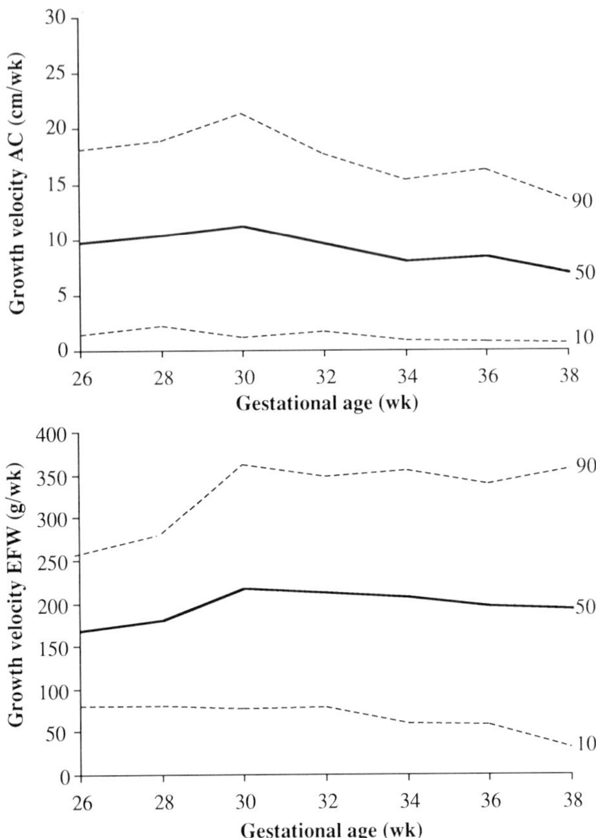

Fig. 12.3. Reference ranges (10th, 50th, 90th centiles) for growth velocity of abdominal circumference (*top*) and estimated fetal weight (*bottom*) derived from 43 fetuses measured every 2 weeks.

Finally, several authors have used growth model coefficients to define normal fetal growth rates. Deter and colleagues have published extensively on the Rossavik growth model. The general equation for this model is: $P = c(t)^{k+s(t)}$ where P is the ultrasound parameter, t is the duration of growth and c, k and s the model coefficients. The coefficient k is specified by the anatomical parameter being studied and is thought to be the same for all fetuses. The coefficient c relates to genetic regulators of growth and s to an unknown regulatory system that modifies genetically determined growth (Rossavik & Deter, 1984). Values for k have been established for AC and EFW from serial scans in 20 normal middle-class mothers of different ethnic backgrounds. Values of c and s may be determined from two scans before 27 weeks gestation allowing the derivation of an individual fetal growth curve. A fetus who consistently departs from this curve may therefore be regarded as having an abnormal growth pattern. This method may be of particular value in the prospective assessment of fetuses at risk of growth abnormalities, although the fact that growth retardation may start in the second trimester poses obvious difficulties. However, rarely in clinical practice is information from two second-trimester scans available at the time when a fetus is referred because of concern about growth. Furthermore, the only group who have independently verified the use of the model reported a systematic overestimation of AC and EFW in the third trimester (Simon et al., 1989).

An alternative approach, reported by Chang et al. (1992*a*) is to compare growth rates using quadratic coefficients. This technique takes account of all the available ultrasound information and is less likely to be affected by one erroneous measurement. Chang et al. (1992*a*) compared mean values of the *a*, *b* and *c* coefficients for $\log_{10}$(AC) and $\log_{10}$(EFW) in Caucasian and Bangladeshi fetuses studied serially between 20 and 38 weeks gestation. The authors hypothesized that differences in growth between the two ethnic groups would be reflected by differences in the quadratic coefficients, in particular the *b* coefficient (representing the slope or growth velocity). However, despite significant differences in mean EFW at 28, 32 and 36 weeks gestation there were no differences in the quadratic coefficients. This suggests that this method may be rather insensitive.

Other ultrasonic parameters used in the assessment of fetal size and growth

Morphometric ratios

Campbell and Thoms (1977) first proposed the head–abdomen circumference ratio (HC/AC) as a means of identifying genuine growth retardation. Mean values decrease linearly from 16 to 40 weeks reaching unity around 36 weeks gestation. Thereafter, the HC/AC falls below unity. Ratios relating weight to length are widely used by neonatologists to assess growth. Comparable ratios can be calculated in the fetus. Hadlock et al. (1983) proposed the use of the FL/AC ratio. This has the advantage of being independent of gestational age after 21 weeks with a mean value [2 SD] of 22 [2]. A more complex ratio is the fetal ponderal index which is calculated as EFW/[length]^3 (Vintzileos et al., 1986). Fetal length is derived from femur length ($6.18 + 5.9 \times$ FL). The rationale for using morphometric ratios is to predict the fetus with a disproportionately small liver (and hence AC) compared with head size or body length. It is suggested that asymmetrical growth retardation results from utero-placental insufficiency with brain sparing while fetuses with aneuploidy or infection are symmetrically small. This distinction is rather misleading as most symmetrically small fetuses are perfectly normal. Furthermore, euploid fetuses with severe early-onset uteroplacental insufficiency often show an asymmetrical pattern.

Amniotic fluid volume

Oligohydramnios may complicate IUGR and results from decreased urine production secondary to redistribution of fetal cardiac output. The two most widely used ultrasonic methods for quantifying amniotic fluid volume are the maximum vertical pocket (MVP) and the four-quadrant amniotic fluid index (AFI). Definitions of oligohydramnios based on MVP have ranged from 1 to 3 cm. A value of 3 cm corresponds to the fifth centile after 30 weeks gestation (Moore, 1990). The fifth centile for AFI decreases from 9 cm at 30 weeks gestation to 7 cm at 40 weeks (Moore, 1990).

Total intrauterine volume (TIUV)

The TIUV represents the sum of the volumes of all intrauterine products (fetus, amniotic fluid and placenta). Measurements are made using a static B-mode scanner and volumes are calculated using a parallel planimetric method (Geirsson et al., 1985). Median TIUV increases from 1006 ml at 20 weeks of pregnancy to 4420 ml at 40 weeks (Geirsson et al., 1985). Respective values for the third centile are 688 and 3457 ml. It is not possible to perform TIUV measurements with real time scanners, and therefore this indirect method of assessing fetal size is rarely used today.

Placental imaging

Fetal growth retardation is often associated with morphological changes in the placenta and a reduction in placental weight. The ultrasonic appearance of the placenta may be graded (Grannum, Berkowitz & Hobbins, 1979). The finding of a mature [grade 3] placenta, i.e. one in which there are complete indentations from the chorionic plate to the basal layer of the placenta combined with calcification is normal in late pregnancy but can occur prematurely in growth-retarded fetuses. This method may only be of value in the prediction of the preterm fetus with IUGR. Ultrasonic measurements of placental size are unreliable.

Doppler flow velocity waveforms

Flow velocities can be obtained from several maternal and fetal vessels. Use of flow velocity indices avoids the major sources of error inherent in the measurement of flow. These indices are independent of the angle of insonation and give information about the impedance in the distal vascular bed. Three indices are in common use: the systolic/diastolic ratio, the Pourcelot resistance index and the pulsatility index (PI). All three indices are highly correlated and there is no clear clinical advantage in one over the others. Resistance index (RI) in the uterine artery falls in early pregnancy but then remains relatively constant from 26 weeks gestation with values greater than 0.56 being abnormal (Pearce et al., 1988). Histopathological studies on placental bed biopsies suggest that the RI of the uteroplacental waveforms reflects the depth of trophoblastic invasion. Abnormal flow velocity waveforms in the uterine arteries, particularly persistent notching, are associated with pre-eclampsia and SGA (Bower, Schuchter & Campbell, 1993). Fetal waveforms may be obtained from several sites although the umbilical artery is the most extensively studied. Umbilical artery PI falls from a mean value of 1.2 at 16 weeks to around 0.8 at term (Pearce et al., 1988). Clinical and experimental evidence suggests that abnormal waveforms are primarily a reflection of occlusion of the small placental vessels. An abnormal umbilical artery PI, particularly if associated with absent end-diastolic frequencies, appears to be useful in predicting the compromised fetus (Low, 1991). Doppler studies of the fetal cerebral circulation, aorta and renal arteries appear to be able to identify cardiovascular redistribution in response to hypoxia (the so-called 'brain-sparing' effect). These changes may precede abnormalities in the umbilical artery.

Soft tissue measurements

Thigh circumference is measured at the junction of the upper and middle thirds of the thigh. Values increase linearly after 24 weeks gestation but may be reduced in small fetuses (Hill et al., 1989). Quantitative assessment of fetal fat is difficult and there is little evidence that it is a useful predictor of fetal growth.

Prediction of the small-for-gestational age infant

Which ultrasound measurement is best?

Many ultrasound parameters have been used to predict the SGA infant at birth. The results of these studies are generally reported using sensitivity, specificity and predictive values (positive and negative). While sensitivity and specificity are independent of the prevalence of SGA in the population studied, this is not the case for predictive value. Although it is possible to standardize the positive predictive value for a population prevalence of 10% using Bayes theorem, a more appropriate prevalence-independent method is to calculate the odds ratio (OR) (the ratio of the odds that a fetus that is SGA on ultrasound measurement will actually have a birthweight less than the tenth percentile, to that of a fetus AGA on ultrasound having a birthweight greater than the tenth centile).

The extensive literature on this subject has recently been reviewed by the authors with the aim of determining the most appropriate ultrasonic measurement for the prediction of a SGA infant (birthweight less than the tenth centile) (Chang et al., 1992*b*). Studies were included in the analysis if antenatal and postnatal criteria for diagnosis were clearly defined and data for SGA and normal fetuses were reported allowing the construction of a 2 × 2 table. Providing there was more than one study with the same criteria, these were grouped according to whether the population was high or low risk and the sensitivity, OR and false-positive rates calculated for each study. Although the intention was to derive summary statistics for each ultrasound parameter, this frequently proved impossible because of statistically significant differences between individual studies. This heterogeneity may reflect differences in the ultrasonic and birthweight standards used and the interval between the ultrasonic measurement and delivery. Despite the statistical limitations of such an analysis, some important conclusions can be drawn.

Abdominal circumference and EFW appear to be better predictors of an SGA infant at birth than BPD, HC/AC and FL/AC ratios, TIUV, amniotic fluid volume and placental grading. The limited data on other parameters precludes meaningful comparisons. In high-risk women, an AC below the tenth centile predicts 84% of SGA fetuses with an overall or common OR of 18.4 [95% CI 9.8, 34.3], compared with a common OR of 39.1 [95% CI 28.9, 52.8] for an EFW below the tenth centile. These ultrasonic measurements have comparable false-positive rates [20–25%]. In low-risk women sensitivities and ORs are lower for all morphometric parameters although the same trend is seen. An AC below the tenth centile has sensitivities ranging from 48 to 64% and a common OR of 13.5 [95% CI 11.5, 15.9]. Sensitivities of an EFW below the tenth centile range from 31 to 73% with ORs of 10.7–28.8. False-positive rates are again comparable [44–47%].

Umbilical artery and uteroplacental Doppler waveforms are inferior to AC and EFW in the prediction of SGA infants at birth. In a high-risk population, the sensitivity and common OR for umbilical artery systolic/diastolic (S/D) ratio ≥ 3 is 52.6% and 6.9 [95% CI 4.8, 10.0], respectively. The common OR for an S/D above the 95th centile is 5.8 [95% CI 4.8, 7.0]. False-positive rates are 43–47%. Abnormal uteroplacental waveforms have a lower common OR [2.3, 95% CI 1.2, 4.3]. Limited data on fetal Doppler waveforms from the aorta and cerebral circulation suggest these may be more predictive. In a low-risk population, Doppler waveforms perform very poorly (sensitivities typically <35% and ORs < 5). Of the six studies in which AC or EFW measurements were compared with Doppler measurements in the same group of women, the Doppler ORs were significantly lower in three studies. In the remaining three studies the same trend was seen although the differences were not statistically significant.

Thus screening with AC below the tenth centile will detect the highest percentage of SGA fetuses, but the odds of SGA in any individual fetus are greatest if the EFW is below the tenth centile. The value of Doppler ultrasound appears not to be in the prediction of SGA but in the detection of serious compromise in high-risk pregnancies, including those which are SGA.

Does detection of SGA improve perinatal outcome?

Five randomized controlled trials of ultrasound in late pregnancy have been published (Table 12.1). In the study of Bakketeig et al. (1984) women whose fetuses had ultrasound measurements of BPD at 32 weeks gestation were admitted to hospital more often than unscreened women [OR 1.92 (95% CI 1.37, 2.68) with no reduction in the incidence of adverse perinatal outcome. In contrast the trial conducted by Eik-Nes et al. (1984) showed that fewer women who had measurements of fetal BPD and abdominal diameter at 32 weeks gestation were admitted to hospital compared with controls [OR 0.60 (95% CI 0.49, 0.75); this did not lead to any reduction in neonatal morbidity or mortality. No significant effects on admission rates, neonatal morbidity or mortality were noted in the study of Neilson, Munjaja and Whitfield (1984) where measurements of

Table 12.1. *Randomized controlled trials of ultrasound measurement of fetal size in late pregnancy and perinatal outcome*

Outcome	Reference	Measurement	Ultrasound	Control	OR (95% CI)
Low Apgar Score	Bakketeig et al.	BPD	34/510	23/499	1.47 (0.86, 2.51)
	Eik-Nes et al.	BPD, AD	41/809	35/819	1.20 (0.75, 1.89)
	Neilson et al.	TA, CRL	37/433	40/444	0.94 (0.59, 1.51)
	Secher et al.	EFW, AD	8/96	10/88	0.71 (0.27, 1.99)
	Larsen et al.	EFW	22/484	22/481	0.99 (0.52, 1.89)
NICU admission	Bakketeig et al.	BPD	21/510	25/499	0.81 (0.45, 1.47)
	Eik-Nes et al.	BPD, AD	68/809	66/819	1.05 (0.74, 1.49)
	Secher et al.	EFW, AD[a]	8/96	8/88	0.91 (0.33, 2.53)
	Larsen et al.	EFW	75/484	48/481	1.66 (1.11, 2.49)
Perinatal deaths	Bakketeig et al.	BPD	5/510	5/499	0.98 (0.28, 3.40)
	Eik-Nes et al.	BPD, AD	3/809	7/819	0.45 (0.13, 1.57)
	Neilson et al.	TA, CRL	0/433	0/444	1.00 (1.00, 1.00)
	Secher et.	EFW, AD	0/96	0/88	1.00 (1.00, 1.00)
	Larsen et al.	EFW	5/484	3/481	1.67 (0.35, 8.83)

[a]Based on small fetuses (EFW <85% expected weight).
Abbreviations: AD, abdominal diameter; TA, trunk area; CRL, crown rump length; EFW, estimated fetal weight; NICU, neonatal intensive care unit.

CRLs and trunk areas were performed between 34 and 36 weeks of pregnancy.

In the study of Secher et al. (1987), 184 of 1570 screened women were found to have a small fetus at 32 and 34 weeks gestation (EFW > 85% below the expected mean). This group were then randomized into those in whom the results of a subsequent scan at 37 weeks were revealed to the clinician and those in whom the results were concealed. The incidence of induction of labour was increased in the revealed group [OR 3.55, 95% CI 1.87, 6.75] with no reduction in neonatal morbidity or mortality. In the recent study of Larsen et al. (1992) the group in which EFWs obtained after 28 weeks gestation were revealed to the clinicians had more elective deliveries based on the diagnosis of smallness [OR 2.37, 95% CI 1.32, 4.29] and more healthy preterm babies admitted to the neonatal intensive care unit [OR 1.66, 95% CI 1.11, 2.49] without any improvement in perinatal morbidity or mortality.

The results of these trials suggest that isolated measurements of fetal size by ultrasound in late pregnancy, whether in low-risk or selected women, do not improve fetal outcome or obstetric management. However, these trials do not address the benefit of serial measurements. This is important as fetal size is not the most important determinant of perinatal outcome; some SGA babies are constitutionally small, while some AGA babies have failed to reach their growth potential and are growth retarded.

Prediction of the growth-retarded infant

Definition of IUGR

Although a proportion of SGA infants are growth retarded, the majority exhibit no symptoms or signs associated with IUGR. These infants have no subcutaneous fat or muscle wasting, are well proportioned and may be constitutionally small (Walther & Raemaker, 1982). Several neonatal morphometric measurements have been used to detect wasting or malnutrition at birth (Table 12.2). Ponderal index has been the most widely used, although the weight/length appears to correlate more closely with fat content. The mid-arm to head circumference ratio (MAC/HC) assesses muscle and fat wasting while newborn fat content may be more directly assessed by measurement of skinfold thickness. Skinfold measurements show a close inverse correlation with lean body mass (Petersen, Larsen & Greisen, 1992). Alternative methods of defining IUGR include biochemical indices, which either reflect the metabolic

Table 12.2. *Neonatal morphometric measurements used to define IUGR*

Weight/length
Weight/length^2
Weight/length^3 (ponderal index)
Body mass index
Mid-arm circumference/head circumference ratio
Skinfold thickness (triceps, subscapular)
Percentage body fat

consequences of or the endocrine changes in IUGR, and measures of adverse perinatal outcome associated with IUGR (operative delivery for fetal distress, acidaemia, low Apgar scores, admission to neonatal intensive care). The limitations of these definitions have been extensively reviewed (Chang, 1993). No single measure reliably defines IUGR but there are several arguments in favour of adopting abnormal morphometric indices as the criteria against which ultrasound parameters should be evaluated:

1. They provide quantitative measures of wasting and lack of fat, evidence that the neonate has suffered some degree of impaired growth in utero.
2. Ponderal index, MAC/HC ratio and skinfold thickness are superior to birthweight in predicting neonatal complications associated with IUGR (Walther & Raemaker, 1982; Patterson & Pouliot, 1987) and SGA infants with a low PI have a 5.7 fold increased risk of perinatal mortality compared with those with a normal ponderal index (Haas, Balcazor & Caulfield, 1987).
3. Neonatal reference standards for ponderal index, MAC/HC ratio and skinfold thickness exist.

Prediction of abnormal neonatal morphometry

Few studies have reported data on ultrasound measurements in the prediction of neonatal morphometry. The results of studies that have reported data relating to the prediction of a neonatal ponderal index < tenth centile are shown in Table 12.3. In high-risk women the highest sensitivity was achieved with a fetal ponderal index < tenth centile although the false positive rate was 64.3% (Vintzileos et al., 1986). One further study evaluated umbilical artery Doppler waveforms (Trudinger et al., 1991). Neonatal ponderal index was lower in fetuses with absent

Table 12.3. *Ultrasound measurements in the prediction of abnormal neonatal morphometry (ponderal index < 10th centile) subdivided by population studied*

Reference	Gestation (wk)	Ultrasound criteria	Se (%)	OR (95% CI)
High risk				
Ott (1985)	20–42	FL/AC > 23.0	51.5	2.8 (1.3, 6.2)
		FL/AC > 24.0	33.3	3.3 (1.4, 7.9)
Patterson et al. (1987)	II/III	Reduced AF diameter[a]	65.8	6.3 (1.6, 27.6)
Vintzileos et al. (1986)	26–40	Ponderal index < 10th centile[b]	76.9	14.7 (3.8, 72.1)
Low risk				
Weiner & Robinson (1989)	28–43	AC < 2.5th centile	81.8	7.7 (1.6, 38.1)
		EFW < 10th centile	36.4	3.3 (0.9, 13.0)
		HC/AC > 95th centile	16.7	2.2 (0.2, 21.4)
		FL/AC > 24.0	55.6	3.3 (0.8, 13.6)
Sijmons et al. (1989)	34	Umbilical artery PI > 1.46	19.4	4.5 (1.7, 12.0)
		Umbilical artery PI > 1.27	24.1	3.8 (1.5, 10.1)
Sarmandal & Grant[c] (1990)	34–36	AC < 25th centile	62.0	5.7 (2.5, 12.7)
		Ponderal index < 25th centile[b]	51.7	3.7 (1.7, 8.2)

[a] Average amniotic fluid diameter <3.2 cm, [b] EFW/FW^3, [c] Ponderal index or MAC/HC ratio < 10th centile.
Abbreviations: Se, sensitivity; OR, odds ratio; CI, confidence interval; FL, femur length; AC, abdominal circumference; AF, amniotic fluid; EFW, estimated fetal weight; ΔSDS, change in standard deviation score; MC, middle cerebral; PI, pulsability index; UA, umbilical artery.

end-diastolic frequencies compared to those with a normal S/D ratio but insufficient information was provided to construct contingency tables.

In low-risk women the highest sensitivity was obtained using an AC < 2.5th centile; however, this cut-off resulted in a false-positive rate of 80.8% (Weiner & Robinson, 1989). Increasing the antenatal cut-off to an AC < 25th centile reduced the sensitivity to 62%, although the false-positive rate remained high (72%) (Sarmandal & Grant, 1990). Comparable results were found for an AC < 25th centile for the prediction of MAC/HC < 10th centile (sensitivity 67%, OR 6.7) (Sarmandal & Grant, 1990). One further study has reported data on umbilical artery Doppler waveform indices although insufficient information was provided to construct contingency tables (Beattie & Dornan, 1989). Measurements at 28, 34 and 38 weeks of pregnancy did not predict IUGR (defined as either a low ponderal index, MAC/HC ratio or skinfold thickness).

Very limited data are available from serial ultrasound studies. Petersen et al. (1992) calculated fetal growth velocity in a group of 378 fetuses from a minimum of three measurements of EFW and weight at birth. Individual growth velocities were compared with gender-specific population curves and expressed as a standard deviation score per 28 days. Mean fetal growth velocity was significantly different in SGA infants (−0.32 [SD 0.33]) compared with appropriate-for-gestational age (−0.04 [0.32]) and large-for-gestational age (0.31 [0.37]) infants. Fetal growth velocity was related to ponderal index ($r = 0.40$, $p < 0.001$) and skinfold thickness ($r = 0.46$, $p < 0.001$) at birth. However the correlations disappeared when birthweight relative to gestational age was accounted for.

In an attempt to define whether serial measurements of fetal size are superior to isolated morphometric and Doppler measurements prior to delivery, the authors studied 104 small fetuses with an AC < 10th centile from the time of diagnosis until delivery (Chang et al., 1993*b*). The median gestational ages at the first and last scans were 220 days (range 182–270) and 269 days (range 238–294) respectively. Initial comparisons were carried out using receiver-operating characteristic (ROC) curves to determine which methods of quantifying serial measurements of EFW were the best predictors of IUGR (defined as a ponderal index, MAC/HC ratio and subscapular skinfold thickness more than 2SDs below the mean for gestational age). For all three neonatal indices, the area under the ROC curve was greatest using the change in standard deviation score (SDS) compared with either the quadratic *b*-coefficient or the fetal growth velocity, expressed in g/week (Chang, 1993). Comparable results were obtained for AC measurements.

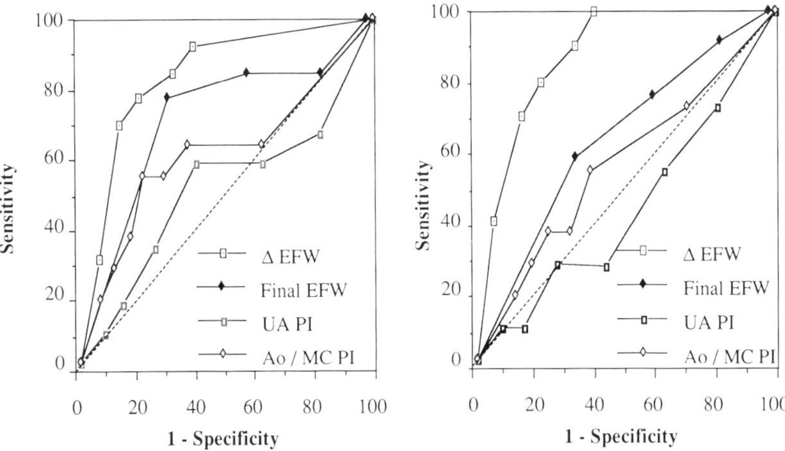

Fig. 12.4. Receiver-operating characteristic curves in the prediction of abnormal neonatal ponderal index (*left*) and mid-arm circumference/head circumference ratio (*right*). Abbreviations: ΔEFW, change in standard deviation score of estimated fetal weight; UA, umbilical artery; Ao, aortic; MC, middle cerebral; PI, pulsatility index.

The ROC curves for change in EFW (expressed as SDS), final EFW, umbilical artery Doppler PI and the aortic/middle cerebral artery Doppler PI ratio in the prediction of an abnormal ponderal index and MAC/HC ratio are shown in Fig. 12.4. For both neonatal indices, the best antenatal predictor, as determined by the area under the ROC curve, was the change in EFW (Chang et al., 1993*b*). Furthermore the optimal cut-off for EFW, defined from the ROC curve as the point closest to a sensitivity of 100% and (l-specificity) of 0%, was found to be change in SDS of ≥ -1.5. Adoption of this cut-off led to the detection of 76.9% of babies with an abnormal ponderal index with a specificity of 80.3% and an OR of 13.6 [95% CI 3.3, 56.2]. Comparable values for an abnormal MAC/HC ratio were 80%, 78.5%, 14.6 [95% CI 2.8, 76.5].

The results suggest that serial measurement of EFW, and to a lesser extent AC, during the third trimester can be used to predict IUGR. These measurements are superior to single estimates of fetal size prior to delivery, morphometric ratios and umbilical artery Doppler.

Does antenatal detection of IUGR predict perinatal outcome?

Randomized trials of ultrasound during pregnancy have not addressed the value of serial measurements of fetal size. Danielian, Allman and

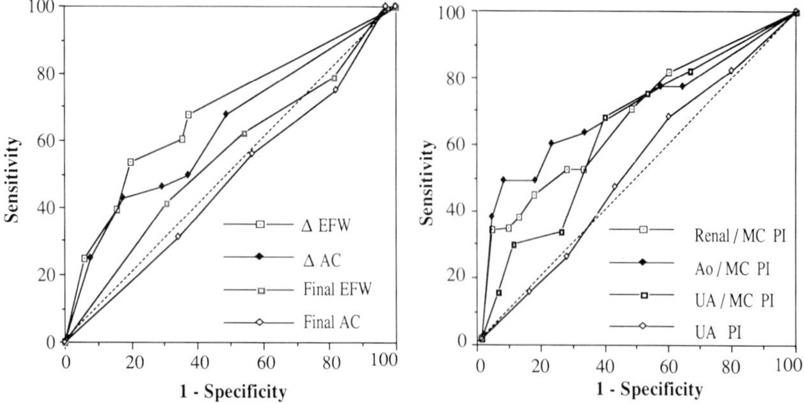

Fig. 12.5. Receiver-operating characteristic curves in the prediction of suboptimal perinatal outcome (see text for definition) using (*left*) estimated fetal weight (EFW) and abdominal circumference (AC) and (right) Doppler waveform indices. Abbreviations: ΔEFW, change in standard deviation score of EFW; ΔAC, change in standard deviation score of AC; MC middle cerebral; Ao, aortic; UA, umbilical artery; PI, pulsatility index.

Steer (1992) measured EFW between 28 and 34 weeks gestation in 197 fetuses. Actual and expected birthweight, calculated from a projection of EFW, were then compared; the authors found that a difference of greater than 5% was associated with a significantly increased incidence of cardiotocographic abnormalities and need for operative delivery. This was the first study to assess the relation between change in size and perinatal outcome, although serial ultrasound measurements were not performed.

In the same group of 104 small fetuses discussed above, we compared the ability of serial measurements of EFW and AC, expressed as SDS, with predelivery measurements of fetal size and Doppler measurements from the umbilical and fetal arteries to predict suboptimal perinatal outcome at term (Chang et al., 1994). Suboptimal outcome included acidaemia at birth (umbilical arterial pH < tenth centile), fetal distress requiring emergency Caesarean section, and admission to the neonatal intensive care unit with complications related to IUGR (hypoglycaemia, necrotizing enterocolitis, and neurological abnormalities). Ultrasound parameters were again compared using the area under the ROC curve (Fig. 12.5). Changes in EFW and AC, together with the predelivery Doppler ratios reflecting cardiovascular redistribution (renal/middle cerebral PI and aortic/middle cerebral PI) were significantly better predictors of suboptimal perinatal outcome than predelivery size and umbilical artery PI. However, the sensitivities and ORs were low; for change in EFW, using a SDS cut-off of $\geqslant -1.5$, the sensitivity was 54%, specificity 81% and OR 3.6 [95% CI 1.3–9.5]. It is important to emphasize that there were no perinatal deaths in this group of small babies delivered at term. There is an urgent need for much larger studies to address the value of serial measurements in the prediction of perinatal mortality.

Conclusions

Ultrasound has been reported to be useful in the diagnosis of IUGR. However, most of the parameters reported have been assessed in their ability to predict SGA at birth. Measurements of AC and EFW appear to be the most reliable indicators of a small fetus although this knowledge does not appear to improve perinatal mortality. This is perhaps not surprising as most SGA babies are constitutionally small and have not suffered pathological growth retardation. Serial measurements of fetal size can be used to assess growth, although the most appropriate method of quantifying changes remains to be determined. Individual measurements of AC or EFW can be expressed as standard deviation scores from the population mean. The simple method is superior to isolated measurements of fetal size in predicting wasting at birth and perinatal morbidity. Future work needs to address the value of serial ultrasound measurements and fetal Doppler waveforms in the prevention of perinatal death.

References

Adelstein, P. & Fedrick, J. (1978). Antenatal identification of women at increased risk of being delivered of a low birth weight infant at term. *British Journal of Obstetrics and Gynaecology*, **85**, 8–12.

Altman, D.G. & Chitty, L.S. (1994). Charts of fetal size: 1. Methodology. *British Journal of Obstetrics and Gynaecology*, **101**, 29–34.

Bakketeig, L.S., Jacobsen, G., Brodtkorb, C., Eriksen, B.C., Eik-Nes, S.H., Ulstein, M.P. & Jorgansen, N.P. (1984). Randomized controlled trial of ultrasonographic screening in pregnancy. *Lancet,* **ii**, 207–10.

Beattie, R.B. & Dornan, J.C. (1989). Antenatal screening for intrauterine growth retardation with umbilical artery Doppler ultrasonography. *British Medical Journal*, **298**, 631–35.

Bower, S., Schuchter, K.& Campbell, S. (1993). Doppler ultrasound screening as part of routine antenatal screening: prediction of pre-eclampsia and intrauterine growth retardation. *British Journal of Obstetrics and Gynaecology*, **100**, 989–94.

Campbell, S. & Thoms, A. (1977). Ultrasound measurement of the fetal head to abdomen circumference ratio in the assessment of growth retardation. *British Journal of Obstetrics and Gynaecology*, **84**, 165–70.

Chang, T.C., Robson, S.C., Spencer, J.A.D. & Gallivan, S. (1992*a*). Fetal growth: a comparison between Bangladeshi and Caucasian women. *British Journal of Obstetrics and Gynaecology*, **99**, 1027–8.

Chang, T.C. (1993). Diagnosis of growth retardation in small fetuses: serial ultrasound assessment of abdominal circumference and fetal weight. MD Thesis, University of London.

Chang, T.C., Robson, S.C., Boys, R.J.& Spencer, J.A.D. (1992*b*). Prediction of the small-for-gestational age baby; which ultrasound measurement is best? *Obstetrics and Gynecology*, **80**, 1030–38.

Chang, T.C., Robson, S.C., Spencer, J.A.D.& Gallivan, S. (1993*a*). Ultrasonic fetal weight estimation: analysis of inter- and intra-observer variability. *Journal of Clinical Ultrasound*, **21**, 515–19.

Chang, T.C., Robson, S.C., Spencer, J.A.D. & Gallivan, S. (1993*b*). Identification of fetal growth retardation: comparison of Doppler waveform indices and serial ultrasound measurements of abdominal circumference and fetal weight. *Obstetrics and Gynecology*, **82**, 230–6.

Chang, T.C., Robson, S.C., Spencer, J.A.D.& Gallivan, S. (1994). Prediction of perinatal morbidity at term in small fetuses: comparison of fetal growth and Doppler ultrasound. *British Journal of Obstetrics and Gynaecology*, **101**, 422–7.

Chard, T. (1989). Hormonal control of growth in the human fetus. *Journal of Endocrinology*, **123**, 3–9.

Chitty, L.S., Altman, D.G., Henderson, A.& Campbell, S. (1994*a*). Charts of fetal size: 2. Head measurements. *British Journal of Obstetrics and Gynaecology*, **101**, 35–43.

Chitty, L.S., Altman, D.G., Henderson, A.& Campbell, S. (1994*b*). Charts of fetal size: 4. Femur length. *British Journal of Obstetrics and Gynaecology*, **101**, 132–5.

Danielian, P.J., Allman, A.C.J.& Steer, P.J. (1992). Is obstetric and neonatal outcome worse in fetuses who fail to reach their own growth potential? *British Journal of Obstetrics and Gynaecology*, **99**, 452–4.

Daya, S. (1993). Accuracy of gestational age estimation by means of fetal crown–rump length measurement. *American Journal of Obstetrics & Gynecology*, **168**, 903–8.

Deter, R.L. & Harrist, R.B. (1992). Growth standards for anatomic measurements and growth rates derived from longitudinal studies of normal fetal growth. *Journal of Clinical Ultrasound*, **20**, 381–8.

Deter, R.L., Harrist, R.B., Hadlock, F.P. & Pointdexter, A.N. (1982). Longitudinal studies of fetal growth with the use of dynamic image ultrasonography. *American Journal of Obstetrics and Gynecology*, **143**, 545–54.

Divon, M.Y., Chamberlain, P.F., Sipos, L., Manning, F.A.& Platt, L.D. (1986). Identification of the small for gestational age fetus with the use of gestational-age independent indices of fetal growth. *American Journal of Obstetrics and Gynecology*, **155**, 1197–201.

Eik-Nes, S.H., Okland, O., Aure, J.C.& Ulstein, M. (1984). Ultrasound screening in pregnancy: A randomised controlled trial. *Lancet*, **i**, 1347.

Fescina, R.H., Ucieda, F.J., Cordano, M.C., Nieto, F., Fenzer, S.M.& Lopez, R. (1982). Ultrasonic patterns of intrauterine growth in a Latin American country. *Early Human Development*, **6**, 239–42.

Gallivan, S., Robson, S.C., Chang, T.C., Vaughan, J.& Spencer, J.A.D. (1993). An investigation of fetal growth using serial ultrasound data. *Ultrasound in Obstetrics and Gynaecology*, **3**, 109–14.

Geirsson, R.T. (1991). Ultrasound instead of last menstrual period as the basis of gestational age assignment. *Ultrasound in Obstetrics and Gynaecology*, **1**, 212–19.

Geirsson, R.T., Ogston, S.A., Patel, N.A.& Christie, A.D. (1985). Growth of total intrauterine, intra-amniotic and placental volume in normal singleton pregnancy measured by ultrasound. *British Journal of Obstetrics and Gynaecology*, **92**, 46–53.

Grannum, P.A.T., Berkowitz, R.L.& Hobbins, J.C. (1979). The ultrasonic changes in the maturing placenta and their relation to fetal pulmonary maturity. *American Journal of Obstetrics and Gynecology*, **133**, 915–19.

Haas, J., Balcazor, H.& Caulfield, L. (1987). Variation in early neonatal mortality for different types of fetal growth retardation. *American Journal of Physical Anthropology*, **73**, 467–73.

Hadlock, F.P., Deter, R.L., Harrist, R.B., Roecker, E. & Park, S.K. (1983). A date-independent predictor of intrauterine growth retardation: femur length/adbominal circumference ratio. *American Journal of Roentgenology*, **141**, 979–84.

Hadlock, F.P., Harrist, R.B., Sharman, R.S., Deter, R.L.& Park, S.K. (1985). Estimation of fetal weight with the use of head, body, and femur measurements – A prospective study. *American Journal of Obstetrics and Gynecology*, **151**, 333–7.

Hill, L.M., Guzick, D., Thomas, M.L., Kislak, S.L., Hixson, J.L.& Peterson, C.S. (1989). Thigh circumference in the detection of intrauterine growth retardation. *American Journal of Perinatology*, **6**, 349–52.

Larsen, T., Larsen, J.F., Petersen, S. & Greisen, G. (1992). Detection of small-for-gestational age fetuses by ultrasound screening in a high risk population: a randomized controlled study. *British Journal of Obstetrics and Gynaecology*, **99**, 469–74.

Larsen, T., Petersen, S., Greisen, G.& Larsen, J.F. (1990). Normal fetal growth evaluated by longitudinal ultrasound examinations. *Early Human Development*, **24**, 37–45.

Low, J.A. (1991). The current status of maternal and fetal blood flow velocimetry. *American Journal of Obstetrics and Gynecology*, **164**, 1049–63.

Moore, T.R. (1990). Superiority of the four-quadrant sum over the single-deepest-pocket technique in ultrasonographic identification of abnormal amniotic fluid volumes. *American Journal of Obstetrics and Gynecology*, **163**, 762–7.

Neilson, J.P., Munjaja, S.P. & Whitfield, C.R. (1984). Screening for small-for-dates fetuses: a controlled trial. *British Medical Journal*, **289**, 1179–82.

Ott, W.J. (1985). Fetal femur length, neonatal crown-heel length, and screening for intrauterine growth retardation. *Obstetrics and Gynecology*, **65**, 460–4.

Patterson, R.M. & Pouliot, R.N. (1987). Neonatal morphometrics and perinatal outcome: who is growth retarded? *American Journal of Obstetrics and Gynecology*, **157**, 691–3.

Patterson, R.M., Prihoda, T.J.& Pouliot, M.R. (1987). Sonographic amniotic fluid measurement and fetal growth retardation: a reappraisal. *American Journal of Obstetrics and Gynecology*, **157**, 406–10.

Pearce, J.M., Campbell, S., Cohen-Overbeek, T., Hackett, G., Hernandez, J.& Royston, J.P. (1988). Reference ranges and sources of variation for indices of pulsed Doppler flow velocity waveforms from the uteroplacental and fetal circulation. *British Journal of Obstetrics and Gynaecology*, **95**, 248–56.

Petersen, S., Gotfredsen, A. & Knudsen, F.U. (1988). Lean body mass in small-for-gestational age and appropriate-for-gestational age infants. *Journal of Pediatrics*, **113**, 886–9.

Petersen, S., Larsen, T. & Greisen, G. (1992). Judging fetal growth from body proportions at birth. *Early Human Development*, **30**, 139–46.

Robson, S.C., Gallivan, S., Walkinshaw, S.A., Vaughan, J.& Rodeck, C.H. (1993). Ultrasonic estimation of fetal weight: use of targeted formulas in small for gestational age fetuses. *Obstetrics and Gynecology*, **82**, 359–64.

Rossavik, I.K. & Deter, R.L. (1984). Mathematical modelling of fetal growth: I. Basic principles. *Journal of Clinical Ultrasound*, **12**, 529–33.

Sabbagha, R.E., Minogue, J., Tamura, R.K. & Hungerford, S.A. (1989). Estimation of birth weight by use of ultrasonographic formulas targeted to large- , appropriate- , and small-for-gestational age fetuses. *American Journal of Obstetrics and Gynecology*, **160**, 854–62.

Sarmandal, P. & Grant, J.M. (1990). Effectiveness of ultrasound determination of fetal abdominal circumference and fetal ponderal index in the diagnosis of asymmetrical growth retardation. *British Journal of Obstetrics and Gynaecology*, **97**, 118–23.

Secher, N.J., Hansen, P.K., Lenstrup, C., Eriksen, P.S., Thomsen, B.L. & Keiding, N. (1987). On the evaluation of routine ultrasound sereening in the third trimester for the detection of light for gestational age infants. *Acta Obstetrica Gynecologica Scandinavica*, **66**, 463–71.

Shepard, M.J., Richards, V.A., Berkowitz, R.L., Warsof, S.L. & Hobbins, J.C. (1982). An evaluation of two equations for predicting fetal weight by ultrasound. *American Journal of Obstetrics and Gynecology*, **142**, 47–54.

Sijmons, E.A., Reuwer, P.J.H.M., van Beek, E. & Bruinse, H.W. (1989). The validity of screening for small-for-gestational age and low-weight-for-length infants by Doppler ultrasound. *British Journal of Obstetrics and Gynaecology*, **96**, 557–61.

Simon, N.V., Deter, R.L., Shearer, D.M. & Levinsky, J.S. (1989). Prediction of normal fetal growth by the Rossavik growth model using two scans before 27 weeks, menstrual age. *Journal of Clinical Ultrasound*, **17**, 237–43.

Simon, N.V., Levisky, J.S., Shearer, D.M., O'Lear, M.S. & Flood, J.T. (1987). Influence of fetal growth patterns on sonographic estimation of fetal weight. *Journal of Clinical Ultrasound*, **15**, 376–83.

Thomson, A.M., Billewicz, W.Z. & Hytten, F.E. (1968). The assessment of fetal growth. *Journal of Obstetrics and Gynaecology of the British Commonwealth*, **75**, 903–16.

Trudinger, B.J., Cook, C.M., Jones, L. & Giles, W.B. (1991). A comparison of fetal heart rate monitoring and umbilical artery waveforms in the recognition of fetal compromise. *British Journal of Obstetrics and Gynaecology*, **98**, 378–84.

Vintzileos, A.M., Lodeiro, J.G., Feinstein, S.J., Campbell, W.A., Weinbaum, P.J. & Nochimson, D.J. (1986). Value of fetal ponderal index in predicting growth retardation. *Obstetrics and Gynecology*, **67**, 584–8.

Walther, F.J. & Raemaker, L.H.J. (1982). The ponderal index as a measure of the nutritional status at birth and its relation to some aspects of neonatal morbidity. *Journal of Perinatal Medicine*, **10**, 42–7.

Weiner, C.P. & Robinson, D. (1989). Sonographic diagnosis of intrauterine growth retardation using postnatal ponderal index and the crown–heel length as standards of diagnosis. *American Journal of Perinatology*, **6**, 380–3.

13

Assessment of fetal well-being in growth-retarded fetuses

GERARD H.A. VISSER

Introduction

At present, there are many ways of assessing fetal health. When comparing the various tests it becomes obvious that no one is superior, but that all contribute to a better understanding of the actual fetal condition. Combination of tests, therefore, gives more information than relying solely on one assessment technique. When interpreting the test results, it is possible to combine them into one scoring result (biophysical profile score; 'Apgar score' in utero) or to analyse them separately and to relate the individual results to the stage in the process of deterioration of the fetal conditon. The latter procedure is more informative than a combined score, especially in intrauterine growth retardation (IUGR) in which there is a specific sequence of changes occurring with respect to the various assessment tests.

In this chapter the diagnostic value of the various (non-invasive) assessment techniques is discussed in the light of pathophysiological changes occurring with progressive deterioration of the condition of the IUGR fetus. Special attention is paid to the issue of whether changes in biophysical variables are a sign of fetal adapatation or of organ damage. The interpretation of some of the tests is discussed. Finally, the question as to the timing of delivery of the IUGR fetus is addressed.

Changes in blood velocity waveforms, fetal movements, amniotic fluid volume and fetal heart rate patterns

Figure 13.1 shows the rank order in which changes occur in the various assessment tests, with progressive deterioration of the condition of the IUGR fetus. This rank order is based on longitudinal and cross-sectional

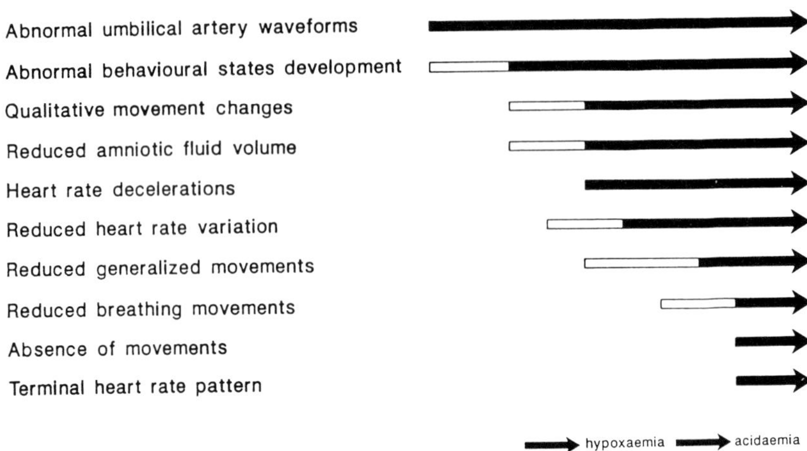

Fig. 13.1. Suggested rank ordering in which blood velocity waveforms, amniotic fluid volume, movements and heart rate changes occur in growth-retarded human fetuses with progressive deterioration of the fetal condition. Interfetal variation in first occurrence of an abnormal test result is indicated by the open part of the arrow.

studies in which fetal parameters were related to blood gases at cordocentesis or Caesarean section. The ordering shown applies to the population of IUGR fetuses and individual fetuses may show different patterns. The individual papers that have resulted in the rank ordering have been reviewed before (Visser, 1991). In this chapter only the conclusions and interpretations are emphasized.

From Fig. 13.1 we can see that abnormal Doppler waveform patterns of the umbilical artery (and of fetal vessels) are usually the first signs of fetal deterioration. They reflect inadequate growth of the placenta and are most likely to be an indication of increased impedance to blood flow. Abnormal Doppler waveforms occur before the onset of fetal hypoxaemia. Since abnormal Doppler waveforms occur rather early in the process of deterioration, this technique has been shown to be useful in a risk population for identifying fetuses at risk of becoming hypoxaemic (e.g. Omtzigt, Reuwer & Bruinse, 1994) and to distinguish 'low-risk' small-for-gestational age fetuses from IUGR fetuses (Beattie & Dornan, 1989).

FHR abnormalities coincide with the occurrence of fetal hypoxaemia. This holds both for a reduction of FHR variation below the normal range and for the occurrence of late FHR decelerations (Bekedam et al., 1987; Visser, Sadovsky & Nicolaides, 1990). In the weeks preceding the onset of FHR abnormalities (and fetal hypoxaemia) FHR variation usually

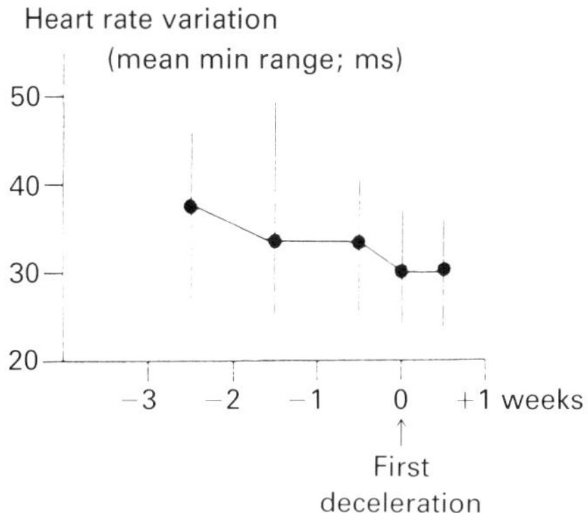

Fig. 13.2. Fetal heart rate (FHR) variation (median and interquartile range; expressed as mean minute range, in ms) in IUGR fetuses followed longitudinally. On average, FHR variation fell below the norm (30 ms) at the same time as decelerations occurred. (Reproduced with permission from Snijders et al., 1992.)

gradually decreases (Snijders et al., 1992) (Fig. 13.2); longitudinal FHR recordings may, therefore, give an indication of gradual deterioration of the fetal condition, even before the onset of hypoxaemia. However, a single recording will not identify the small fetus at risk of becoming hypoxaemic, since FHR variation is still within the normal range. This indicates that antenatal FHR monitoring is not a useful screening test. It should be applied longitudinally in a high-risk population. The best indication for FHR monitoring is the IUGR fetus with abnormal Doppler waveform patterns, in whom hypoxaemia is likely to occur in due course.

In IUGR fetuses the interval between first abnormal Doppler finding and the onset of FHR abnormalities/hypoxaemia differs considerably. This interval is shorter in late than in early gestation and also shorter in IUGR complicated by pre-eclampsia than in IUGR without pre-eclampsia (Bekedam et al., 1990; Arduini, Rizzo & Romanini, 1993) (Fig. 13.3). Apparently, a tiny fetus in early gestation can cope with a reduced placental supply for much longer than a bigger IUGR fetus later in pregnancy. This seems logical, taking into account the higher oxygen demand in the latter case. In line with these findings is the fact that, in early gestation, fetuses can survive for a considerable time in utero with absent end-diastolic velocities in the umbilical artery, whereas during the later part of pregnancy FHR abnormalities usually occur when end-diastolic velocities are still present. From these findings, one may also conclude that in pre-eclampsia deterioration of the placental function

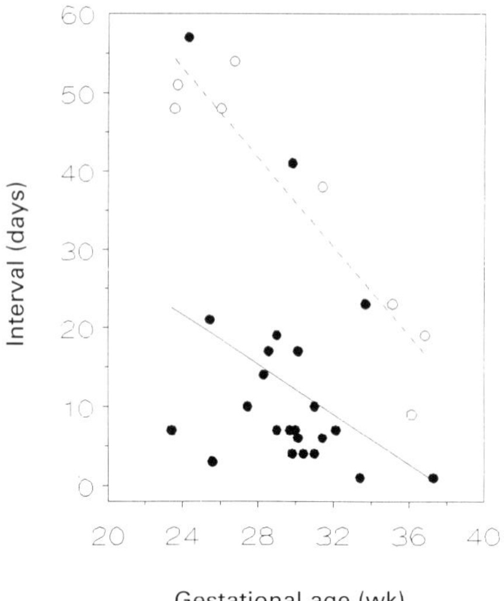

Fig. 13.3. Interval between first abnormal blood velocity waveform pattern in the umbilical artery and the occurrence of FHR abnormalities in IUGR fetuses followed longitudinally. Open dots: pre-eclampsia, closed dots: no hypertensive disease. (Unpublished data from our institute: Pal, R., Reuwer, P.J.H.M., Bruinse, H.W., Bekedam, D.J. & Visser, G.H.A.)

occurs more rapidly than in IUGR fetuses without pre-eclampsia. Clinically, these data imply that, once Doppler waveforms become abnormal, FHR monitoring should be especially frequent beyond 30 weeks and/or in the case of pre-eclampsia.

Disturbances in the development of fetal behavioural (sleep) states usually precede occurrence of FHR abnormalities and the same holds for abnormalities in the quality of fetal movements (monotonous, reduced speed and amplitude) (Van Vliet et al., 1985; Sival, Visser & Prechtl, 1992). This indicates that in IUGR fetuses these disturbances in development of the fetal nervous system are more likely to be the result of chronic malnutrition rather than merely the result of hypoxaemia. This is in line with data obtained by cordocentesis, which show that hypoglycaemia and deprivation of essential amino acids precede the occurrence of hypoxaemia.

In IUGR fetuses oligohydramnios is most likely to be due to a reduced renal blood flow (due to blood flow redistribution) and decreased urine output (Arduini & Rizzo, 1991). In most third-trimester IUGR fetuses oligohydramnios occurs before the onset of FHR abnormalities (and hypoxaemia) (Ribbert et al., 1993). Therefore, its occurrence is an important finding which warrants intensive fetal monitoring. However, before 32 weeks of gestation, oligohydramnios usually occurs after the onset of FHR abnormalities (Ribbert et al., 1990, 1993). Data from immature sheep fetuses indicate that induced hypoxaemia does not result in a decrease of blood flow to the kidneys (Iwamoto et al., 1989); this is in contrast to findings in term fetuses. Relative immaturity in chemoreceptor functioning and in adaptation might explain this difference.

The incidence of fetal movements usually only falls below the normal range after the occurrence of FHR abnormalities and this reduction is associated with (impending) acidaemia (Ribbert et al., 1990, 1993). In IUGR fetuses a reduction in movements is therefore a late sign of compromise, and quantification of fetal movements is of restricted value. From subjective fetal movement records kept by pregnant women, it is also known that, before the sudden decline in movements which may indicate impending fetal death, the movement incidence is still within the normal range (Sadovsky, Yaffe & Polishuk, 1974; Pearson & Weaver, 1976). Recording of movements by pregnant women ('kick chart') does not have a high sensitivity or specificity with regards to fetal compromise or otherwise; however, it is cheap and may identify the small and compromised fetus, who was not identified by normal prenatal care.

Do we identify fetal adaptation or organ damage?

Fetal movements consume significant amounts of oxygen. In fetal sheep, oxygen consumption fell by 17% after neuromuscular blockade (Rurak & Gruber, 1983) and PO_2 values rose by a similar percentage (Nathanielsz, Yu & Calabum, 1982; Rurak & Gruber, 1983). Reduction of fetal movements when oxygen supply is limited therefore aids in maximizing delivery of oxygen to vital organs. Such a reduction can be considered as adaptation. This adaptation can be nicely seen from longitudinal records made in IUGR fetuses (Ribbert et al., 1993) (Fig. 13.4). In these fetuses, heart rate variation gradually decreases until it reaches the lower limit of the normal range, i.e. until the fetuses are likely to have become hypoxaemic. Thereafter, FHR variation usually remains constant for a certain period of time, but body movements are reduced in incidence. In other words, it seems likely that the fetal PO_2 is maintained over a certain period by the reduction of the body movements. Finally, FHR variation is

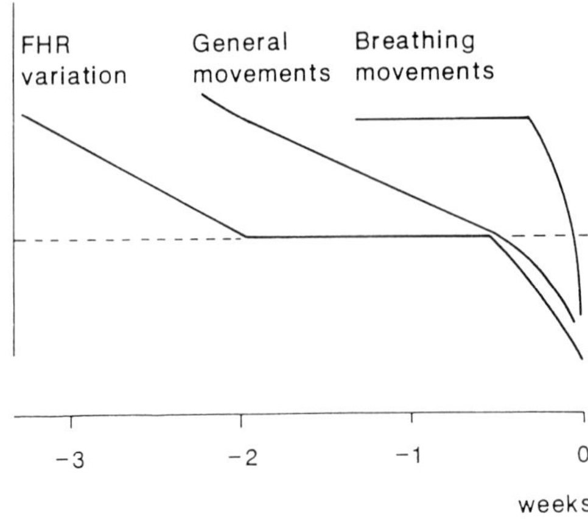

Fig. 13.4. Diagram of the time-related changes in % of fetal general movements, breathing movements and FHR variation with progressive deterioration of the fetal condition. Broken line represents lower limit of normal range for the biophysical variables studied. (Data extracted from the longitudinal study of Ribbert et al., 1993.)

reduced further and body and also breathing movements disappear: the fetus becomes progressively hypoxaemic and acidaemic.

Redistribution of blood to organs such as the heart and brain may also be considered as adaptation. Redistribution has been demonstrated to occur in hypoxaemic conditions in fetal sheep (Peeters et al., 1979; Goetzman, Itskovitz & Rudolph, 1984). In human IUGR fetuses, redistribution of blood in favour of the brain has been suggested by blood flow-velocity waveform studies (Wladimiroff, Tonge & Stewart, 1986; Arduini et al., 1988). Both in humans and in sheep this adaptation can be reversed by maternal hyperoxygenation (Goetzman et al., 1984; Arduini et al., 1988). The reduction in amniotic fluid volume may, at least in part, be considered as a consequence of redistribution of blood flow.

The usefulness of reduction of movements and of blood flow redistribution has been demonstrated nicely by an experiment in which oxygen was administered to women carrying an IUGR fetus (Bekedam et al., 1991). During hyperoxygenation, fetal movements and heart rate variation increased. However, after discontinuation of oxygen there was a temporary impairment of the fetal heart rate pattern with an increase of heart rate decelerations. The increase in movements (and oxygen demand) and possibly a reversal of blood redistribution are likely to have caused this impairment. In the clinical situation this implies that when oxygen administration is considered as a 'treatment', it should be administered continuously without interruption.

Movements and heart rate accelerations are linked together. A reduction in the size and number of accelerations – and, therefore, of heart rate variation – as a consequence of a reduction of fetal movements fits the concept of adaptation. It is hard, however, to consider the occurrence of late heart rate decelerations as a sign of adaptation. It is more likely that they are just signs of fetal hypoxaemia. There are only a few studies concerning the relationship between antepartum heart rate abnormalities and neurological outcome. In all, however, a definite relationship between heart rate decelerations and neurological morbidity was found (see Visser, 1988). This stresses the impact of prenatal hypoxaemia on brain development. In IUGR fetuses hypoxaemia is associated with chronic hypoglycaemia and deprivation of essential amino acids (Soothill, Nicolaides & Campbell, 1987; Economides et al., 1989). In these fetuses brain damage is, therefore, more likely to be due to chronic malnutrition (including hypoxaemia), rather than simply to hypoxaemia. This reasoning can to a large extent be supported by the morphological findings in human IUGR fetuses (Dobbing, 1974) and in animal models (Bedi, 1984), where a smaller brain size, fewer cells, deficits in synapse-to-neurone ratios and reduced dendritic growth are found, rather than distinct localized lesions. The latter are often found after (acute) asphyxia. In IUGR fetuses the occurrence of antepartum decelerations might be considered as a sign of chronic malnutrition, a sign related to impaired brain development.

The abnormal quality of fetal movements and the disturbance in the development of behavioural states are also likely to be indicators of impaired development, rather than signs of adaptation. They already occur before the development of evident hypoxaemia and have also been described in growth-retarded newborn infants in whom the metabolic state was restored and adequate (Michaelis, Schulte & Nolte, 1971; Schulte, Schremf & Hinze, 1971; Sival et al., 1992). This suggests that impairment of neurological development occurs before hypoxaemia develops.

Interpretation of the antenatal assessment tests

With the interpretation of antenatal test results I restrict myself to the most widely used tests, i.e. Doppler recording of the umbilical artery flow–velocity waveform, FHR monitoring and assessment of the biophysical profile score. Since cordocentesis is also promoted in the management of the IUGR fetus, some remarks will be made on the (restricted) value of this invasive technique.

Doppler recordings of the umbilical artery

Flow velocity waveform patterns in the umbilical artery are abnormal if there is a decrease in end-diastolic velocities. This probably reflects increased downstream resistance. It may be quantified by relating the peak systolic velocities to the end-diastolic velocities (A/B ratio), or by calculating the pulsatility index ($V_{max} - V_{min}/V_{mean}$). During the course of normal pregnancy (and growth of the placenta), the flow velocity during diastole increases, which results in a decrease of the pulsatility index (PI). Abnormal waveform patterns may be classified into three categories:

1. present but decreased end-diastolic velocities (PI > 2 SD above mean for gestation),
2. flow velocities absent during end-diastole, and
3. reversed velocities (and blood flow) during diastole.

The first category is the most benign situation and also includes some false positive cases (especially in the case of a low fetal heart rate); confirmation is therefore necessary. The second category will almost invariably result in FHR abnormalities, which may already be present at the first occurrence of absent end-diastolic blood flow. The third category indicates poor fetal condition. Reversed end-diastolic velocities may be due to a further increase in placental vascular resistance; however, in my opinion it is more likely that this severe waveform abnormality is due to cardiac failure, since cardiac contractility decreases concomitantly (De Vore, 1988), FHR patterns become 'terminal' (which is indicative of myocardial hypoxaemia) and hence outcome is poor.

Normal Doppler findings in small-for-gestational age fetuses are reassuring and usually indicate that the growth delay is not due to an insufficient feto-placental exchange. However, near-term FHR abnormalities sometimes precede Doppler abnormalities; a normal Doppler pattern in the umbilical artery in a small near-term fetus does therefore not exclude forthcoming impairment.

Antenatal FHR monitoring

There are four randomized trials in which the effects of antenatal FHR monitoring have been investigated in high-risk pregnancies (see Mohide & Keirse, 1989). All four trials are from the 1970s/early 1980s and have a relatively small size. Meta-analysis showed no positive predictive effects for perinatal death or poor condition at or after birth. Do these data imply that antenatal FHR monitoring is of no use, despite the fact that earlier in this chapter it was stated that with FHR monitoring fetal hypoxaemia/acidaemia or otherwise could reliably be assessed? An answer to this question is not easy. In my opinion the lack of any benefit of FHR, as found in the randomized trials, indicates that proper knowledge of FHR patterns, both normal and abnormal, is required before any benefit will emerge. In the 1980s such knowledge was still largely absent and it may well be that possible beneficial effects were counterbalanced by inappropriate interpretations and actions.

Knowledge essential for adequate interpretation of FHR patterns includes among others the following aspects:

1. Gestational changes. In the course of normal pregnancy FHR variation increases and accelerations become larger in size. Accelerations of more than 15 beats per minute, generally thought to indicate fetal well-being, are not a consistent phenomenon before 35 weeks of gestation. Before 30 weeks, small decelerations are even more numerous than accelerations. The small size of the accelerations and the frequently occurring decelerations make the FHR pattern difficult to interpret between 26 and 30 weeks (Visser, Dawes & Redman, 1981).
2. Development of fetal rest–activity cycles and behavioural states. From about 28 weeks onwards there is a progressive patterning of FHR into episodes of low and high heart rate variation. These patterns are related to the developing sleep states, with episodes of low variation corresponding to quiet (non-REM) sleep. When interpreting FHR and movement recordings, the presence of these rest–activity cycles has to be taken into account. During a normal quiet sleep episode, movements may be absent and the FHR pattern may be more or less flat ('non-reactive') for up to 40 minutes near term, and for up to 30 minutes earlier during the third trimester (Visser et al., 1981; Nijhuis et al., 1982).
3. Fetal reactions following external stimulation. Since a flat FHR pattern may indicate quiet sleep but also poor fetal health, all kinds of

stimuli have been applied in an effort to 'arouse' the fetus. However, it has been shown that widely used stimuli such as shaking of the maternal abdomen and application of sound at close distance from the abdomen do not change fetal heart rate or quiet sleep. Fetuses do react to vibro-acoustic stimulation; however, the reactions are sometimes so excessive that it is unclear if this test should be employed (for review, see Visser, 1991).

4. Effects of drugs. Sedative drugs reduce FHR variation, but also other medication may have effects. For instance, it has recently been shown that betamethasone, given to enhance fetal lung maturation, temporarily reduces FHR variation by about 30%, fetal body movements by 50% and fetal breathing movements by almost 100%. This effect lasts about 3 days. Dexamethasone may not have such effects (at least not on FHR variation) (Derks, Mulder & Visser, 1995).

FHR patterns may be assessed visually and recently also by numerical analysis. Computer analysis is to be preferred since inter- and intra-observer variation hamper the former. However, up to now, most FHR patterns are still assessed by eye. There are two visual classification methods: one in which the different aspects are analysed separately and given a score, whereafter the total score (usually 0–10, like the Apgar score) is used to quantify the FHR pattern. The second classification is more global and descriptive and describes the total pattern. One of the latter classifications, extensively evaluated in clinical research, will be described (Visser et al., 1980; Bekedam et al., 1987; Visser et al., 1990).

Classification of the FHR pattern into normal, flat (or non-reactive), decelerative and 'terminal' is as follows:

1. Normal (reactive) FHR pattern: basal heart rate between 110 and 160 beats per minute, bandwidth > 10 beats per minute, frequent accelerations, absence of (late) FHR decelerations and flat episodes (without accelerations) lasting < 45 minutes. Interpretation: no signs of fetal hypoxaemia at the time of recording.
2. Flat (non-reactive) FHR pattern: bandwidth < 10 beats per minute, no accelerations and no decelerations for more than 45 minutes. This heart rate pattern is difficult to interpret: prolonged episode of quiet sleep in a healthy fetus?, fetal hypoxaemia/acidaemia?, effects of drugs?, congenital or acquired fetal brain abnormality? Advice: repeat recording and perform additional examinations (ultrasound, Doppler, fetal movements).

3. Decelerative FHR pattern: isolated or repetitive late or variable decelerations (not following each Braxton Hicks contraction), with FHR variability during the decelerations, small accelerations and reduced overall variability. Interpretation: periodic hypoxaemia, usually not yet acidaemia.
4. Terminal FHR pattern: completely flat with late decelerations (usually shallow) after each Braxton Hicks contraction. Interpretation: hypoxaemia and acidaemia.

It has taken Dawes and Redman almost 10 years to develop a computer program that analyses the different aspects of the antenatal FHR pattern (Dawes, Redman & Smith, 1985). Assessment of the basal heart rate, from which FHR variation, accelerations and decelerations are calculated, appeared to be the most difficult problem. Computer analysis of FHR patterns has several advantages: it is objective, reproducible, can be used for trend analysis and facilitates exchange of data between centres. Data on FHR variation are clinically of greatest value.

Biophysical profile score (BPS)

The biophysical profile includes several variables known to be important with respect to the assessment of the fetal condition: fetal heart rate variation, amount of amniotic fluid, fetal breathing and body movements and fetal tone. The advantage of the BPS is that several variables are assessed. Combination of these variables into a single score obscures, however, the underlying abnormality. For instance, reduced amniotic fluid volume and absence of breathing movements (score 6) may clinically have different implications than presence of heart rate decelerations with a reduced amniotic fluid volume (score also 6). Some of the variables of the BPS change early in the process of deterioration of the fetal condition (amniotic fluid volume, FHR pattern), others change later. The BPS correlates well with the fetal pH, as determined by cordocentesis (Ribbert et al., 1990). It is obvious that, with the interpretation of the BPS, due account has also to be taken of the presence of fetal rest–activity cycles.

Cordocentesis

There is one invasive antenatal assessment technique which is also promoted in the management of the IUGR fetus, namely cordocentesis.

With this technique, fetal blood gases and pH, haematological parameters, glucose and amino acids can be measured and the fetal karyotype can also be determined. The use of this technique has provided a wealth of information concerning changes occurring under patho-physiological conditions and has also been of great help in validating non-invasive assessment techniques. However, this technique is not without risk and in IUGR fetuses it may lead to emergency Caesarean section or result in fetal death in up to 5% of cases. Moreover, cordocentesis only gives information on the current fetal situation and longitudinal monitoring may require repeated sampling from the umbilical cord, with repeated risks for the fetus.

In the opinion of this author and in that of others (Fisk & Bowes, 1993), there is little (if any) need for measurement of blood gases in IUGR fetuses, since non-invasive tests give quite reliable results. When non-invasive tests are compared with cordocentesis data, the false positive and false negative results are usually emphasized. However, by doing so, it is assumed that cordocentesis data are always correct, whereas spasms of the umbilical vessels, supine hypotension syndrome, or prolonged uterine contractions, may influence the results. Moreover, action on the basis of abnormal results of non-invasive tests is not, or should not be, taken on one test result, but only when repeated tests show similar results. Finally, in IUGR fetuses the false negative and false positive results of non-invasive tests are low, even when only one test result is related to cordocentesis data (Visser et al., 1990; Ribbert et al., 1991; Pardi et al., 1993).

Cordocentesis may be considered in IUGR fetuses for karyotyping, if the risk for chromosomal abnormalities is thought to be substantial. This holds especially if:

1. there are fetal abnormalities;
2. there is inappropriately normal or increased volume of amniotic fluid;
3. there is no evidence of impaired perfusion in the uteroplacental or feto-placental circulation.

In IUGR fetuses without additional anatomical abnormalities and with evidence of uteroplacental insufficiency and reduced amniotic fluid, the risk of a chromosomal abnormality is low (2%). In such cases, parents may wish to avoid invasive tests for fetal karyotyping, given the relatively high risk of cordocentesis (Snijders et al., 1993).

Timing of delivery of the IUGR fetus

When should the small fetus, in which growth restriction is likely to be caused by a reduced supply line, be delivered? At present, it is impossible to answer this question as randomized trials, in which early versus late delivery are compared, are lacking. There is evidence that IUGR fetuses delivered when severe waveform abnormalities of fetal vessels are present have a greater morbidity and mortality than those with end-diastolic frequencies still present (Hackett et al., 1987; Bekedam et al., 1990). IUGR fetuses with antepartum decelerations are more likely to develop a severe degree of intraventricular haemorrhage or show abnormal neurological signs during the newborn period than those without decelerations (Westgren, Malcus & Svenningsen, 1986; Dijxhoorn et al., 1987; Visser, 1988). Fetuses delivered before 34 weeks of gestation have a poorer cognitive development at the age of two years when antenatal FHR abnormalities had been present, than when only abnormal Doppler results had been obtained (Todd et al., 1992). Moreover, IUGR fetuses who were acidaemic at cordocentesis (Soothill et al., 1992) or at elective Caesarean section (Visser, 1988) have a poorer neonatal and subsequent neurodevelopment than non-acidaemic fetuses. These data may lead to the conclusion that IUGR fetuses should be delivered before severely abnormal antenatal tests are present (Hackett et al., 1987). However, in none of these studies were patients randomized, and gestational age was lower and growth retardation more severe in the populations with the poorest outcome. When we matched IUGR fetuses with and without end-diastolic velocities in the umbilical artery for gestational age and birthweight, no differences in outcome were found (Bekedam et al., 1990). This seems to indicate that absence of end-diastolic velocities is a marker of early and severe IUGR – which by itself has an effect on outcome – rather than a marker purely related to outcome.

So, when should the small fetus, in which growth restriction is likely to be caused by a reduced supply line, be delivered, taking into account the fact that delivery at an earlier age may increase the risk of prematurity-related neonatal complications? A small fetus with an estimated weight of 900 g at 31 weeks is bound to be at risk for neurological handicap. The obstetrician may decide to deliver this fetus before signs of hypoxaemia occur, let us say at about 29 or 30 weeks, but handicap may then result from pulmonary problems during the neonatal period. He may also decide to leave the fetus in utero longer, in the hope of improving

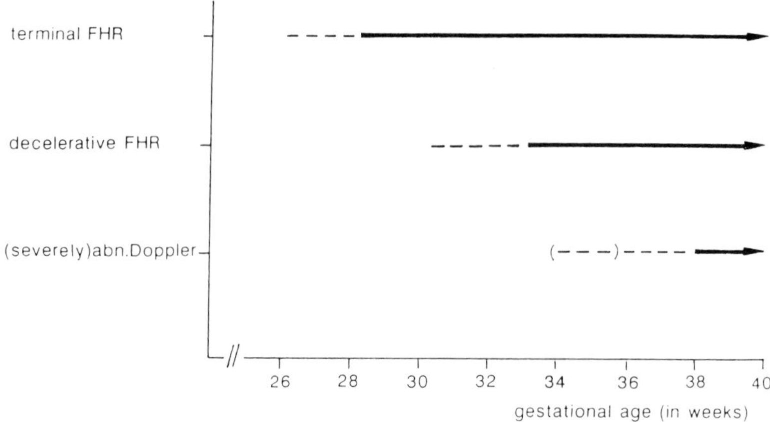

Fig. 13.5. Timing of delivery of intrauterine growth-retarded fetuses, according to gestational age and fetal heart rate and Doppler waveform abnormalities. Uninterrupted line: delivery indicated; interrupted line: delivery may be considered. (From Visser et al., 1991; reproduced with permission.)

maturation, but then the impact of prolonged malnutrition on the brain may offset these benefits.

The timing of delivery of IUGR fetuses depends on many aspects: gestational age, degree of growth retardation, growth rate at subsequent ultrasound scans, amount of amniotic fluid, FHR pattern and Doppler waveforms and, last but not least, on the severity of a possible coexisting maternal disease (e.g. pre-eclampsia). The presence of so many variables requires individualization of management and of the timing of delivery. A proposal for the timing of delivery of the IUGR fetus, based on only three of these variables (gestational age, FHR and Doppler), is shown in Fig. 13.5. This scheme has been discussed extensively elsewhere (Visser, Stigter & Bruinse, 1991). Although it is very rigid, given the complexity of the problem and absence of controlled trials, it may be helpful in decision-making or at least in stimulating discussion.

Signs of impaired neurological development emerge early in the process of deterioration of the condition of the IUGR fetus. Moreover, brain damage is more likely to be the result of chronic malnutrition rather than simply the result of hypoxaemia. Therefore, research directed towards the prevention of IUGR would seem to hold more promise, with respect to the prevention of neurological handicaps, than further refinement of the assessment techniques for studying fetal condition. Fetal monitoring saves fetal lives – at least when it is done properly – since it is possible to deliver the fetus before it will die in utero; its impact on the prevention of (neurological) handicap may, however, be limited.

Conclusions

In this review a possible rank order is presented concerning changes in FHR patterns, body and breathing movements and Doppler waveform patterns of the umbilical artery. The data are restricted to IUGR fetuses and do not apply to the whole population. The rank order might contribute to our understanding of changes which occur under pathological conditions. It might also be helpful in establishing the diagnostic value of the various assessment techniques, of assessing effects of treatment modalities, and of determining the timing of delivery. However, as to the latter there are still many uncertainties.

In IUGR fetuses changes in heart rate and motility are rather late signs of impairment. In general, a growth-retarded fetus will be found to have a normal heart rate pattern and a normal incidence of movements. It is not growth retardation that is detected with these assessment techniques but presumably in the first instance hypoxaemia and the beginning of acidaemia. The lack of identification of fetuses with a PO_2 in the (lower) normal range indicates that antepartum FHR monitoring is not a reliable screening method for future impairment. With progressive deterioration of the fetal condition, the different components of FHR pattern (accelerations, baseline variation, decelerations) change at about the same time as decelerations occur. However, there are large interfetal differences. As both in normal and in IUGR fetuses FHR variation in the same individual remains within a far narrower range (Visser et al., 1981; Snijders et al., 1992), it is advisable to follow IUGR fetuses longitudinally, and to consider each fetus as its own control. This is facilitated by (objective) computer analysis of FHR variation.

The incidence of movements usually falls below the normal range after the occurrence of FHR abnormalities. This implies that monitoring of movements is of restricted value. Possible applications include assessment of fetal well-being in case of suspect (suboptimal) FHR patterns and in assessing the degree of impairment in fetuses with abnormal FHR patterns in whom further maturation in utero must be considered (at early gestation).

The fact that changes in the quality of fetal movements and impairment in the development of fetal behavioural states precede the occurrence of 'hypoxaemia' (antenatal FHR decelerations) suggests that impairment of neurological development occurs before evidence of hypoxaemia presents itself. These data emphasize the fact that in IUGR fetuses brain damage is more likely to be the result of chronic malnutrition than simply the result of hypoxaemia.

Doppler recordings are useful in a high-risk population to identify fetuses at risk of becoming hypoxaemic and to distinguish 'low-risk' small-for-gestational age fetuses from IUGR fetuses. Abnormal Doppler recordings form a strict indication for intensive FHR monitoring. After 34 weeks, delivery of IUGR fetuses may be considered before signs of hypoxaemia and/or acidaemia (e.g. abnormal FHR patterns) occur, when Doppler waveform patterns are abnormal.

With proper knowledge of the various non-invasive assessment techniques, the condition of the IUGR fetus can be assessed quite accurately. A combination of tests always gives more information than relying solely on one assessment technique and recordings should be repeated and expanded if results are equivocal. There are, however, still many uncertainties as to the optimal timing of delivery of these fetuses as controlled trials in which 'early' versus 'late' delivery are compared are lacking. The impact of adequate management of IUGR is likely to be limited since possibilities for in utero treatment of fetal growth retardation, i.e. of restoration of oxygen and nutrient supply, are limited. Given the abnormal (reduced) development of the placenta in such cases, in utero treatment may never become adequate. Therefore, all attention should be directed towards prevention of this disease entity. This requires early and effective identification of pregnancies at risk for IUGR and development of treatment modalities more effective than low dose aspirin. There is evidence that the incidence of cerebral palsy is increasing in the Western world (Hagberg & Hagberg, 1989). This is mainly caused by increased survival of low birthweight infants. This once more underlines the importance of prevention of IUGR.

References

Arduini, D. & Rizzo, G. (1991). Fetal renal artery velocity waveforms and amniotic fluid volume in growth-retarded and post-term fetuses. *Obstetrics and Gynecology*, **72**, 370–3.

Arduini, D., Rizzo, G., Mancuso, S. & Romanini, C. (1988). Short-term effects of maternal oxygen administration on blood flow velocity waveforms in healthy and growth-retarded fetuses. *American Journal of Obstetrics and Gynecology*, **159**, 1077–80.

Arduini, D., Rizzo, G. & Romanini, C. (1993). The development of abnormal heart rate patterns after absent end-diastolic velocity in umbilical artery. *American Journal of Obstetrics and Gynecology*, **168**, 43–8.

Beattie, R.B. & Dornan, J.C. (1989). Antenatal screening for intrauterine growth retardation with umbilical artery Doppler ultrasonography. *British Medical Journal*, **298**, 631–5.

Bedi, K.S. (1984). Effects of undernutrition on brain morphology: a critical review of methods and results. In *Current Topics in Research on Synapses, Volume 2*. pp. 93–163. A.R. Liss, New York.

Bekedam, D.J., Mulder, E.J.H., Snijders, R.J.M. & Visser, G.H.A. (1991). The effects of maternal hyperoxia on fetal breathing movements, body movements and heart rate variation in growth retarded fetuses. *Early Human Development*, **27**, 223–32.

Bekedam, D.J., Visser, G.H.A., Mulder, E.J.H. & Poelmann-Weesjes, G. (1987). Heart rate variation and movements incidence in growth-retarded fetuses: the significance of antenatal late heart rate decelerations. *American Journal of Obstetrics and Gynecology*, **157**, 126–33.

Bekedam, D.J., Visser, G.H.A., van der Zee, A.G.J., Snijders, R.J.M. & Poelmann-Weesjes, G. (1990). Abnormal velocity waveforms of the umbilical artery in growth retarded fetuses: relationship to antepartum late heart rate decelerations and outcome. *Early Human Development*, **24**, 79–90.

Dawes, G.S., Redman, C.W.G. & Smith J.H. (1985). Improvements in the registration and analysis of fetal heart rate records at the bedside. *British Journal of Obstetrics and Gynaecology*, **92**, 317–25.

De Vore, G.R. (1988). Examination of the fetal heart in the fetus with intrauterine growth retardation. *Seminars in Perinatology*, **12**, 66–79.

Derks, J.B., Mulder, E.J.H. & Visser, G.H.A. (1995). The effects of maternal betamethasone administration on fetal heart rate variation rest–activity cycle and eye movements. *British Journal of Obstetrics and Gynaecology*, **102**, 40–6.

Dijxhoorn, M.J., Visser, G.H.A., Touwen, B.C.L. & Huisjes, H.J. (1987). Apgarscore, meconium and acidaemia at birth in small-for-gestational age infants born at term, and their relationship to neonatal neurological morbidity. *British Journal of Obstetrics and Gynaecology*, **94**, 873–79.

Dobbing, J. (1974). The later development of the brain and its vulnerability. In *Scientific Foundations of Paediatrics*. ed. J.A. Davis and J. Dobbing. pp. 565–87. Heinemann, London.

Economides, D.L., Nicolaides, K.H., Gahl, W.A., Bernardini, I., Bottoms, S. & Evans, M. et al. (1989). Cordocentesis in the diagnosis of intra–uterine starvation. *American Journal of Obstetrics and Gynecology*, **161**, 1004–8.

Fisk, N.M. & Bowes, S. (1993). Fetal blood sampling in retreat. *British Medical Journal*, **307**, 143–4.

Goetzman, B.W., Itskovitz, J. & Rudolph, A.M. (1984). Fetal adaptations to spontaneous hypoxaemia and responses to maternal oxygen breathing. *Biology of the Neonate*, **46**, 275–84.

Hackett, G.A., Campbell, S., Gamsu, H. et al. (1987). Doppler studies in the growth retarded fetus and prediction of neonatal necrotising enterocolitis, haemorrhage and neonatal morbidity. *British Medical Journal*, **294**, 13–6.

Hagberg, B. & Hagberg, G. (1989). The changing panorama of infantile and cerebral palsy over forty years: a Swedish survey. *Brain Development*, **11**, 368–73.

Iwamoto, H.S., Kaufman, T., Keil, L.C.& Rudolph, A.M. (1989). Responses to acute hypoxemia in fetal sheep at 0.6–0.7 gestation. *American Journal of Physiology*, **256**, 613–20.

Michaelis, R., Schulte, F.J. & Nolte, R. (1971). Motor-behaviour of small for gestation infants. *Journal of Pediatrics*, **76**, 208–21.

Mohide, P. & Keirse, M.J.N.C. (1989). Biophysical assessment of fetal well-being. In *Effective Care in Pregnancy and Childbirth*. ed. I. Chalmers, M. Enkin & M.J.N.C. Keirse. pp. 477–92. Oxford University Press, Oxford.

Nathanielsz, P.W., Yu, H.K. & Calabum, T.C. (1982). Effect of abolition of fetal movements on intravascular PO_2 and incidence of tonic myometrial contractures in the pregnant ewe at 114 to 134 days gestation. *American Journal of Obstetrics and Gynecology*, **144**, 614–18.

Nijhuis, J.G., Prechtl, H.F.R., Martin, C.B.Jr. & Bots, R.S.G.M. (1982). Are there behavioural states in the human fetus? *Early Human Development*, **6**, 177–95.

Omtzigt, A.W.J., Reuwer, P.J.H.M. & Bruinse, H.W. (1994). A randomized controlled study on the clinical value of umbilical Doppler velocimetry in antenatal care. *American Journal of Obstetrics and Gynecology*, **170**, 625–35.

Pardi, G., Cetin, I., Marconi, A.M., Langranchi, A., Bozzeti, P., Ferrazzi, E., Buscaglia, M. & Battaglia, F.C. (1993). Diagnostic value of blood sampling in fetuses with growth retardation. *New England Journal of Medicine*, **328**, 692–6.

Pearson, J.F. & Weaver, J.B. (1976). Fetal activity and fetal well-being; an evaluation. *British Medical Journal*, **1**, 1305–7.

Peeters, L.L.H., Sheldon, R.E., Jones, M.D. et al. (1979). Blood flow to fetal organs as a function of arterial oxygen content. *American Journal of Obstetrics and Gynecology*, **135**, 637–43.

Ribbert, L.S.M., Snijders, R.J.M., Nicolaides, K.H. & Visser, G.H.A. (1990). Relationship of fetal biophysical profile and blood gas values at cordocentesis in severely growth-retarded fetuses. *American Journal of Obstetrics and Gynecology*, **163**, 569–71.

Ribbert, L.S.M., Snijders, R.J.M., Nicolaides, K.H. & Visser, G.H.A. (1991). Relation of fetal blood gases and data from computer-assisted analysis of fetal heart rate patterns in small for gestation fetuses. *British Journal of Obstetrics and Gynaecology*, **98**, 820–3.

Ribbert, L.S.M., Visser, G.H.A., Mulder, E.J.H., Zonneveld M.F. & Morssink, L.P. (1993). Changes with time in fetal heart rate variation, movement incidences and haemodynamics in intrauterine growth retarded fetuses; a longitudinal approach to the assessment of fetal wellbeing. *Early Human Development*, **31**, 195–208.

Rurak, D.W. & Gruber, N.C. (1983). Effect of neuromuscular blockade on oxygen consumption and blood gases in the fetal lamb. *American Journal of Obstetrics and Gynecology*, **145**, 258–62.

Sadovsky, E., Yaffe, H. & Polishuk, W.Z. (1974). Fetal movement monitoring in normal and pathologic pregnancy. *International Journal of Obstetrics and Gynecology*, **12**, 75–9.

Schulte, F.J., Schremf, G. & Hinze, G. (1971). Maternal toxemia, fetal malnutrition and motor behaviour in the newborn. *Pediatrics*, **48**, 871–9.

Sival, D.A., Visser, G.H.A. & Prechtl, H.F.R. (1992). The effect of intrauterine growth retardation on the quality of general movements in the human fetus. *Early Human Development*, **28**, 119–32.

Snijders, R.J.M., Ribbert, L.S.M., Visser, G.H.A. & Mulder, E.J.H. (1992). Numeric analysis of heart rate variation in intrauterine growth-retarded fetuses: a longitudinal study. *American Journal of Obstetrics and Gynecology*, **166**, 22–7.

Snijders, R.J.M., Sherrod, C., Gosden, C.M. & Nicolaides, K.H. (1993). Severe fetal growth retardation: associated malformations and chromosomal abnormalities. *American Journal of Obstetrics and Gynecology*, **168**, 547–55.

Soothill, P.W., Ajaji, R.A., Campbell, S., Ross, E.M., Candy D.C.A., Snijders, R.J.M. & Nicolaides, K.H. (1992). Relationship between fetal acidaemia at cordocentesis and subsequent neurodevelopment. *Ultrasound in Obstetrics and Gynecology*, **2**, 80–4.

Soothill, P.W., Nicolaides, K.H. & Campbell, S. (1987). Prenatal asphyxia, hyperlacticaemia, hypoglycaemia and erythroblastosis in growth-retarded fetuses. *British Medical Journal*, **294**, 1051–3.

Todd, A.L., Trudinger, B.J., Cole, M.J. & Cooney, G.H. (1992). Antenatal tests of fetal welfare and development at age 2 years. *American Journal of Obstetrics and Gynecology*, **167**, 1661–71.

Van Vliet, M.A.T., Martin, C.B., Nijhuis, J.G. & Prechtl, H.F.R. (1985). Behavioural states in growth-retarded fetuses. *Early Human Development*, **12**, 183–98.

Visser, G.H.A. (1988). Abnormal antepartum fetal heart rate patterns and subsequent handicap. In *Antenatal and Perinatal Causes of Handicap. Baillière's Clinical Obstetrics and Gynaecology, 2(1)*, ed. N. Patel. pp. 117–24, Baillière Tindall, London.

Visser, G.H.A. (1991). Fetal health assessment. *Current Opinion in Obstetrics and Gynecology*, **3**, 242–7.

Visser, G.H.A., Dawes, G.S. & Redman, C.W.G. (1981). Numerical analysis of the normal human antenatal fetal heart rate. *British Journal of Obstetrics and Gynaecology*, **88**, 792–802.

Visser, G.H.A., Redman, C.W.G., Huisjes, H.J. & Turnbull, A.C. (1980). Non-stressed antepartum heart rate monitoring: implications of decelerations after spontaneous contractions. *American Journal of Obstetrics and Gynecology*, **128**, 429–35.

Visser, G.H.A., Sadovsky, G. & Nicolaides, K.H. (1990). Antepartum heart rate patterns in small-for-gestational-age third trimester fetuses: correlations with blood gas values obtained at cordocentesis. *American Journal of Obstetrics and Gynecology*, **162**, 698–703.

Visser, G.H.A., Stigter, R.H. & Bruinse, H.W. (1991). Management of the growth-retarded fetus. *European Journal of Obstetrics, Gynecology and Reproductive Biology*, **42**, S73–8.

Westgren, L.M.R., Malcus, P. & Svenningsen, N.W. (1986). Intra-uterine asphyxia and long-term outcome in preterm fetuses. *Obstetrics and Gynecology*, **67**, 512–16.

Wladimiroff, J.W., Tonge, H.M. & Stewart, P.A. (1986). Doppler ultrasound assessment of cerebral blood flow in the human fetus. *British Journal of Obstetrics and Gynaecology*, **93**, 471–8.

Index

Note: **bold** type denotes illustrations